Psychology Revivals

Neural Repair, Transplantation and Rehabilitation

Originally published in 1999, this book begins with a synopsis of experimental work underlying degeneration and recovery in the nervous system, which is then discussed in the context of strategies to repair the central nervous system (CNS) and peripheral nervous system (PNS). The major part of the book is given over to the approach involving the use of transplanted tissues to replace and restore disrupted neural networks. This experimental work has formed the basis for the emerging clinical trials employing neural grafts for diseases such as Parkinson's and Huntington's, which are discussed in detail. The book then goes on to discuss newer cellular strategies involving the manipulation of neural cells both in culture and genetically, an approach that may ultimately be employed in the clinical situation.

Neural Repair, Transplantation and Rehabilitation is unique in bridging the gap from experimental studies to clinical trials, whilst also providing the non-specialist with a background in rehabilitation strategies as well as basic neuroscience. It is recommended for all those involved in the management of patients with degenerative and traumatic injuries to the nervous system. Today it can be read in its historical context.

Neural Repair, Transplantation and Rehabilitation

Roger A. Barker and Stephen B. Dunnett

Routledge
Taylor & Francis Group
LONDON AND NEW YORK

First published in 1999
by Psychology Press

This edition first published in 2026 by Routledge
4 Park Square, Milton Park, Abingdon, Oxon, OX14 4RN

and by Routledge
605 Third Avenue, New York, NY 10158

Routledge is an imprint of the Taylor & Francis Group, an informa business

A Library of Congress record exists under ISBN: 9780863776281

ISBN: 978-1-041-24449-3 (hbk)
ISBN: 978-1-003-74196-1 (ebk)
ISBN: 978-1-041-24452-3 (pbk)

Book DOI 10.4324/9781003741961

Neural repair, transplantation and rehabilitation

Roger A. Barker and Stephen B. Dunnett
Departments of Neurology and Experimental Psychology, and the MRC Cambridge Centre for Brain Repair, University of Cambridge, UK

Psychology Press
a member of the Taylor & Francis group

Psychology Press Ltd, Publishers
27 Church Road
Hove
East Sussex, BN3 2FA
UK

British Library Cataloguing in Publication Data
A catalogue record for this book is available from the British Library

ISBN 0-86377-628-0 (hbk)
ISBN 0-86377-629-9 (pbk)

ISSN 1466-6340

Typeset by Graphicraft Limited, Hong Kong
Printed and bound in the UK by Biddles Ltd, Guildford and King's Lynn

Contents

Series preface

Rehabilitation is a process whereby people, who have been injured by injury or illness, work together with health service staff and others to achieve their optimum level of physical, psychological, social and vocational well-being (McLellan, 1991). It includes all measures aimed at reducing the impact of handicapping and disabling conditions and at enabling disabled people to return to their most appropriate environment (WHO, 1986; Wilson, 1997). It also includes attempts to alter impairment in underlying cognitive and brain systems by the provision of systematic, planned experience to the damaged brain (Robertson & Murre, in press). The above views apply also to neuropsychological rehabilitation, which is concerned with the assessment, treatment and natural recovery of people who have sustained an insult to the brain.

Neuropsychological rehabilitation is influenced by a number of fields both from within and without psychology. Neuropsychology, behavioural psychology and cognitive psychology have each played important roles in the development of current rehabilitation practice. So too have findings from studies of neuroplasticity, linguistics, geriatric medicine, neurology and other fields. Our discipline, therefore, is not confined to one conceptual framework; rather, it has a broad theoretical base.

We hope that this broad base is reflected in the modular handbook. This first book by Roger Barker and Stephen Dunnett sets the scene by talking about 'Neural repair, transplantation and rehabilitation'. The second, by Josef Zihl, addresses visual disorders after brain injury. Forthcoming titles include volumes on specific cognitive functions such as language, memory and motor skills, together with social and personality aspects of neuropsychological rehabilitation and behavioural approaches to rehabilitation. Other titles will follow as this is the kind of handbook that can be added to over the years.

Although each volume will be based on a strong theoretical foundation relevant to the topic in question, the main thrust of a majority of the books will be the development of practical, clinical methods of rehabilitation arising out of this research enterprise.

The series is aimed at neuropsychologists, clinical psychologists and other rehabilitation specialists such as occupational therapists, speech and language pathologists, rehabilitation physicians and other disciplines involved in the rehabilitation of people with brain injury.

Neuropsychological rehabilitation is at an exciting stage in its development. On the one hand, we have a huge growth of interest in functional imaging techniques to tell us about the basic processes going on in the brain. On the other hand, the past few years have seen the introduction of a number of theroetically driven approaches to cognitive rehabilitation from the fields of language, memory, attention and perception. In addition to both the above, there is a growing recognition from health services that rehabilitation is an integral part of a health care system. Of course, alongside the recognition of the need for rehabilitation is the view that any system has to be evaluated. To those of us working with brain injured people including those with dementia, there is a feeling that things are moving forward. This series, we hope, is one reflection of this move and the integration of theory and practice.

REFERENCES

McLellan, D.L. (1991). Functional recovery and the principles of disability medicine. In M. Swash & J. Oxbury (Eds.), *Clinical neurology*. Edinburgh: Churchill Livingstone.

Robertson, I.H., & Murre, J.M.J. (in press). Rehabilitation of brain damage: Brain plasticity and principles of guided recovery. *Psychological Bulletin*.

Wilson, B.A. (1997). Cognitive rehabilitation: How it is and how it might be. *Journal of the International Neuropsychological Society*, *3*, 487–496.

World Health Organisation (1986). Optimum care of disabled people. *Report of a WHO meeting*, Turku, Finland.

BARBARA A. WILSON

IAN H. ROBERTSON

Preface

The last two decades have seen radical and rapid new advances in our understanding of the mechanisms of damage and disease in the nervous system, opening up the vision of completely new approaches to treatment that were unforeseen until very recently. In this book, we attempt to draw together the latest progress in our knowledge of the principles that underlie development and cell death in the nervous system as the basis for a new science of neural protection, transplantation, and repair. The scientific advances will produce major new clinical opportunities for novel treatments in a range of neurodegenerative diseases and insults, which will in turn require major changes in our provision of rational rehabilitation programmes if the efficacy of the new treatments is to be optimised.

The book begins with a discussion of the processes that underlie both normal development as well as the plasticity in the mature nervous system. This plasticity, whilst being seen as a normal physiological response to the environment in which the individual finds itself, is also recruited at the time of neural damage, which can be in the form either of an acute insult (such as head injury) or of a chronic degenerative process (such as Parkinson's disease). The capacity for compensation and regeneration differs markedly depending on whether the damage occurs in the central or in the peripheral nervous system. However, whereas it was formerly believed that the central nervous system (CNS) of adults is fixed and immutable, one of the major new principles now emerging is that the mature CNS can also show a considerable degree of dynamic remodelling. Whilst this has for many years been implicitly exploited in the field of clinical rehabilitation, it is only now that the cellular and molecular bases of brain plasticity are being defined. Understanding these principles can lead in turn to identifying completely novel strategies for repair and rehabilitation which utilise and amplify innate regenerative processes. Furthermore, spontaneous repair processes can be dramatically enhanced by using transplanted tissues in the brain to supplement and replace that which is lost.

Neural transplants into the brain are most successful when the donor tissue is taken from a developing embryo and used to replace dying or dead neurones within the mature host CNS. This approach has been used in a number of CNS disorders, but most notably in Parkinson's disease. Functional neural tissue transplants were first developed in animal models of parkinsonism and shown to survive and receive and form connections with the host as well as ameliorate a range of behavioural deficits. These experimental studies then provided the basis for the development of clinical transplants for patients with Parkinson's disease, for which there is now over 10 years of clinical experience and the beginnings of an understanding of the critical principles for successful transplantation therapy. The discussion in Parkinson's disease then provides a prototype for considering the problems that will need to be overcome if a similar strategy is to lead to therapy in a variety of other neurodegenerative conditions including Huntington's and Alzheimer's disease as well as spinal cord injury.

Although these programmes have shown that grafts of embryonic tissue can be successful in such patients, and provide the gold standard for what is possible, therapies based on human foetal tissues are always going to be controversial. A number of key ethical, immunological, and practical issues need to be addressed before neural transplantation is likely to be widely available in clinical practice. In particular, there is now a vigorous search for alternative sources of tissue and transplantation strategies that do not rely on a regular supply of human foetal donors, and research interest is exploring several options including engineering ethically neutral cells, maintaining and expanding cells in tissue culture, and use of non-human (e.g. pig) donors. This then raises issues of how grafts best work in the diseased brain, so that the search can be based on a rational understanding of the critical requirements that any novel tissue must fulfil rather than simply on an empirical sampling of all the possibilities.

Finally, as physiological psychologists join with their neurobiological colleagues in analysing the functional consequences of cell transplantation, both in experimental animals and in patients, it is becoming increasingly clear that successful recovery involves more than simply anatomical repair and reconstruction. Changes in behaviour, experience, and environment influence the integration of graft tissues into host neural circuits, and restoration of complex cognitive and motor skills requires not just replacement of lost neurones but also relearning and retraining of the reconstructed brain systems. As the surgical technology comes of age, we are only now beginning to realise that the reconstructive skills of the cell biologists and neurosurgeons will need to be combined with the rehabilitative skills of clinical psychologists and physiologists if a fully functional repair is ever to be achieved. It is our belief that a field that has until now been dominated by cellular technology will only be translated into successful new therapies when traditional clinical boundaries are dismantled and a true multidisciplinary approach to structural and functional reconstruction is adopted.

We hope that this review will not only convey some of our excitement for recent progress in basic research, but also will provide the background information necessary to start a debate on how to develop clinical programmes of rehabilitation to accompany surgical and medical advances in brain repair. We are convinced that these new strategies will become progressively more common in the fields of neurological and neurosurgical treatment in the first decades of the new century.

We thank Ms Amy Abraham for her excellent assistance during preparation of the manuscript.

ROGER BARKER AND STEPHEN DUNNETT
Cambridge, October 1998

CHAPTER ONE

The limits of regeneration in the central nervous system

All things are possible until they are proved impossible—and even the impossible may only be so, as of now

—Pearl Buck, *A Bridge for Passing* (1962)

INTRODUCTION

The human brain and spinal cord (which together comprise the central nervous system, CNS) is a delicate structure of immense complexity that is susceptible to many damaging insults from the time of its early development before birth to the time of its senescence in the ageing adult. Since the brain controls all higher mental and cognitive functions, damage in the brain has a profound impact on all aspects of human function. Opportunities for treatment or alleviation of such damage are a major theme of this series of books. However, in contrast to many of our other clinical colleagues, neurologists and neuropsychologists confront a profound problem when addressing the consequences of damage in the brain, namely its limited ability to repair itself. If, for example, a fibre pathway is cut in the CNS, then the cut fibres have only limited potential for regrowth. If a population of nerve cells (neurones) are damaged and most of the neurones lost, they cannot divide or be rescued. By contrast, the peripheral nervous system (PNS) is capable of significant regeneration so that if a peripheral nerve is damaged, regrowth of the damaged nerve and recovery of function will occur over a period of time.

This lack of spontaneous recovery in the CNS from injury or disease presents a number of challenges to the health care professional. One involves the lengthy programmes of rehabilitation required by the patient and his/her family that take account of the likely need for long-term support. A second, the area that this book will concentrate on, is the development of new therapeutic strategies for slowing down or even reversing the clinical course of neurological disease or damage. Finally, health care professionals have to act as a source of balanced information and advice about the realistic long-term prospects and opportunities of new treatments and therapies that patients and their families read about in the media and hear about in support groups.

The last two decades have produced steady advances in understanding the causes and processes involved in cell degeneration and death in the nervous system. This includes a greater knowledge of the reasons why neurones of the CNS are not spontaneously replaced when damaged as well as their meagre capacity to re-grow when their fibre connections are cut. Coupled to this has been an increase in our ability to stimulate CNS neuronal survival and restoration of their connections experimentally. However, many problems still exist. The area of neurobiology concerned with regeneration and repair constitutes one of the most vigorous and active areas of biological research today, stimulated not only by the scale of the human and economic burden of brain damage, but also by the fact that the prospects of radically new therapies are now considered a realistic objective.

At present, the latest scientific insights still have made little impact on day-to-day clinical services. It is our belief, however, that the next decade will see a change. We can expect the introduction into clinical practice of new strategies for halting degenerative diseases and stimulating repair processes in the damaged brain and spinal cord. In the first instance this will be through clinical trials of novel growth factors and surgical treatments, many of which will, by the very nature of things, not be fully effective on the first attempt. Consequently, we can expect alternating periods of enthusiasm and optimism interspersed with dashed hopes and calls for retrenchment into old ways. It is our hope that this book may provide an introduction for clinical neurologists and neuropsychologists to the recent developments coming out of the research laboratories into the mechanisms of brain damage, degeneration, and disease, and how this can be translated into the development of new therapies. The aim of this book is therefore to provide a bridge from the currently available techniques of rehabilitation to ones that incorporate some of the newer possibilities for CNS repair. Whereas our particular focus is on repair by replacement of damaged cells and tissue by neural transplantation, this approach opens up many new avenues and strategies for repair and remediation that are likely to have progressively greater impact in the first decades of the next century.

In this first chapter we discuss some of the problems that the CNS presents in terms of recovery and regeneration.

THE ABSENCE OF REGENERATION WITHIN THE CNS

Cells of the nervous system

If we are to understand the principles of degeneration and regeneration of cells in the nervous system, we must start by reviewing the major types of cell that exist in the CNS and PNS (see Fig. 1.1). The peripheral nervous system (PNS) is defined as those nerves that lie outside the brain, brainstem, or spinal cord, whilst the central nervous system (CNS) embraces those cells that lie within these structures. The CNS can be further subdivided into the spinal cord, brainstem, cerebellum, and the cerebral hemispheres, which have an outer cerebral cortex,

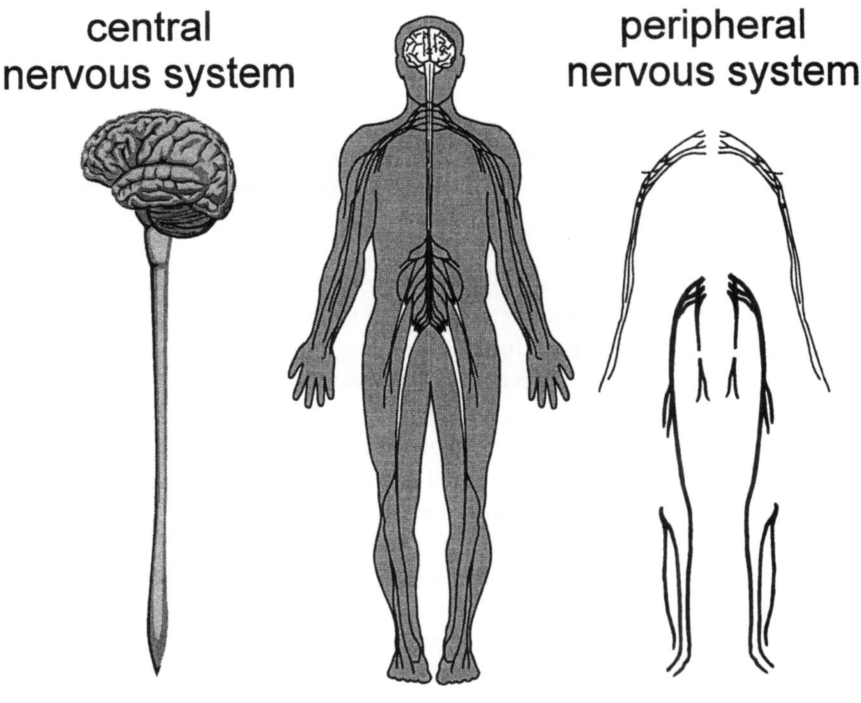

Central Nervous System	Peripheral Nervous Systems
Neurones	Neurones
Astrocytes	Schwann cells
Oligodendrocytes	
Microglia	
Ependyma	

FIG. 1.1. The peripheral and central nervous systems and their major cellular components.

which overlies the interconnected nuclei of the basal ganglia and limbic systems, and a core comprising the thalamus and hypothalamus (which together make up the "diencephalon").

The autonomic nervous system (ANS) makes up the third major component of the nervous system. It has both a central and peripheral component and is concerned with the innervation of internal and glandular organs. The ANS therefore consists of a complex of fibre connections and nerve ganglia that regulate the smooth muscles controlling a wide range of automatic and visceral functions (breathing, heart rate, vasoconstriction and dilation, gut motility, sweat gland activity, etc.) which are largely outside voluntary control.

The peripheral nervous system consists of nerves (bundles of nerve fibres, or "axons") comprising both afferent fibres (conducting sensory information into the spinal cord and brainstem) and efferent fibres (transmitting impulses primarily out to the muscles). The cell bodies of sensory nerves lie outside the spinal cord in the "dorsal root ganglia", whilst the cell bodies of the motor neurones lie within the CNS, located in the anterior horn of the spinal cord and in specialised brainstem nuclei. The PNS is more susceptible to physical damage when compared to the CNS in that it not only lacks the protection of a bony mantle but also does not possess as tight a barrier to circulating factors in the bloodstream—a barrier that in the CNS is represented by the relatively impermeable blood–brain barrier.

The CNS and PNS differ not only in gross features, such as the level of bony protection and separation from other tissues of the body, but also in their cellular compositions and responses to injury.

The nervous system is composed of two main populations of cells, the neurones and the glia. The neurones are the electrically excitable cells that encode and relay information in the form of action potentials and communicate with each other through synapses (see Fig. 1.2). These synapses are discrete points of contact between neurones, and the arrival of an action potential at the presynaptic terminal leads to the release of a chemical neurotransmitter that diffuses across the synaptic cleft to the postsynaptic membrane. The neurotransmitter binds to the postsynaptic membrane at specific protein sites called receptors. This in turn leads to a change in the membrane potential that subsequently is integrated by the postsynaptic cell and results in an action potential being generated and propagated in the majority of cases. Synapses onto a neurone are primarily located on the cell body (or "soma") or dendrites that feed into it, although they can occasionally also be found on axons (so-called "axo-axonic" synapses).

The postsynaptic cell integrates all the afferent inputs converging on the cell body and the new action potential so generated originates from the most excitable part of the proximal axon—the axon hillock. Once initiated, an action potential is conducted down the axon away from the cell body of the neurone. This conduction requires that the axon is well insulated so that the action potential signal is not lost due to current leakage. Whilst this is not a major problem for

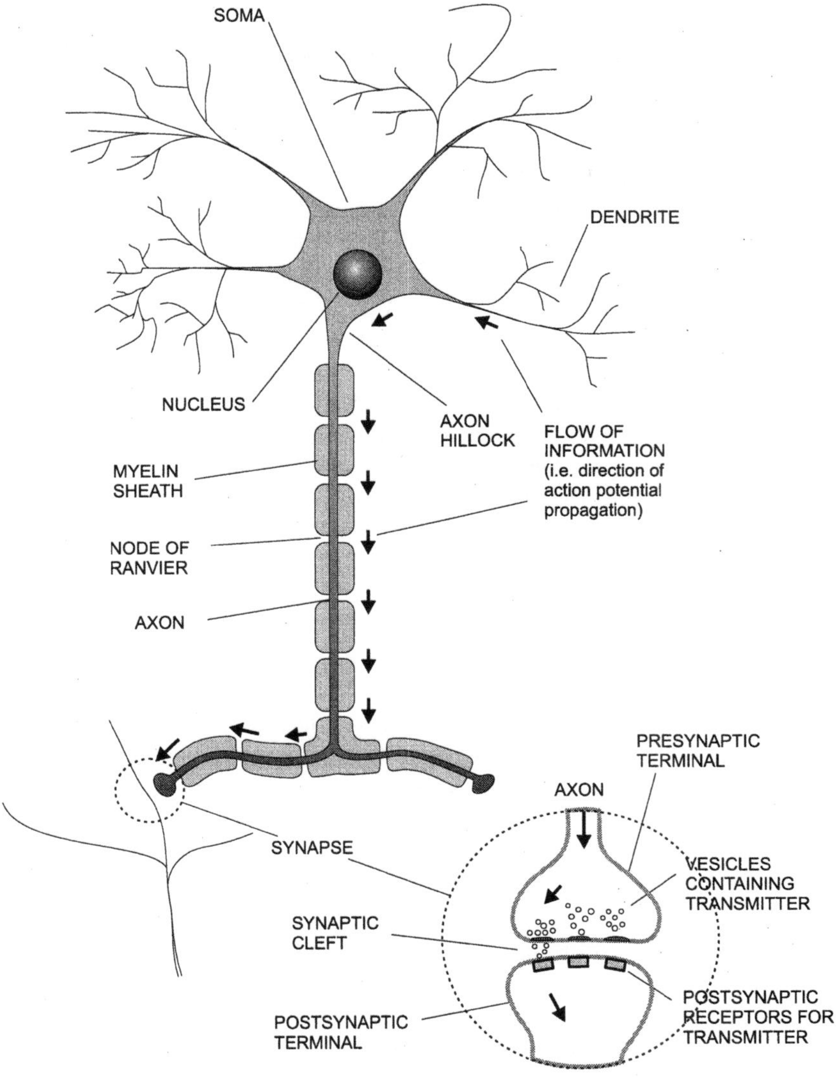

FIG. 1.2. Schematic figure of a neurone with a myelinated axon forming a chemical synapse with another (postsynaptic) neurone.

neurones with small diameter axons, it is a significant factor in the conduction of nerve impulses by neurones with large diameter axons that project over long distances. This problem is overcome in these neurones by the use of fatty insulation around the axon in the form of a "myelin sheath". Because the mode of conduction in myelinated fibres is more rapid and reliable than in non-myelinated fibres, these nerve fibres are the predominant type found in both the CNS and PNS.

The second main class of cells found in both the CNS and PNS are the glia, which are different for the CNS and PNS (see Fig. 1.1). In the CNS there are four main types of glia whilst in the PNS there is only one, the Schwann cell which is responsible for myelination of the nerve fibres, a role subserved by the oligodendrocyte in the CNS. Astrocytes, on the other hand, are found only in the CNS and have a number of different structural and regulatory functions which include the maintenance of the blood–brain barrier and nutritive, metabolic, and energy homeostasis of the CNS extracellular environment. Astrocytes also play a role in immunological reactions, inflammation, and the response to damage within the CNS, a function they share with the microglia. This third type of glial cell, the microglia, can best be viewed as the main immunologically active cells of the CNS, analogous to the macrophage and antigen presenting cells found in the rest of the body. The final class of CNS glia, the ependymal cells, line the cerebrospinal fluid-filled ventricular system. In addition, the glial population as a whole have an important role in the development of the nervous system which includes regulating the differentiation of neurones and the guidance of their developing axons to their targets. Many of these development processes are reactivated after injury and influence the capacity and extent of neurones to regenerate.

Degeneration and regeneration in the PNS

If an axon is cut or crushed in the PNS then it has the capacity to regenerate. Peripheral axons not only have the capacity to grow over long distances to find their appropriate targets in this process, they can also restore the sensory or motor function associated with the initial damage (reviewed in Fawcett & Keynes, 1990).

When a peripheral nerve is damaged, the distal aspect of the axon is lost by a process of "Wallerian degeneration". When the distal segment of the cut nerve fibre is separated from its cell body, it loses all the nutrients and metabolic regulation necessary for its survival, and so dies. Macrophages invade the area to remove the axonal and myelin-derived debris, but leave in place the Schwann cells inside the basal lamina tube that surrounds the nerve fibres. These columns of Schwann cells surrounded by basal lamina are known as "endoneurial tubes", and provide the favourable substrate necessary for successful axon regrowth (see Fig. 1.3).

In addition to their scavenging function, the macrophages release a number of chemical signals (cytokines) which provide a "mitogenic" signal (the signal to divide) to the Schwann cells. The proximal end of the cut axon, i.e. the segment still connected to the cell body, starts to sprout within hours of injury. The regenerating stump of the cut axon forms a growth cone which contacts the Schwann cell basal lamina on one side, and the Schwann cell membrane on the other. Contacts between the growth cone and these surfaces are fundamental to enabling the axon to grow back down the endoneurial tube to its distant targets.

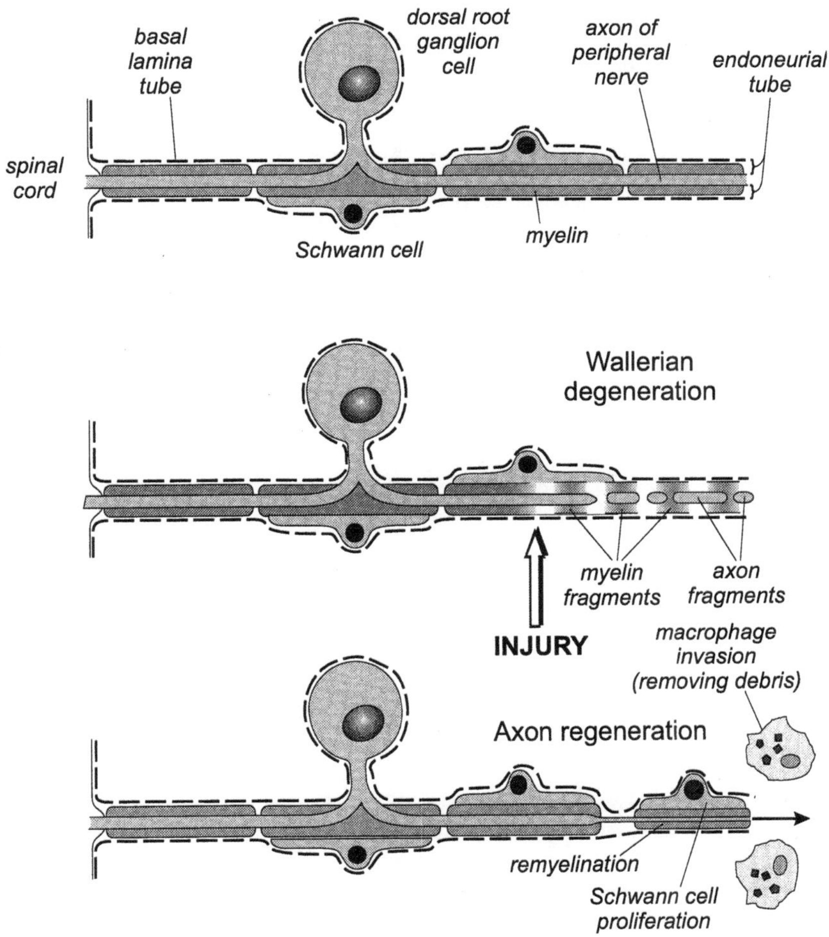

FIG. 1.3. Regeneration of a cut PNS axon along the endoneurial tube of Schwann cells and their basal laminae.

The Schwann cell basal lamina express a number of surface molecules (such as laminin and fibronectin) that are known to be effective substrates across which axons can grow in tissue culture. The Schwann cells also produce a number of "neurotrophic factors" which promote the survival and stimulate the growth of neurones (see Chapter Two). Thus, Schwann cells provide a rich neurotrophic environment to stimulate axon growth, a favourable substrate to which the growing axons can adhere, and a guidance channel along which the regenerating axons can grow. All of these features combine to permit and facilitate the ordered regeneration of peripheral neurones and reconnection of cut axons with even distant somatosensory and muscular targets.

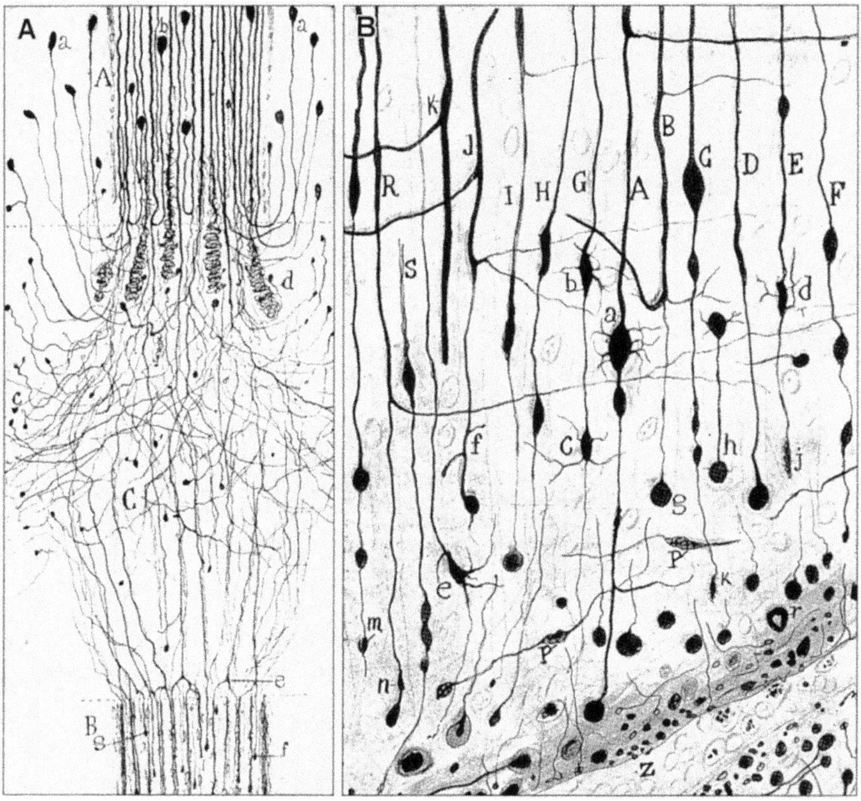

FIG. 1.4. Regeneration of the neurones in the PNS and CNS. (A) Cut PNS axons regenerate across the injury in the PNS (sciatic nerve). (B) Cut CNS neurones (in the neocortex) undergo abortive attempts at regeneration and then die back. (Reproduced from Cajal, 1928, with permission © Oxford University Press.)

Abortive regeneration in the CNS

There are two aspects of the failure of regeneration in the CNS that need to be addressed. First, as a general principle, CNS neurones are formed during embryonic or early postnatal development, and are not capable of subsequent division later in life. Consequently, once lost through death or disease, there is no mechanism for their replacement in the adult mammalian CNS.[1] The second principle

[1] The inability of CNS neurones to undergo cell division in adulthood is a general principle, but is not an absolute rule. There remain a small population of "stem cells" in restricted areas of the brain that retain a capacity to divide and form new neurones throughout life. Although only recently identified, these may provide an important alternative source of cells for transplantation (see Chapter Nine).

is that, in contrast to the capacity for regrowth seen in the PNS, cut or crushed axons of the CNS have an extremely limited capacity to regenerate. Consequently, once a fibre pathway is damaged, the axons do not regrow.

The great classical Spanish anatomist Santiago Ramon y Cajal (1928) provided some of most elegant descriptions of the events that follow fibre damage in the CNS. Using silver staining methods, he recorded how the distal parts of central axons also undergo degeneration, as in the PNS. Similarly, the proximal ends of the cut axons form a club-like ending, now known as growth cones, which appear to send out fine processes in initial attempts to regrow, again just the same as in the PNS. However, the growth cones fail to adhere and draw themselves forward and so, after several abortive attempts, the axons finally retract. Over a period of weeks and months the cut axon continues to die back, leading eventually to degeneration and death of the cell itself and disappearance of the cell soma.

This led to a perspective that the neurones of the CNS are not capable of regeneration, a view encapsulated by the classical quotation of Cajal (1928, p. 750): "Once development was ended, the founts of growth and regeneration of axons and dendrites dried up irrevocably. In adult centres, the nerve paths are something fixed and immutable; everything may die, nothing may be regenerated".

It is important to note that the situation is probably not as bleak as suggested by this quotation. Cajal himself recognised the prospect for sprouting in restricted circumstances in the CNS and undertook some important early studies involving transplantation in the CNS. However, many of his followers did adopt the absolute dictum that regeneration simply did not occur in the CNS. Until recently, the predominant *Zeitgeist* has been that repair in the CNS simply is not possible, and any search for new strategies to repair nervous system damage was doomed to failure.

In recent years, our understanding of the general principles of cell death in the nervous system has expanded considerably. Thus, one of the main reasons for the dying back of cut axons (so-called "axotomy") is now known to be loss of trophic support from the targets to which the neurones project (see Chapter Two). Moreover, cell death is not inevitable, in particular if the neurones can receive additional support from collateral branches that are not damaged. Indeed recent studies have provided a considerably more detailed analysis of the changes that occur in neurones in response to axotomy, such as atrophy and the down-regulation of cell metabolism, which offers the opportunity to rescue these neurones before they die (Sofroniew et al., 1990b).

It is therefore clear that the impossibility of regeneration in the CNS is not absolute, although situations where effective regeneration occurs are extremely rare. The normal response of the CNS therefore remains that damaged axons neither regrow nor reconnect appropriately to distant targets, but the therapeutic manipulation of the CNS may affect this response characteristic.

What is the difference between the PNS and CNS?

The key question that first must be addressed is whether the bar to regeneration is intrinsic to the neurones of the CNS or is a feature of the glial environment in which they find themselves. Several lines of evidence point towards the latter answer.

The ability of peripheral axons to regenerate indicates that many of the cellular behaviours associated with growth persist in mature neurones. Since many of the cell bodies which give rise to axons in peripheral nerves are actually located in the CNS (such as the large motor neurones of the ventral horn of the spinal cord), the limited capacity for regeneration of axons in the CNS cannot be due to a limited capacity of all central neurones to regenerate. Rather it suggests that the peripheral nerve environment is more conducive to the regrowth of axons than is the CNS environment.

This view is supported by two main lines of evidence. First are experiments which have investigated the regenerative capacity of sensory nerves, whose neuronal cell bodies are located in the dorsal root ganglia of the PNS but which innervate both peripheral targets in the skin and central targets in the dorsal horn of the spinal cord (Carlstedt et al., 1989; Liuzzi & Lasek, 1987). When these axons are crushed (see Fig. 1.5) both the peripheral and central axon branches undergo Wallerian degeneration. The peripheral branch will regenerate back to its distal target, like all other peripheral nerves. By contrast, axons of the central branch regenerate back to the transition zone in the dorsal root where they would normally enter the CNS, but they will grow no further within the CNS environment, and they do not re-innervate their central targets. Thus, the axons of the same nerve cell body can regenerate within the glial environment of the PNS, but not within that of the CNS.

The second set of experiments have used transplants to provide different glial environments for central neurones. In a classic experiment exploring the possibilities of spinal cord regeneration, David and Aguayo (1981) first transected the spinal cord of rats, and then implanted a segment of peripheral nerve across the transection with one end inserted into the brainstem and the other into the distal stump of the spinal cord (see Fig. 1.6).

Brainstem axons were seen to regenerate into the peripheral nerve graft, to grow the full length of the graft, and to grow out into the host spinal cord at the far end. However, whereas these axons of central neurones would grow several centimetres through the peripheral nerve graft, they penetrated no more than a few hundred microns back into the host CNS environment. Further long-distance growth within the CNS was not possible, and the axons did not connect up with appropriate target cells such as the motor neurones in the ventral horn of the spinal cord. Similarly, neurones of the distal segments of the spinal cord were able to grow long distances in the reverse (ascending) direction through the

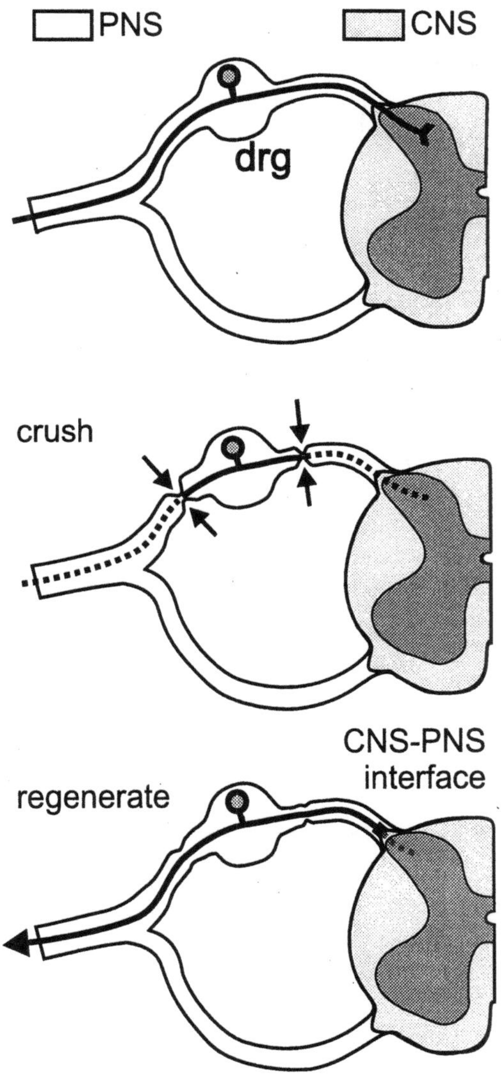

FIG. 1.5. Crushed peripheral nerves regenerate in the PNS but not in the CNS. drg, Dorsal root ganglia. (After Carlstedt et al., 1989.)

peripheral nerve graft, but further regeneration was again abortive once the axon terminals re-entered the CNS environment of the brainstem. This study shows that cells of the CNS have the clear capacity to regenerate, and their axons can grow effectively over long distances when confronted by a PNS environment, but not when the same axons meet a CNS environment. Complementary studies by Hall and Kent (1987) have shown that if CNS tissue is grafted into a peripheral

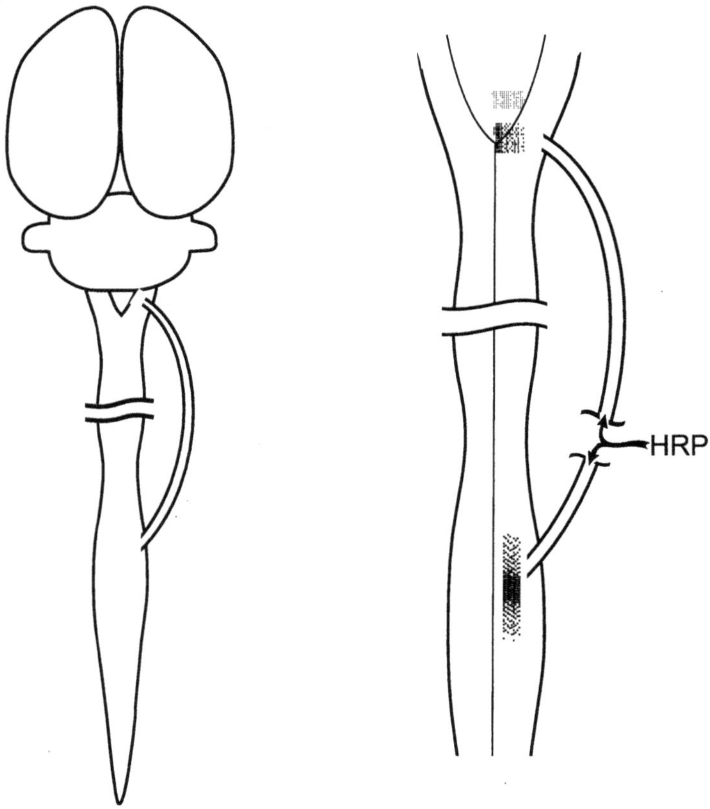

FIG. 1.6. Regeneration of central axons through a peripheral nerve bridge spanning a spinal cord injury. The tracer horseradish peroxidase (HRP) is applied to cut axons in the middle of the bridge to demonstrate that CNS neurones in both the brainstem and peripheral stump of the spinal cord regenerate into and through the bridge. Axon terminals exiting at the far ends of the bridge show only a few hundred microns further growth back in the host CNS. (After David & Aguayo, 1981, reprinted with permission © 1981 American Association for the Advancement of Science.)

nerve, it prevents the regeneration of cut axons that would otherwise have taken place through that nerve.

Thus, there is clear evidence for the view that the poor regeneration observed in the CNS is due to the non-permissive nature of the CNS environment for regrowth rather than to any inherent limitation of CNS neurones. Attention therefore turns naturally to differences in central and peripheral glial populations.

Recovery in the CNS: The glial component

There is increasing evidence for the view that the critical differences in the regenerative capacities of the CNS and PNS relate to the different glia populations in the two parts of the nervous system. In the CNS, the environment provided by both central astrocytes and oligodendrocytes appears to be inhibitory to axonal outgrowth whilst in the PNS the Schwann cell environment is permissive, or indeed actually facilitatory, to regrowth.

The simplest experiments to demonstrate this conclusion are undertaken in tissue culture systems where the neurones either of a peripheral ganglion (such as the dorsal root ganglion) or from the embryonic nervous system (such as the dopamine cells of the substantia nigra) are grown on a substrate of glial cells that have previously been established as a confluent monolayer in the culture dish. Schwann cells provide a good substrate for axon growth, whereas CNS astrocytes and oligodendrocytes are relatively poor. In fact, although a limited regrowth of axons can be seen over a surface of astrocytes grown in monolayer culture, the impermeability of astrocytes is particularly apparent when the glial cells are grown in a three-dimensional matrix, more akin to the packing density of the normal nervous system (Fawcett et al., 1989).

In order to identify the particular cellular components that inhibit regeneration in the CNS, there have been many subsequent studies in tissue culture, investigating the cellular and molecular substrates over which axons will grow and those that are inhibitory for growth. Without elaborating the details of what turns out to be a very complex field, it is apparent that a wide variety of molecules are expressed on the surfaces of glial cells and within the extracellular matrix that facilitate the growth of axon terminals. Many of these molecules are now known (such as laminin, fibronectin, tenascin, proteoglycans, etc.) and differences in their expression may account for the more permissive nature of PNS over CNS glia.

In addition to the molecules that promote growth, migration, penetration, and adhesion of growth cones through a matrix of glial cells, recent attention has turned to the possibility that glial cells in the CNS also express molecules that are actually inhibitory for axon growth. For example, time lapse photography of axons growing across a culture dish indicates that growth cones can appear to collapse or be actively repulsed on making contact with the surface of scattered oligodendrocytes. Schwab (1990) and colleagues have sought to identify inhibitory molecules derived from central myelin. They succeeded in making a monoclonal cell line that secretes an antibody (known as IN-2) against the hypothesised inhibitory molecules. This antibody blocks the inhibitory effects of oligodendrocytes on axon growth in tissue culture.

Even more remarkably, Schnell and Schwab (1990, 1993) have shown that blocking the inhibitory activity *in vivo* can promote regeneration in the damaged spinal cord. They first made partial transections of the dorsal column of the spinal cord to cut the descending corticospinal axons. These axons will not spontaneously regrow across the cut ends of the damaged cord. However, they then implanted cells secreting the IN-2 antibody into the brain ventricles, so that the antibodies can diffuse via the cerebrospinal fluid throughout the CNS. In contrast to controls, corticospinal axons were seen to cross the area of transection and to regrow into the distal segment of the spinal cord in a substantial proportion of antibody-treated animals. Although the density and extent of the regeneration induced by this treatment is still extremely limited, these studies clearly demonstrate the importance of inhibitory factors in the limited regeneration observed in damaged CNS and open up new possibilities for promoting improved regenerative response.

Glial scars

The limits to regeneration as so far outlined are made more complicated by the formation of glial scars in response to CNS injuries. In general, CNS trauma results in a vigorous glial response (proliferation and activation), characterised as a glial scar and associated with the production of a number of extracellular molecules which are capable of further inhibiting axonal growth (Eddleston & Mucke, 1993; McKeon et al., 1991). This glial scar is age-dependent; in very young animals little scar tissue is deposited in wounds in the CNS (Berry & Henry, 1975), whilst in older animals the response is more marked (Berry et al., 1983). This may also help explain the more marked recovery seen in younger animals with CNS injury. The situation is not as simple as this, however, since the glial scar can in some circumstances promote axonal growth rather than inhibit it, possibly by the elaboration of neurotrophic factors (Reier & Houle, 1988).

Overall, though, the glial environment within the resting CNS is not permissive for axonal outgrowth, and in the case of CNS injury and glial scar formation the inhibitory influences can be even more apparent. Therefore any strategy to promote regeneration and recovery in the adult CNS must take into consideration the inhibitory nature of the glial environment, a point to which we shall return when we consider glial responses to intracerebral grafts.

Neurogenesis in the nervous system

The second aspect of the absence of regeneration within the nervous system is the inability of mature neurones to divide. Consequently, once neurones are lost they are not replaced, and the loss of critical populations of neurones results in dysfunction that cannot recover.

During development all cells of the body originate by progressive division from multipotential precursor cells. However, as the embryo/foetus grows and develops, the cells become progressively more specialised as the dividing cells become committed to particular lineages from which only restricted types of cells can derive, until cells ultimately divide into their final phenotypic state. Neurones and glia originate from precursor cells with limited differentiation capacity, and for most cells of the nervous system the final steps of the lineage are still poorly understood. Furthermore, it is clear that there is no general principle of “neurogenesis” (i.e. birth of new neurones) within the adult CNS.

However, there are two particular populations of neural cells that have been studied and which prove to be particularly instructive when considering plasticity in the CNS and PNS. The first of these is found within the PNS. The noradrenergic neurones of the sympathetic nervous system and the adrenaline-secreting neuroendocrine chromaffin cells of the adrenal medulla both originate from the same precursor cells found in the neural crest. The differentiation into these two different cell types is dependent on the neurochemical environment in which the developing sympathoadrenal cells finds themselves—a high concentration of corticosteroids drives the cells into the chromaffin cell phenotype whereas the presence of nerve growth factor (NGF) and a low corticosteroid environment drives the cells into a sympathetic neuronal phenotype. Furthermore, even when the cells have adopted their mature form they may be induced to switch phenotype by changing the environment in which they are grown and maintained. Moreover, the cells can not only switch their phenotype but also can be induced to undergo further cell division even in the postnatal state (Lillien & Claude, 1985).

The other well-worked-out cell lineage relates to the "O-2A" progenitor cells of the CNS, from which are derived both oligodendrocytes and type-2 astrocytes. The determining factor in their differentiation again appears to be an exogenous signal, from the axon in this case. However, unlike the case of the sympathoadrenal lineage, the number of O-2A progenitors in the adult brain is very small, and the regulation and ability of these cells to change their phenotype in the adult state is not known.

The lineages that give rise to neuronal phenotypes are not so well characterised for any population of CNS cells. It is generally believed that virtually all CNS neurones are born prenatally or in the very early postnatal period, although there are small populations of precursor cells that survive into adulthood. These cells are located in the lining of the ventricles and support a turnover of neurones in the dentate gyrus of the hippocampus (see later) and olfactory bulb throughout life (Suhonen et al., 1996). Although rare, these exceptions have recently been attracting particular attention because of the possibility that they reveal new sources of cells for regeneration of neurones and novel strategies for repair (see Chapter Nine).

In the developing CNS one of the simplest way of determining the birth dates of neurones and identifying the levels of neurogenesis at different stages of development is to label dividing neurones. Classically, this was done by observing chromatin accumulation as the dividing chromosomes separate within the nucleus of a dividing cell. This technique is extremely laborious as it requires cell by cell analysis under high magnification microscopy in very carefully stained sections of brain tissue. However, the task has become much easier with the advent of specific labelling techniques, such as by using radioactive thymidine. A dividing cell constructs a duplicate copy of its DNA by taking up molecules of the four essential amino acids that make up the genetic code, cytosine, guanidine, adenosine, and thymidine. If [^{3}H]thymidine is injected into a living animal, this radio-labelled amino acid can substitute for the normally available thymidine in newly synthesised DNA. The brain is then fixed and sectioned at a later time and either placed against an X-ray film or actually coated with an X-ray photographic emulsion. All cells that were dividing at the time of injection of the label remain radioactive and can be clearly identified on the film. Since ^{3}H has a half-life of several thousand years, the cells remain radioactive throughout their lifespan.

In a series of studies undertaken over two decades, Altman and Bayer have used [^{3}H]thymidine autoradiography to provide a comprehensive analysis of the times of birth of the main cell populations of the nervous system in the rat. From this comes the clear outcome that virtually all CNS neurones are born during the second half of embryogenesis, extending into the first weeks of postnatal life in only a few instances such as subpopulations of neocortical neurones and in the dentate gyrus of the hippocampus. There are only two populations of neurones that continue to divide after the immediate postnatal period throughout adult life—a group of olfactory neurones in the heart of the olfactory bulb, and scattered granule cells in the hippocampal dentate gyrus. The latter population is of particular interest because of the possible role of the hippocampus in the hypothesised plastic processes (e.g. long-term potentiation) involved in the laying down of new memories. The appealing aspect of this hypothesis has been tempered by the fact that neurogenesis in the dentate gyrus may be a particular feature of the rat. Thus, detailed studies by Rakic (1985) in rhesus monkeys using thymidine labelling have failed to find any evidence for a similar process in primates. However, more recent work has shown that precursor stem cells can be identified and shown to divide in the adult human and primate brain (Suhonen et al., 1996; Svendsen et al., 1997; Eriksson et al., 1997).

Of course, the critical issue is not so much whether neurogenesis takes place in the normal adult CNS, but whether it occurs in response to injury. Whilst traumatic injury in the brain can induce a massive increase in cell division, double-labelling studies suggest that this is entirely attributable to dividing precursor cells and glial cells, that differentiate into different classes of reactive glia, and not new neurones. Thus, the reactive response to injury includes the induction of glial cell division within the CNS, as well as migration of glia, macrophages, and immune cells into the nervous system, but it does not include the formation of new neurones as part of any natural repair process.

Thus, to summarise, there are two distinct aspects to the limited capacity of the CNS to regenerate. First, damaged axons cannot reform disrupted connections, and second, once lost, neurones are not replaced. Consequently, there is extremely limited capacity for self-repair. We might therefore expect to observe very limited recovery following damage or disease in the CNS. In practice, this expectation does not always turn out to be as gloomy as the neurobiology might predict.

SPONTANEOUS RECOVERY AFTER CNS DAMAGE

The limited capacity of the CNS to repair itself seems to be contradicted by clinical observation. After a stroke, a patient may initially manifest profound loss of sensation and paralysis on the contralateral side of the body and yet it is a common observation that substantial remission of symptoms can develop over subsequent weeks. Indeed, many aspects of practice lead the clinician to know that on some occasions a remarkable degree of spontaneous recovery can occur, especially in young patients.

Damage to the CNS can broadly be thought of in terms of either an acute fixed insult at a single point in time (e.g. birth trauma, or stroke in adulthood), or a chronic ongoing degenerative process that progresses over time (e.g. Parkinson's disease; see Table 1.1). It turns out that the opportunities for apparent spontaneous recovery occur primarily in situations of acute injury.

The processes involved in recovery after acute injury in the nervous system have been a major topic for speculation for at least a century and are still not well understood. However key concepts involve "compensation", "adaptation", and "diaschisis" (reviewed by Gage et al., 1982).

Compensation

Compensation depends on only part of a system being damaged. Over a period of time, the remainder of that system up-regulates to take over the function of the lost neurones and thereby compensates for their damage. Clear experimental evidence for such a process has been identified after damage of forebrain dopamine systems in rats. Thus, acute bilateral lesions of the ascending dopaminergic nigrostriatal pathways in the rat brain induce a profound aphagia, adipsia, and akinesia (cessation of eating, drinking, and all spontaneous activity, respectively) that resembles the classical lateral hypothalamic syndrome. Provided that there is sparing of at least a few of the midbrain dopamine neurones that project to the striatum, the acute stage is followed by a period of recovery that can take place over a period of days, weeks, and even months. These remaining neurones

TABLE 1.1
Some of the major CNS insults and diseases in humans

Examples of acute lesions	*Examples of progressive lesions*
Head injury	Parkinson's disease
Spinal cord trauma	Alzheimer's dementia
Stroke	Motor neurone disease
Birth trauma/cerebral palsy	Huntington's disease
Toxic insult (e.g. MPTP)	Inherited cerebellar ataxia
	Multiple sclerosis

increase their synthesis and turnover of dopamine and by so doing promote the recovery of function (Zigmond et al., 1990). In other words, the few remaining neurones undergo a dramatic up-regulation that restores a similar level of dopaminergic tone in the striatum as was originally provided by the full normal population of neurones functioning at a lower level of neuronal activity and neurotransmitter turnover.

This compensation within a given biochemical pathway implies that there is considerable redundancy in the forebrain dopamine system, such that residual neurones are capable of compensating fully for up to 90–95% of neuronal loss before permanent deficits are apparent. This is paralleled clinically in Parkinson's disease. In the human disease, symptoms are only apparent when the number of lost dopamine neurones exceeds 70%. At this stage of cell loss, dopa replacement therapy is required and is effective. However, once the dopamine cell loss exceeds 95% then side effects and other problems with the therapy arise, including the rapid switching of the patient from an "on", often dyskinetic, state to an "off" akinetic one. The similar ranges of depletions in the animal lesion and in the human disease suggest that in the early stages of Parkinson's disease plasticity of the spared neurones is fully able to compensate for the early cell loss. The symptoms then only become apparent once the dopaminergic cell loss is already quite advanced. Thus, it is not that recovery cannot take place in chronic disease, but rather that recovery is only able to keep pace with the slow progression of the disease up to a certain point. Once this critical point is reached the disease becomes manifest. Thereafter, the spontaneous compensation cannot keep up with the disease process, and the symptoms then become evident.

Adaptation

Adaptation is the process that describes the situation in which damage to one system results in another taking over the function of the lost system. In the 1930s Margaret Kennard showed that lesions made in the frontal cortex of infant monkeys produced far fewer deficits once the animals had grown up than did a similar-sized lesion in an adult animal. From this she formulated the hypothesis, frequently referred to as the "Kennard principle", that there is much greater capacity for reorganisation between neural systems when damage is sustained in young as compared to adult brain. Although implicit in classical notions of the multipotential nature of the neocortical mantle, there is limited direct evidence for this plasticity (although see Merzenich studies, discussed later).

However, some more direct evidence may be available from studies in the same subcortical systems as have been discussed in the context of compensation. As in the Kennard studies in the neocortex, injection of toxins that produce a profound loss of dopamine from the neonatal rat brain results in very few deficits in the lesioned animals, when compared to the profound deficits that are seen with similar depletions in the adult brain. Although the neonatal lesioned rats may show subtle deficits in complex learning tasks, they show none of the profound locomotor hypokinesia or regulatory eating and drinking deficits so characteristic of the adult lesion syndrome. Bruno and colleagues (1987) found that the loss of dopamine is accompanied by a marked increase in the density of inputs from another brainstem monoamine system—the serotonin fibres originating from the brainstem raphé nucleus. They suggested that the brain adapted to use the serotonin system in place of the lost nigrostriatal dopamine projection.

This interpretation certainly seems plausible. However, there are two major problems with it. First, the adaptation hypothesis would predict that a lesion or drug which blocks serotonin should have a similar effect in the neonatal lesion rats as does a lesion or drug that blocks dopamine in the normal adult rat (Altman, 1963; Bayer, 1982, 1983); and this has never been shown. Second, rats with neonatal lesions are extremely sensitive to drugs which block the synthesis of dopamine (α-methyl tyrosine; Rogers & Dunnett, 1989) which implies that the reason for the limited response to neonatal lesions is not due to adaptation but to compensation—a process that occurs to a greater extent in the neonatal, as opposed to the adult, dopaminergic system.

Diaschisis

A third process of recovery without regeneration was suggested by von Monakow at the turn of the century. He proposed a process, known as diaschisis, whereby nervous tissue exhibits two types of response to injury. The first is damage, resulting in cell death, from which the brain tissue cannot recover. The second is that the surrounding tissue undergoes a form of neural shock in response to trauma. These changes include inflammation, swelling (oedema), disturbance of blood flow, and reduced tissue oxygenation, which disturbs the biochemical metabolic and energy balance of the cells without killing them. These processes are reversible and can wane as the inflammation and oedema recedes and blood flow returns to normal, which is observed as a recovery of function. Therefore, the symptoms that recover are those which are the consequence of neural shock, whereas the residual deficits that remain are those truly related to the specific neuronal injury. In other words, this theory predicts that there is no recovery from primary neuronal injury resulting in cell death.

Von Monakow's diaschisis model emphasises the distinction between primary neuronal loss that is irreversible and the secondary consequences of the lesion which may in some cases be reversible and in other cases may be actively blocked. For a long time, this model had little direct evidence, but has come into sharp focus in the last decade with the realisation that secondary processes appear to be involved in focal ischaemic injury in the brain, offering new opportunities for neuroprotection from stroke in particular (Choi, 1990). Thus, experimental occlusion of the middle cerebral artery (which innervates the lateral parts of the cerebral hemisphere) produces a rapid loss of cells throughout the area of the brain in which there is a complete loss of vascular perfusion—the focus of the lesion. This focal area is surrounded by a "penumbra" zone in which there is an incomplete reduction in blood perfusion which by itself is not sufficient to kill the neurones. However, depolarisation of the dying neurones in the focus of the lesion results in a massive release of glutamate which causes excitotoxic damage to the cells in the adjacent penumbra. This secondary excitotoxic damage can be reduced or even completely eliminated by new drugs such as MK-801 that block the N-methyl-D-aspartic acid (NMDA) type glutamate receptors on those neurones (Foster et al., 1988).

Other aspects of the diaschisis model have been less well investigated but are coming under increasing research focus because of the additional prospects that may be offered for neuroprotection. Thus, for example, in multiple sclerosis there is increasing evidence that ongoing inflammatory processes within the CNS, causing demyelination of central axons, eventually lead to axonal and neuronal loss (Trapp et al., 1998). Early aggressive immunotherapy may be effective to prevent secondary damage which underlines the long-term disability that is often seen in this disease. Furthermore, in spinal cord trauma, a reduction in the oedema in the immediate aftermath of the injury by the use of high-dose steroids has shown some promise in preserving spinal cord function and thus reducing disability (Bracken et al., 1997).

Recovery and repair

Thus, we see that recovery can take place following damage in the CNS although it remains the case that regeneration does not take place on any reliable or regular basis. The range of situations where recovery is observed is limited and offers little help for many patients with traumatic injury of the nervous system and almost none for those with chronic degenerative disease.

The difference in the expected outcomes of acute injury and chronic disease is not because there are any major differences in the response of the CNS to injury in the two cases. Rather the difference lies in the time course of the degenerative changes yielding differences in the appearance of symptoms and the time available for compensatory processes to mask the initial phases of symptom onset. In acute injuries compensation, adaptation and diaschisis can all reduce the severe response to the initial insult. By contrast, chronic diseases of the nervous system involve ongoing degenerative processes that are initially masked by the same compensatory mechanisms, but that are eventually revealed at the point in disease progress where compensation fails and the symptoms become manifest.

However, in both cases compensation *is possible* even though the CNS neurones in the postnatal state are not capable of dividing. Despite the fact that recovery does occur, it is rarely complete in the adult state, and this, coupled to the progressive deterioration in patients with neurodegenerative conditions, has meant that alternative treatment strategies need to be sought. The new approaches that are being investigated include strategies to replace those cells that are lost, to provide additional support that will enable traumatised cells to survive, and to permit the regrowth of damaged connections in the nervous system. In all cases the aim is to restore neuronal circuitry in the damaged nervous system, and with it function.

LIMITED REGENERATION IN THE CNS

Although we have emphasised the relative inability of the CNS to regenerate, it should nevertheless be realised that the limitations are not absolute. Indeed, studies of those situations where even very limited regeneration can take place reveals opportunities for developing new strategies that stimulate intrinsic repair mechanisms to achieve functionally useful recovery.

Collateral sprouting in the injured CNS

The first major evidence against the dictum that regeneration cannot occur in the adult mammalian CNS was provided by Geoff Raisman (1969) who studied the detailed synaptic rearrangements that took place in response to cutting individual inputs to the septum in the rat. The cells of the lateral septum receive two main inputs from the brainstem via the medial forebrain bundle (MFB) and from the hippocampus via the fimbria (Fig. 1.7). These two inputs can be distinguished in the electron microscope both by the distribution of their contacts on the cell body and dendrites, and by the density of the synaptic vesicles in the two types of nerve terminal. Raisman found that when one input was cut, those terminals degenerated over 1–2 days, leading to a temporary reduction in the total number of synapses on the septal cells. However, over the following 1–2 weeks the numbers of synapses returned to normal, and all the synapses were of the type associated with the spared input. Thus, if the MFB inputs are cut, the fimbria input appears to sprout new terminals to fill the vacated postsynaptic spaces, and vice versa. This interpretation was supported not only by the restoration of total synaptic numbers but also by the appearance of numerous cases of double synapses of a type that are rarely seen in the normal brain.

The impact of these studies is hard to imagine three decades later. Although a number of other authors had explored issues of regeneration and transplantation during earlier years, those studies were widely ignored. At that time the *Zeitgeist* was rigid: regeneration simply did not occur. Raisman's studies provide the first clear and unequivocal evidence that, under some conditions, plasticity can indeed occur in the CNS. The fact that the PNS and CNS have different regenerative capacities was not in doubt, but the CNS is now seen to be capable of some regeneration in some situations, opening the way for the proliferation of research into new possibilities for CNS repair that we have seen in subsequent years.

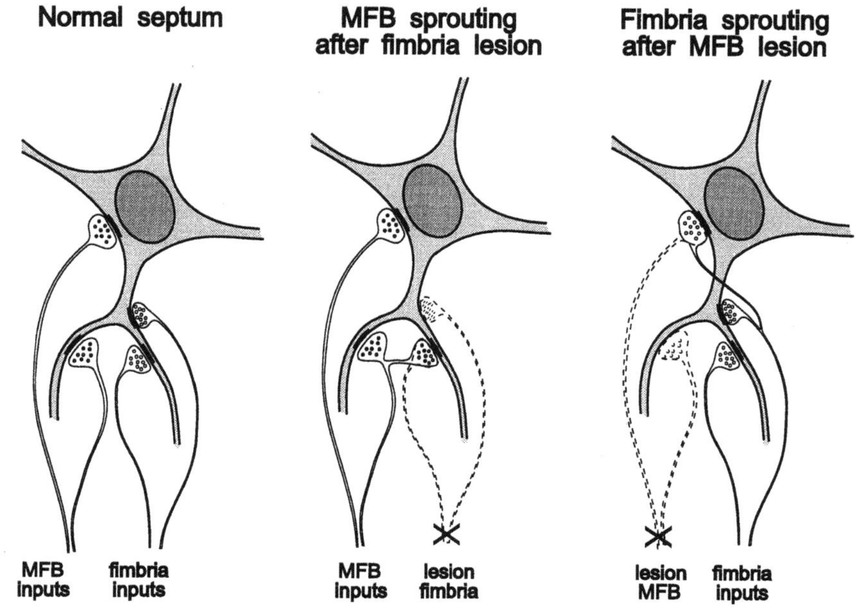

FIG. 1.7. Collateral sprouting in the lateral septum in response to injury. MFB, medial forebrain bundle. (After Raisman, 1969, with permission.)

Functional plasticity in development

Many of the possibilities for regeneration, plasticity, and sprouting in the adult nervous system may represent a recapitulation of developmental processes. It is certainly the case that there is considerably greater plasticity in the developing as compared to the adult nervous system, but studies on the reorganisational capacity of the immature organism can offer important clues as to the limits of what may be induced to occur in maturity.

The extent of plasticity in the developing CNS is well illustrated in the visual system. In their original experiments, Hubel and Wiesel discovered that the visual cortex is organised into columns of cells with similar response properties. The two main principles of columnar organisation are the ocular dominance (which eye has the greatest influence on a given cortical cell) and the preferred orientation of a line stimulus (for review, see Hubel, 1995). They represented these two properties as running orthogonal to each other, and hypothesised that the analysis of a given point in the visual field at the cortical level is by a hypercolumn (see Fig. 1.8), a block of cortex that contains all 360° of line orientations for each eye with corresponding visual fields.

This description of the normal organisation of the primary visual cortex provides the basis for analysing the consequences of disturbance. Hubel and Wiesel found that the normal development of ocular dominance could be altered by

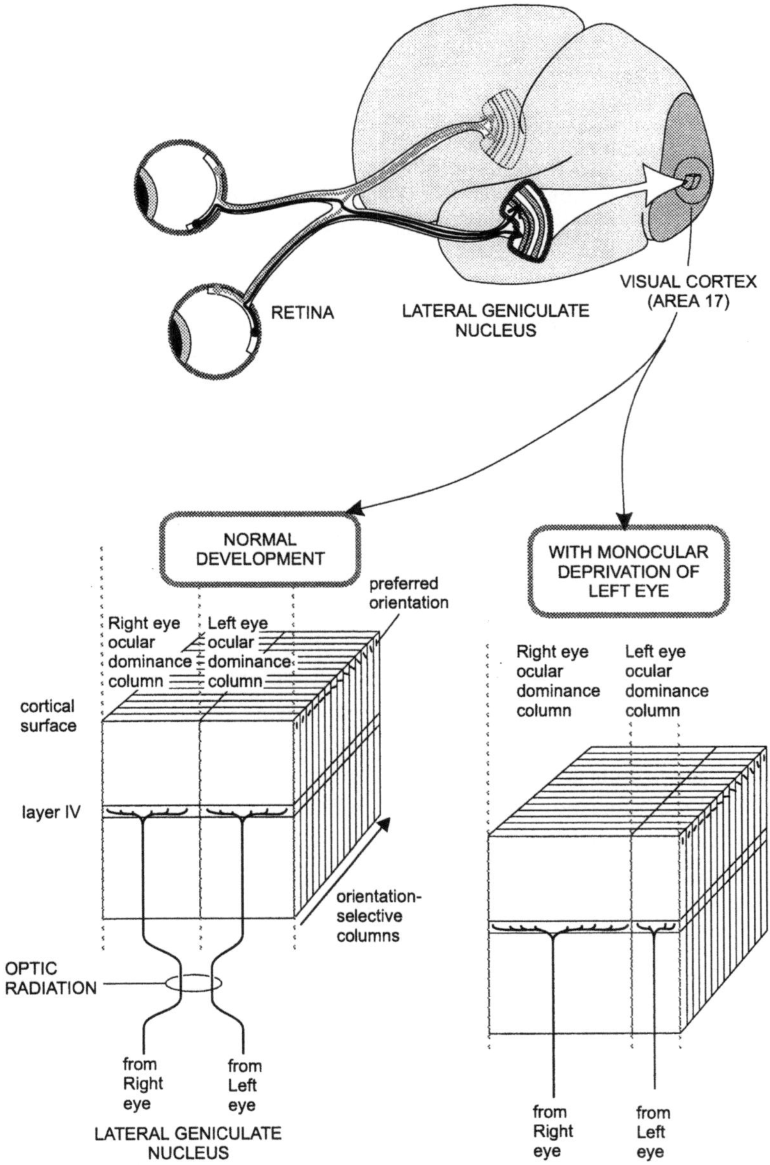

FIG. 1.8. Organisation of the visual cortex. Each eye provides an input via the lateral geniculate nucleus to layer IV of the visual cortex. This input then controls activity in the column of cortex above and below this layer for a particular line orientation and dominance by one eye. A hypercolumn represents a block of visual cortex which has ocular dominance columns for each eye and a complete set of line orientations (i.e. over 180°). Disruption of the thalamic input by monocular deprivation during a critical period in development induces changes in the ocular dominance but not in the orientation columns.

modifying the inputs of the two eyes during a critical postnatal period. For example, they restricted visual inputs into just one eye in a monkey for several months (by suturing the other eyelid shut—so-called monocular deprivation). When it was reopened, the monkey had dramatically reduced acuity in the sutured eye, and the majority of cortical cells were driven by the non-deprived eye. This was seen electrophysiologically as a shift in ocular dominance to the non-deprived eye (Hubel et al., 1977) and anatomically as an expansion of the thalamic input from that eye into layer IV of the primary visual cortex (LeVay et al., 1980). However, the ability of the non-deprived eye to expand its cortical influence was limited to a critical period of postnatal development. Thus, infant macaque monkeys are highly susceptible to monocular deprivation during the first 6 weeks of life. Thereafter, the plasticity of the system declines steadily, and disappears at somewhere between 18 months to 2 years of age. There certainly appear also to be species differences in the duration of the critical period in this system, which Wiesel (1982) has estimated to be in the order of 3–4 months in cats and up to 5–10 years in humans.

These experiments clearly demonstrate that experience, especially in the early postnatal period, can influence the structural organisation of a developing part of the CNS. Hubel and co-workers then went on to analyse the mechanism by which this developmental process may be occurring. They demonstrated that cortical cells could have their preferences further changed in the critical period by a process of "reverse suturing", in which the sutured eye was opened and the normal eye closed. This reversal in preference was again only possible during the critical period. However, importantly, the shift in ocular dominance was seen to take place within days of the reversal procedure and before any significant anatomical reorganisation could have taken place. This suggests that the plasticity of the visual cortex during the critical period involves functional as well as anatomical rearrangements, although it was unclear from these experiments whether plasticity was the result of disuse of an inactive system or competition between the two inputs. Subsequent experiments using binocular deprivation and an experimentally induced squint indicated an answer in favour of competition. In other words, the influence of a given cortical afferent is determined not only by the absolute level of cortical innervation, but also by its influence relative to other competing inputs.

Thus, plasticity is a feature of the developing visual system and it occurs by a process of competition of inputs. We next need to ask whether similar interactions can be seen in the mature central nervous system, as suggested by the earlier work of Raisman.

Functional plasticity in the adult neocortex

In the case of the visual deprivation experiments already described, it would seem that very little plasticity occurs once development has proceeded beyond a critical period. However, importantly, it is not altogether lost, as later experiments have shown (Gilbert & Wiesel, 1992). However, plasticity in the adult state is perhaps best seen in another sensory pathway, the somatosensory system where the plasticity of the neuronal connections that constitute this system has clearly been shown at all levels from the spinal cord to the cortex.

Merzenich and Kaas demonstrated in the early 1980s that the primary somatosensory cortex of the monkey reorganises itself following peripheral nerve injury (reviewed in Jenkins & Merzenich, 1987). They used electrophysiological recordings to examine the responsiveness of areas of somatosensory cortex following section of the peripheral nerves that projected to that cortical area. What they found was that the cortex does not lose its responsiveness to cutaneous stimuli, but rather that adjacent areas of skin (which would normally project to adjacent areas of neocortex) come to provoke a response in the area of cortex that has lost its previous inputs (see Fig. 1.9). This response is apparent immediately after nerve sectioning, although it takes several weeks before the whole cortical area is fully reorganised. Conversely, prolonged stimulation of a sensory

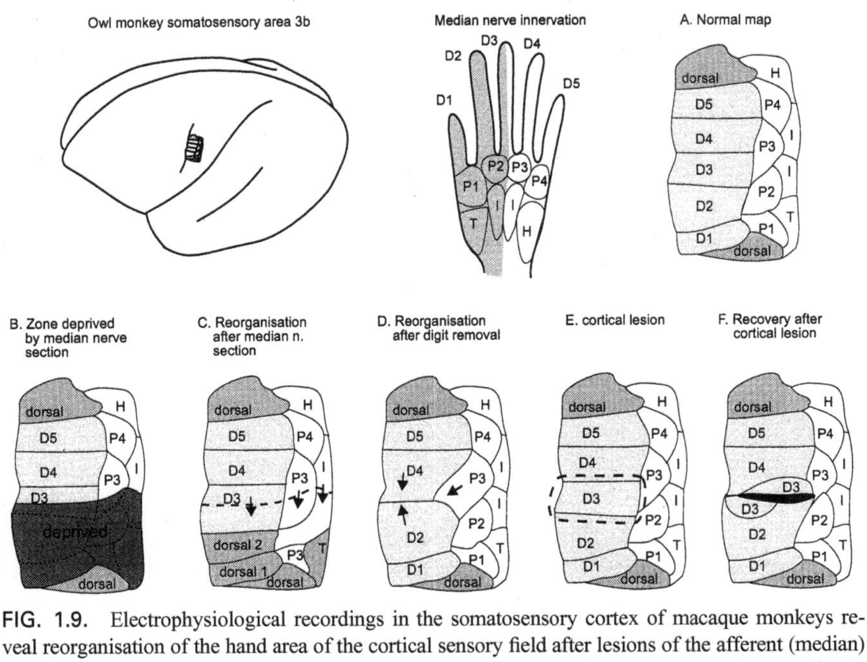

FIG. 1.9. Electrophysiological recordings in the somatosensory cortex of macaque monkeys reveal reorganisation of the hand area of the cortical sensory field after lesions of the afferent (median) nerve, removal of the digit, or lesions of parts of the cortical field itself. (Redrawn from Jenkins & Merzenich, 1987, with permission © Elsevier Science.)

afferent can induce not only an increase in the cortical target area (Diamond et al., 1993; Jenkins et al., 1990), but also an enhancement of tactile frequency discrimination (Recanzone et al., 1992). These studies therefore clearly indicate the capacity for reorganisation of topographical connections in the mature somatosensory cortex in response to altered sensory inputs.

This capacity for reorganisation of the central sensory pathways in response to altered sensory inputs is not just a cortical phenomenon, however, as similar effects have also been reported at the level of the spinal cord and thalamus (Garraghty & Kaas, 1991a). Indeed, this ability of the somatosensory system to reorganise itself in the adult state is not unique to this sensory modality and is seen in other sensory and motor systems, thus implying that plasticity of mature neuronal systems may be a widespread property of the whole CNS. This therefore leads on to questions of how the CNS reorganises itself under such circumstances and why it is so limited in others.

There are several possible mechanisms by which plasticity in the mature CNS can be achieved. First is the notion of "silent synapses" (see Fig. 1.10). These are synapses that are already present in the CNS but that are not functional in the normal state. The concept of silent synapses provides one possible neurological substrate for the hypothetical processes of compensation and adaptation described previously. The plausibility of this interpretation is suggested by the rapidity with which the plasticity of the cortical response to cutaneous stimulation after nerve section can occur, i.e. before there is time for any anatomical reorganisation. If the silent collateral connections are already present then the establishment of the reorganisation over subsequent weeks may simply involve changes in the strength of existing synapses.

This slower reorganisation may alternatively occur by the actual collateral sprouting of terminal nerve fibres to form new connections and synapses (see Fig. 1.10), of the type first demonstrated by Raisman (previously discussed). These two mechanisms are not mutually exclusive, although as yet there is no direct evidence for either. Importantly, there is no suggestion in these studies of regenerative regrowth within the CNS that the cut peripheral axons reconnect with their distal receptors.

A final possibility involves the use of corticocortical connections as the compensatory mechanism that underlies recovery when there is a major loss of afferent sensory information, as occurs with whole limb deafferentation (see Fig. 1.10; Pons et al., 1991). In these instances, activation of functionally silent synapses or collateral sprouting is inadequate to account for the expansion of neighbouring areas into the denervated cortex.

It is therefore apparent that what occurs in the development of the CNS can also occur in the mature adult state; that is, local plasticity is the rule rather than the exception. However, there are important constraints on the degree to which the CNS can adapt to changes in the sensory afferent inputs, not least being the age of the individual. Moreover, this level of reorganisation has been most

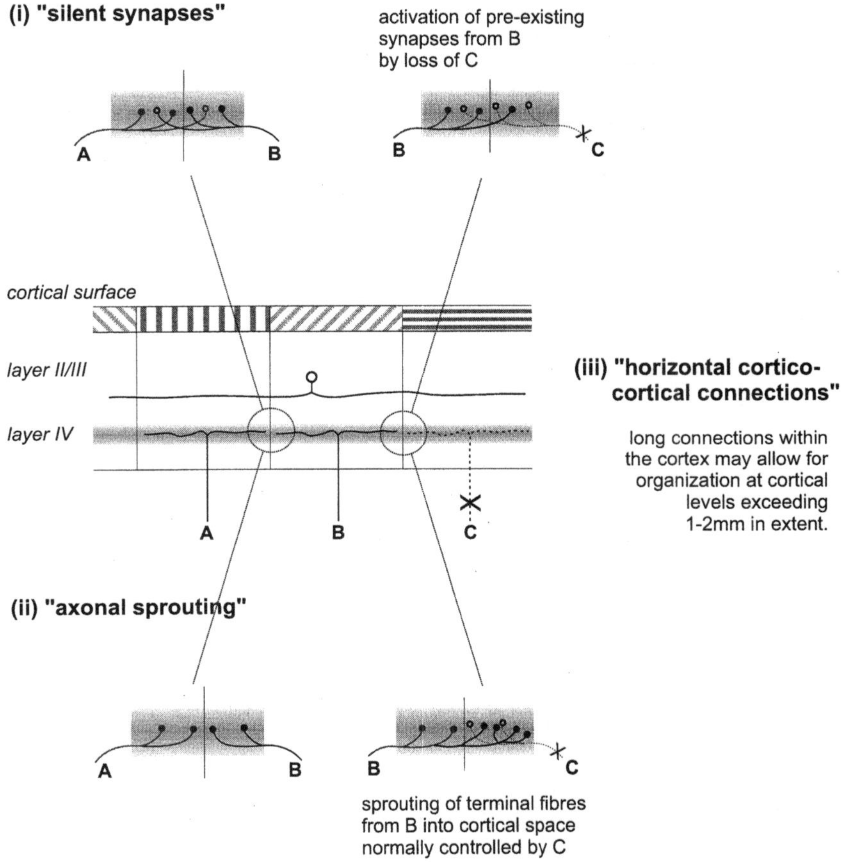

FIG. 1.10. Neuronal mechanisms of functional plasticity. (i) Silent synapses. When one innervation is lost, another innervation that is inactive under normal conditions now becomes active and takes over the function of the lost input. (ii) Axonal sprouting. Following loss of an input, synapses are vacated, other nerve terminals sprout to reoccupy the vacated synaptic spaces. (iii) Local interneurones exert collateral influences to co-ordinate activity in adjacent areas of neocortex.

apparent in the sensory afferent pathways, and clear-cut evidence of a similar capacity for reorganisation is lacking for central processing structures and motor output systems in the brain and spinal cord. This will have important implications for the treatment of disorders of the CNS.

CLINICAL STATEGIES TO DEAL WITH CNS DAMAGE

The current treatment of patients with CNS disease or damage employs minimally invasive strategies and therefore seems far removed from the previous discussion. However, it is probable that in the years ahead this strategy will be

TABLE 1.2
Different time frames for assessing and treating patients with CNS disease

Diagnosis	*Assessment and Stabilisation*	*Therapy and Rehabilitation*
Minutes/hours	Hours/days	Days/years Pharmacological and surgical therapy, psychotherapy, cognitive rehabilitation, physiotherapy, occupational therapy, speech therapy, patient education

replaced by one that is more aggressive and employs some of the principles that we have outlined and which we will be taking up in later chapters.

At present the clinical approach to patients with damage to the CNS can best be thought of as occurring in three temporal stages (see Table 1.2). The initial period represents the time at which the patient presents and the diagnosis is established. There then follows a period during which the situation stabilises and the extent and rate of progression of the insult is ascertained. This period can last for hours in the case of CNS trauma but may involve many months in the case of a neurodegenerative disorder. There then follows a prolonged period of care and rehabilitation that can last for years and which employs a number of different disciplines including speech therapy, occupational therapy, physiotherapy, and psychotherapy, as well as an input from neurologists and neurosurgeons. In this respect the patient may need drug treatments and/or surgical procedures that can alleviate particular symptoms (e.g. L-dopa therapy in Parkinson's disease or ventricular shunts for hydrocephalus) but which will require long-term follow-up and/or modification over years.

Each stage of the management of patients with CNS injury or disease requires different inputs from different specialities. Moreover, the needs of the patient at each stage are different. Overall, though, the goal is the same, namely that the patient is correctly diagnosed, the extent of the damage determined, and the most appropriate package of treatment instigated.

At all stages, but especially at the time of presentation, the condition from which the patient is suffering needs to be accurately diagnosed. This may seem to be a rather obvious comment but only the correct diagnosis will allow for the most appropriate treatment and prognosis. An example of this would be a patient with the motor symptoms of parkinsonism but who is only transiently and variably responsive to dopamine replacement therapy. Such patients may not have true Parkinson's disease but some other "Parkinson-plus" disorder (such as multiple system atrophy) for which a primary dopamine replacement therapy such as cell transplantation would not be appropriate. In addition to accurate diagnosis, techniques of monitoring are required to assess the patient's progress and response to treatment.

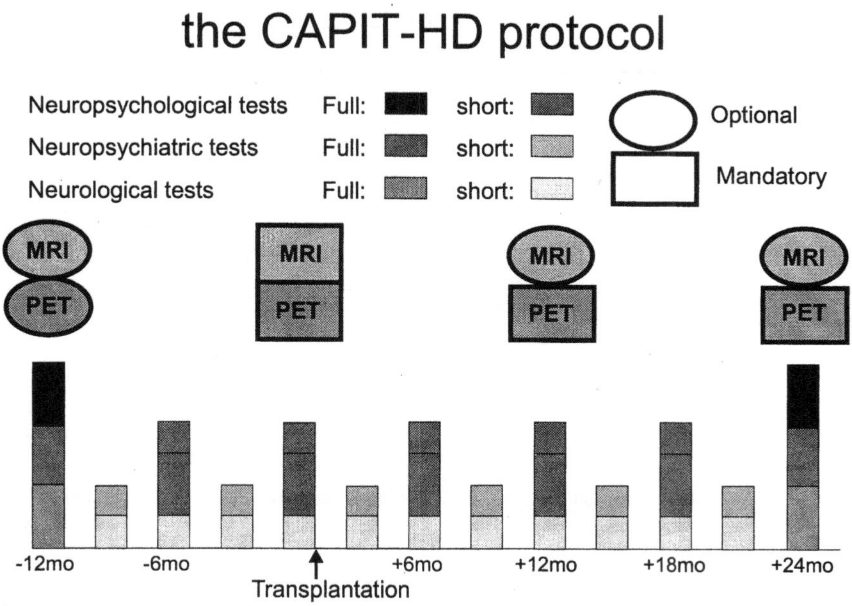

FIG. 1.11. CAPIT-HD core protocol for standardised neurological, neuropsychological, psychiatric, and *in vivo* scanning assessments of intracerebral transplantation trials.

A number of simple scoring systems based on the patient's clinical performance have been available for a long time, such as the Mini-Mental State Examination score for Alzheimer's disease or the United Parkinson's Disease Rating Scale (UPDRS) for Parkinson's disease. These have the advantage of simplicity and are well validated over an extended and widespread period of use.

However, these well-established scales often suffer a relative lack of sensitivity and there is an increasing demand for more sensitive and sophisticated standardised protocols for neurological and neuropsychological assessment of patients that can meet the demands of objectivity and quantification required for the evaluation of new (and often more invasive) therapies. Examples of these newer test batteries are the Unified Huntington's Disease Neurological Rating Scale and the multidimensional Core Assessment Protocols for Intracerebral Transplantation (CAPIT) with separate versions for evaluation in Parkinson's disease and Huntington's disease. For example, the CAPIT-HD protocol is multidimensional in its incorporation of neurological, neuropsychological, psychiatric, and scanning measures to assess the longitudinal progress of the disease at regular defined intervals (Quinn et al., 1996; see Fig. 1.11). The design of the battery has been guided not only by the goal of allowing comparability between centres within one country but also has selected tests that are available in different language versions to allow comparability on a world-wide basis.

TABLE 1.3
Imaging techniques for measuring CNS damage

Scan		*Mode of operation*
CAT	Computerised axial tomography	This uses a computer to reconstruct three-dimensional images of the brain from a series of two-dimensional X-ray images taken from different angles. It outlines the main anatomical structures but gives limited detail on the extent of any damage to the CNS.
MRI	Magnetic resonance imaging	This detects changes in the alignment of charged molecules in a strong magnetic field applied to the brain or spinal cord. It can provide very high resolution images of the extent of damage, as well as functional information of cellular activity under certain conditions of enhancement.
PET	Positron emission tomography	This is based on detecting the pairs of photons emitted as products of radioactive breakdown in the brain. It can provide functional analysis of the brain by selecting appropriate radioactive ligands (e.g. intracellular incorporation, binding to particular receptors, or uptake channels).
SPECT	Single photon emission computerised tomography	This test is useful as a measure of cerebral perfusion, and so can help delineate the extent of ischaemic insults.

The increasing sensitivity and sophistication of modern scanning technologies are also revolutionising the possibilities for direct *in vivo* visualisation and measurement of the progress of underlying neuropathology that was hitherto inconceivable (see Table 1.3).

It is only with the judicious combination of the highest level of clinical judgement with the most valid and sensitive assessment tests that we can expect properly to establish the nature of the problem, the extent of the damage, and the natural prognosis for the patient. At present few options are available, but we expect to see the experimental evaluation, and possibly the clinical introduction, of a variety of radical new therapies in the following decades that will revolutionise options available to clinicians and their patients. At that stage, the validity and rigour of our assessment protocols will become critical, first in selecting those patients most likely to benefit from any particular intervention, and then to monitor and evaluate the benefits (and problems) that arise from such interventions.

The three-stage approach of considered diagnosis and treatment may have served practitioners well in the past; but it is coming under increasing pressure. This is likely to become acute as and when new preventive strategies become available that are only effective when administered rapidly. In particular, the issue has now arisen in the context of both stroke and spinal injury: Experimental evidence is accumulating that rapid administration of acute neuroprotective treatments within minutes or hours of trauma (NMDA antagonists in the case of stroke, steroids in the case of spinal trauma) may significantly alter the degree of subsequent degeneration. However, access to the relevant medical specialists cannot be easily delivered within the present emergency health care system, at least in the UK, although the use of thrombolytic therapy in acute myocardial infarcts has shown that such therapies can be delivered rapidly if the proper infrastructure exists. Another possibility is the use of paramedical personnel for the delivery of such therapy, as occurs in the USA.

SUMMARY

The development of the nervous system involves the birth of neurones, which then send their axons to make synapses with their target structures through a range of neurotrophic factors and chemoattractive/repulsive molecules (see also Chapter Two). After the period of development has been completed no new neurones are born within the CNS, which means that any recovery process must rely on the sprouting of surviving axons. Whilst this is actively encouraged in the PNS, this is generally discouraged in the CNS through inhibitory signals from the glial cells. However, limited recovery can be seen, as, far from being hard-wired, the mature CNS does show a degree of plasticity. Although this is now only beginning to be understood from a biological point of view, it has been exploited for years with clinical programmes of rehabilitation in patients with injury and diseases of the nervous system.

CHAPTER TWO

Strategies for protection and repair of damage in the CNS

INTRODUCTION

The absence of consistent spontaneous repair following CNS injury or disease has heightened the need to identify experimental or therapeutic interventions that can promote recovery. The main strategies under current investigation are summarised in Table 2.1, and involve blocking various aspects of the neurodegenerative process, promoting spontaneous mechanisms of plasticity, and developing new strategies for explicit repair. The different levels of intervention relate to the temporal stages outlined in Table 1.2 and provide a summary of many of the strategies considered in this volume.

These different approaches complement each other, so that a concerted attempt relies on the use of both preventive and reparative strategies. In this respect it is important to consider once again the environment of the neurone, and factors important in its survival *in vivo*.

CELL DEATH IN THE CNS

In order to identify suitable neuroprotective strategies, we first need to identify the reasons why cells die in cases of neuronal trauma and neurodegenerative disease. Cells can die for a number of reasons *in vivo*.

Physical injury

Traumatic injury of neurones is perhaps the most obvious cause of cell death. A physical injury may so disrupt the membranes of the cell that it and its components simply disintegrate. However, this is not an active process of cell death and

TABLE 2.1
Strategies for repair in the damaged CNS (see text for details of each strategy)

- ***Reduce the extent of the original insult***
  - Calcium channel antagonists and NMDA receptor blockers in ischaemia
  - Monoamine oxidase inhibitors in MPTP-induced and idiopathic Parkinson's disease
  - Free radical scavengers in neurodegenerative diseases (e.g. motor neurone disease)
  - High dose corticosteroids in spinal cord trauma.
- ***Reduce the inhibitory influence of the CNS glial environment***
  - Antibodies to glial inhibitory molecules
  - Peripheral nerve grafts or cell lines derived from Schwann cells
- ***Promote the intrinsic plasticity of damaged neurones***
  - Neurotrophic factors, either systemically, topically or in the form of transfected cells
  - Grafts of embryonic or adrenal tissues with neurotrophic actions
- ***Replace the missing biochemical defect***
  - Systemic drug treatments (e.g. L-dopa in Parkinson's disease)
  - Intracerebral drug treatments (e.g. direct infusion into the CNS)
  - Implant cells engineered to secrete the missing transmitter (*ex vivo* gene transfer)
  - Direct transfection of the CNS with vectors (e.g. herpes or adeno-viruses) carrying the genes for the missing transmitter (*in vivo* gene transfer)
- ***Replace the missing neurones***
  - Implantation of the missing neurones from an embryo
  - Implantation of a related population of cells

in fact it is an unusual reason for cells to die in either traumatic injury or disease in the CNS.

Metabolic deficiency

A second obvious source of cell death is nutritive or metabolic deficiency. For example, if a cell loses its local blood supply, through either local or more general cerebrovascular insult, then it will not receive the nutrients and oxygen supply necessary to maintain its integrity and health.

The initial loss of essential nutrients produces a progressive inefficiency of cell membrane pumps which in turn leads to a toxic imbalance of the ionic concentration of cells, such as a major influx of calcium, and it is this that produces cell death (discussed later)—a point which highlights the fact that cells are dependent on a complex range of biochemical and metabolic processes to be kept alive. Indeed dysfunction of particular metabolic enzymes within the cell, such as those in the mitochondria, may be an important initiating cause in some if not all neurodegenerative processes. For example, an impairment in succinate dehydrogenase metabolism has been considered to be the fundamental biochemical deficit that underlies striatal cell death in Huntington's disease (Beal, 1994).

Calcium-mediated toxicity

The normal biochemical, metabolic, and electrochemical processes of neurones require that the cell maintains a stable and precise intracellular environment. The concentrations of a variety of ions, such as potassium, sodium, chloride, and calcium are maintained within narrow ranges by the action of specialised molecular pumps located in the cell membranes as well as a variety of intracellular buffering systems. Any disturbance of these homeostatic mechanisms can have dire consequences for the functioning of the cell: for example, a sustained rise in intracellular calcium level is actively toxic to cells. Indeed, the influx of excessive concentrations of calcium is one of the major final common pathways in cell death triggered by a variety of mechanisms, and any disturbance of enzymes or processes involved in calcium regulation can have a major effect on raising the sensitivity of cells to other toxic influences (see Choi, 1992).

Oxidative stress and free radical formation

Another main class of molecules that are extremely toxic to cells are free radicals—ions that have a high propensity to oxidation (for review see Beal et al., 1993b). These are by-products of many biochemical processes within cells. For example, the metabolism of some neurotransmitters such as dopamine can lead to the formation of hydroxyl ions that can combine to form toxic products. Cells have a variety of active enzymes that neutralise different free radical products (e.g. superoxide dismutase, glutathione peroxidase). However, underactivity in these antioxidant enzymes, or overactivity of other metabolic processes that favour free radical formation can enhance the susceptibility of cells to cell death. Both sides of this process have been proposed to be important in the development of Parkinson's disease (Simonian & Coyle, 1996).

Excitotoxic cell death

A further well-studied cause of cell death relates to the actions of the excitatory amino acid (EAA) glutamate (for reviews see Choi, 1992; Meldrum & Garthwaite, 1990). Glutamate is the most widely distributed excitatory neurotransmitter in the nervous system, and acts at a variety of different receptors characterised by their selective sensitivity to other EAAs—kainic acid, N-menthyl-D-aspartic acid (NMDA), and α-amino-3-hydroxy-5-methyl-4-isoxazol epropionic acid (AMPA)/quisqualate. All of these EAAs are agonists at their respective receptors and have potent excitatory effects that far exceed the stimulatory properties of glutamate itself. It has been known for a long time that several EAAs are toxic to the neurones, by a process of "excitotoxicity". The agonists produce a massive and sustained depolarisation in the postsynaptic cell to the point that the cell membranes and their associated ion pumps collapse and lose their ability to maintain cell homeostasis. The cell is literally stimulated to death. Furthermore, recently it has been discovered that glutamate itself can also directly cause cell death. Although this does not happen at the extracellular concentrations associated with normal intercellular transmission, if the cells are massively depolarised or have leaky membranes as a result of other insults the extracellular release of glutamate can quickly reach toxic concentrations. When this occurs, excitotoxic cell death due to excess glutamate appears to be mediated primarily through the NMDA receptor.

Inflammatory reactions and immunotoxicity

Although the brain has often been considered as immunologically protected ("immunological privilege" is a topic we will need to reconsider in some detail in the context of cell transplantation), inflammatory reactions can occur in the brain in response to injury or infection, resulting not only in the invasion of macrophages and microglial cells to remove debris, but also the invasion of immune cells (T-lymphocytes) with the capacity to attack nerve cells. Although neurones are relatively insensitive to immunological assault, carrying extremely low levels of histocompatibility antigens on their cell surfaces, glial cells are typically more immunogenic, and certain diseases are thought to involve autoimmune reactions within the brain and spinal cord. Thus, for example, multiple sclerosis (MS) is believed to be attributable to a complement-mediated attack on oligodendrocytes, resulting in the demyelination of central axons.

Growth factor deficiency

The first neurotrophic factor to be identified was nerve growth factor (NGF), which has become the prototype for all growth factors (see later). As neurones develop, they initially undertake a period of active outgrowth of neurites towards their targets. Typically, an excess number of cells initially grows towards the target area: Some establish connections with the population of target cells and survive, while others that do not establish appropriate connections regress and die. This process is known as "programmed" cell death and is a normal feature of nervous system development. The mechanism for programmed cell death has been studied in several model systems, at least in the peripheral nervous system (PNS). At a certain time during the peak period of innervation the neurones develop a dependency on growth factor molecules that are secreted by the target. The growth factor is taken up via specific growth factor receptors into the terminals of cells that establish connections with the target. It is then retrogradely transported back to the cell soma, where it acts as a signal for survival of the cell. Cells that do not innervate the target do not receive adequate supplies of the critical factor for their survival, and they undergo an active cell death (see Fig. 2.1).

Certainly, in development, many cells will not thrive in culture unless provided with the critical growth factors for their survival. This is one reason why

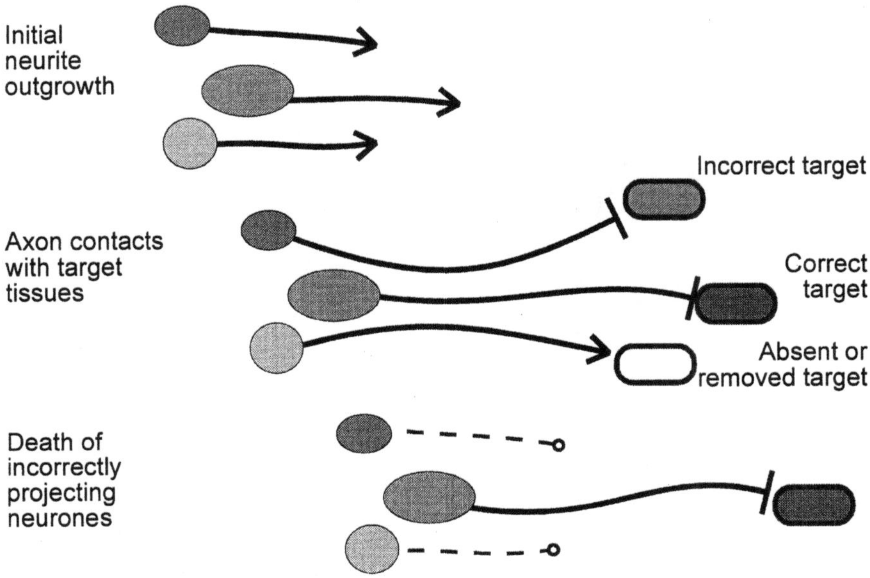

FIG. 2.1. Target dependence and retrograde transport of growth factor molecules is necessary to maintain cell survival, in particular during normal development. Many neurones in the brain retain target dependence for their survival even in adulthood.

serum is added to neuronal cell cultures, in order to provide a general trophic factor cocktail. The specific molecules necessary for the survival of different populations of neurones in development are being progressively identified (see below). For example, NGF itself appears to be important in promoting the survival of peripheral noradrenaline neurones, and central cholinergic neurones, but not of many other cell types. By contrast, developing dopamine neurones are particularly susceptible to glial cell line-derived neurotrophic factor (GDNF), ciliary neurotrophic factor (CNTF), and brain-derived neurotrophic factor (BDNF). It is certainly the case, as will be illustrated throughout this volume, that a variety of growth factors can also influence the survival of neurones in the living adult brain. However, it remains unclear whether this is due specifically to restitution of a target-related molecule that is deficient in particular conditions, or whether the neurotrophic molecule exerts a more general influence on cell survival independent of specific target dependence.

Apoptosis

Wyllie et al. (1980) described how the morphology of cells dying as a result of growth factor deficiency was markedly different to classic forms of cell death associated with trauma or injury. In the classical case, traumatised cells shrivel up, their nuclear and cytoplasmic membranes fragment, and the cells appear to

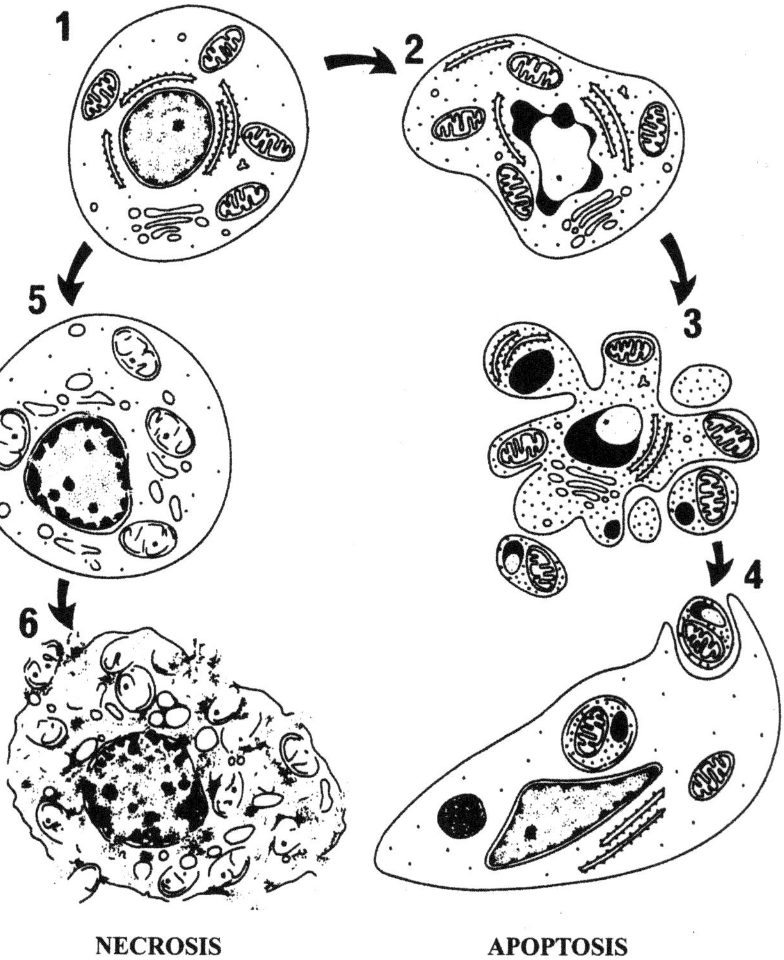

FIG. 2.2. Apoptotic vs. necrotic cell death. (1) A normal cell. (2) Onset of apoptosis is seen by compaction and segregation of chromatin against the nuclear envelope and condensation of the cytoplasm. (3) Rapid progression of apoptosis with nuclear fragmentation, marked convolution of the cellular surface and the development of protuberances. (4) Protuberances separate to produce membrane-bound apoptotic bodies, which are phagocytosed and digested by glial cells. (5) Signs of necrosis include clumping of chromatin into ill-defined masses, gross swelling of organelles, and the appearance of flocculent densities in the matrix of mitochondria. (6) Late stage of necrosis with membrane disintegration. (Reproduced from Kerr & Harmon, 1991, with permission © Cold Spring Harbor Press, after Wyllie et al., 1980.)

die by collapse and disintegration. By contrast, in developmental cell death, the cells swell up to a greater than normal size and the chromatin materials in the cell nucleus aggregate into clumps, before the cells appear to die by explosion. Wyllie described this latter process as "apoptosis" (see Fig. 2.2).

This suggests that although there are common pathways by which different causes of cell death converge, there are at least two different fundamental mechanisms. Apoptosis was initially considered to be primarily an active developmental event whereby cell death was genetically programmed to occur at a specific stage in the elaboration of a complex neuronal organisation. However, it has become increasingly apparent that apoptosis-like processes are widespread and may occur in all cases where there are insufficient extracellular signals to support cell survival. Thus apoptosis has been observed in neurones dying in adulthood, including in some neurodegenerative diseases and as the result of particular forms of insult. However, many dying cells in the context of disease or injury show features of both necrosis and apoptosis and thus raise the question as to whether or not these two processes represent the poles of a continuum of processes (Clarke, 1990).

NEUROPROTECTIVE THERAPIES

As we understand more about the variety of causes and mechanisms of cell death, it becomes apparent that they offer various possible approaches to neural protection. The individual causes of cell death seldom occur in isolation. Rather, many of these factors are closely interrelated and occur together. So, for example, a lack of blood supply to a population of neurones during a stroke not only prevents the adequate supply of oxygen and glucose and the removal of deleterious metabolites but also leads to the generation of toxic free radicals and high extracellular concentrations of excitatory amino acids (EAA), which in turn leads to excessive influxes of calcium ions. Consequently, alternative strategies for protection and treatment may target any individual component or a combination of components in this cascade.

A variety of neuroprotective strategies are under development that address the various causes of cell death at different levels, and many of these are showing considerable promise experimentally. In several cases clinical trials are already well under way.

Anti-inflammatory agents

Corticosteroids are effective in reducing the oedema around brain tumours with symptomatic benefit, as well as reducing the extent of spinal damage following spinal trauma. They appear to work by preventing the excessive leakage of fluid through damaged membranes and must be given at rather high doses. In multiple sclerosis, steroids are used differently, to reduce the inflammation that typifies a relapse in this disease. By so doing, they hasten the recovery, but not the outcome of this relapse.

Reduction of ischaemia

Calcium channel antagonists (e.g. nimodipine) can reduce the degree of cerebral vasospasm (i.e. spontaneous paroxysmal constriction of blood vessels) and thus secondary ischaemia, as well as help prevent the influx of calcium into the cell through its voltage gated channels. Nimodipine has been shown to be of benefit in reducing the sequelae of subarachnoid haemorrhage, although the mechanism by which this is achieved seems to be independent of any effect it has on cerebral vasomotor tone.

NMDA antagonists

A variety of glutamate receptor antagonists have been found to be effective in blocking EAA toxicity in the nervous system. Of particular importance for neuroprotection are antagonists at the NMDA receptor, since this appears to be the major site of excitotoxic action of endogenous glutamate. The most widely studied compound of this class is MK-801. It has been shown experimentally to protect neurones not only against direct glutamate-mediated toxicity (both *in vivo* and *in vitro*), but also against a wide variety of other traumas and forms of injury, suggesting that glutamate toxicity may be an implicit or contributory component in many different forms of cell death in the nervous system.

The most widely studied of these indirect processes is the involvement of glutamate excitotoxicity in stroke. As described in Chapter One, the cells dying within the focal zone of an ischaemic lesion release glutamate, which diffuses into adjacent areas of the brain to cause secondary excitotoxic cell death in the surrounding "penumbra" zone. This secondary excitotoxic damage can be reduced or even completely eliminated by treatment with MK-801 administered not only prior to, but also over several hours after, the ischaemic insult. This will have important implications for strategies to deliver effective treatment in the acute period immediately following a stroke. Although MK-801 itself is unlikely to enter clinical practice because of potential toxic side effects, there is now an active search for safe NMDA antagonists that can be delivered acutely to provide efficient and effective neuroprotection and thus limit the spread of damage in cerebrovascular accidents.

Calcium homeostasis

Two different approaches have been adopted to reduce the final common pathways of calcium toxicity in cells. First has been the development of calcium channel antagonists, such as nimodipine, which reduce calcium influx and have been shown to reduce cell death and enhance revascularisation in experimental models of ischaemic injury. Nimodipine and related compounds are the subject of a number of clinical trials in alleviating the immediate effects of stroke.

The second approach is the identification of the calcium binding and chelating compounds that cells use to maintain calcium homeostasis. Several families of calcium-binding proteins and enzymes have recently been identified (which have been allocated appropriately suggestive names, such as calbindin, calretinin, calcineurin, etc.). As their distribution, expression, and mechanisms of action within the cell, both at rest and in response to injury, become better known, we can expect manipulation of these molecules to provide powerful new options for intervening in the processes of cell death.

Antioxidants

Oxidative stress has only recently been identified as a potentially widespread mechanism of cell death in the nervous system, so antioxidative treatments are at an early stage of development. The primary focus of this research has been into the role of oxidative stress in Parkinson's disease, but its role in other chronic neurodegenerative conditions, such as prion disease, is now also being suggested.

In Parkinson's disease there is a convergence of several factors all promoting oxidative stress. Thus, metabolism of the key neurotransmitter dopamine involves free radical formation as an essential side product. Indeed, injection of free dopamine into the striatum can itself induce striatal cell death by an oxidative mechanism. There are high levels of ferritin (a molecule that promotes free radical formation) in the substantia nigra (the critical area for cell loss in the disease), and there has been seen to be a reduction in the activity of free radical scavenging compounds (such as superoxide dismutase and glutathione peroxidase) in the same area, both of which may contribute to the targeting of cell death in the substantia nigra in Parkinson's disease.

A variety of antioxidants and free radical scavengers are currently under active investigation as neuroprotective agents in animal models of parkinsonism. These include lazaroids, N-acetyl-cysteine and vitamin E, all of which have been found to be effective in promoting dopamine cell survival in tissue culture and protecting against a variety of catecholamine toxins in experimental animals. The first main clinical trial of vitamin E treatment in Parkinson's disease (the DATATOP trial, in which deprenyl, by contrast, was shown apparently to reduce disease progression) did not reveal clear beneficial effects, but other trials with lazaroids, N-acetyl-cysteine, and other related compounds are now under way.

Immunosuppression therapies

For diseases that involve a clear autoimmune component, an immunosuppression treatment is naturally suggested. For example, there is evidence that drug-induced abrogation of the immune response can reduce the rate of demyelinating plaque formation in multiple sclerosis (MS). However, such therapies do not affect the natural history of MS in an individual patient, although this has recently been disputed for β-interferon. The reason for this almost certainly relates to the secondary axonal loss that characterises this disease in the later stages (see Chapter One). Other immune-mediated disorders affect the nervous system both peripherally and centrally and thus antagonists of particular components of the immune response may have a role in a number of other neurological disorders. However, none of the major neurodegenerative disorders at present appears to have a primary immunological basis, although this has been disputed, most notably with motor neurone disease.

NEUROTROPHIC AND OTHER GROWTH FACTORS

The next strategy to be considered is the application of neurotrophic molecules that promote cell survival and growth. They have been considered as potential therapies both to retard the development of neurodegenerative diseases and to promote recovery by enhancing the regenerative capacity of the surviving neurones.

What is a neurotrophic factor?

Nerve growth factor (NGF) was the first neurotrophic molecule to be isolated, and the basic mechanisms of neurotrophic action supporting the survival of sympathetic neurones were largely worked out first for this molecule. So also, the basic principles of dependence of axons on specific target-derived molecules for neuronal survival during development and programmed cell death in the absence of such target-derived support were first worked out in the case of NGF. Over the past decade, many further molecules with similar structures and neurotrophic actions have been identified. These molecules are termed neurotrophic factors, and can now be classified into different classes with common structural and functional properties (see Table 2.2).

Barde (1988) identified three major criteria that a molecule should exhibit to be considered as a neurotrophic factor:

(1) The factor must be able to keep neurones alive *in vitro* and *in vivo*. In the absence of the growth factor, or in the presence of antibodies to it, these same neurones will not survive development.
(2) The molecule must be present in a biologically active form and synthesised in the target tissues of those neurones that need it for survival. In addition, the molecule is released by the target, incorporated into the presynaptic neurone by internalisation of a specific receptor, and retrogradely transported to the cell body, where it acts as an active signal for maintaining survival of the cell.
(3) The amount of the neurotrophic factor in the target tissue is limited and thereby regulates the population of neurones projecting to it.

TABLE 2.2
The main families of neurotrophic factor and some of their members

A. Neurotrophins	***D. Growth factors***
(Factors of the prototypic NGF family)	(Other neurotrophic factors of the CNS)
Nerve growth factor (NGF)	Epidermal growth factor (EGF)
Brain derived neurotrophic factor (BDNF)	Fibroblast growth factor (FGF1-5)
Neurotrophin-3 (NT3)	Glial-cell line derived neurotrophic factor (GDNF)
Neurotrophin-4/5 (NT4/5)	Neurturin
Neurotrophin-6 (NT6)	Insulin
	Insulin-like growth factors (IGF-I, -II)
B. Neuropoietic factors	Transforming growth factor (TGF-α, -β)
(Factors with a predominantly neuronal action, but that can also affect blood cells)	Tumour necrosis factor (TNF-α, -β)
Ciliary neurotrophic factor (CNTF)	***E. Neuropeptides***
Cholinergic differentiation factor (CDF)	(Peptides identified in the PNS, subsequently found to have central neurotrophic actions)
Leukaemia inhibitory factor (LIF)	ACTH
C. Haemopoietic factors	Calcitonin gene-related peptide (CGRP)
(Factors with a primary action in blood cell production, but also affecting neurones)	Cholecystokinin (CCK)
Platelet-derived growth factor (PDGF)	Neuropeptide Y
Interleukins (IL-1, -2, -6, -11)	Neurotensin
Other lymphokines	Substance P, and other tachykinins
	Vasoactive intestinal polypeptide (VIP)
	Vasopressin

Based on Baird, 1993; Patterson & Nawa, 1993; Schwartz, 1992

These criteria must be fulfilled by any molecule for it to be considered as a true neurotrophic factor. However, whilst they are met for NGF within certain parts of the PNS, this is not the case for the action of the majority of proposed neurotrophic molecules acting on neurones within the CNS. Thus, for example, whereas the survival of many populations of neurones in the CNS is promoted by the application of neurotrophic molecules, the neurones do not remain critically dependent upon their presence for survival in adulthood. Similarly, other molecules can promote the neurite outgrowth of neurones, both *in vivo* and *in vitro*, without influencing cell survival *per se*. Varon et al. (1988) drew a useful distinction between "neurotrophic" effects in promoting neuronal survival and "neurotropic" effects on neurite growth. Any particular molecule may exhibit either or both of these properties. In addition, in the present work, we also follow Varon in retaining the term growth factor for any molecule that acts via selective receptors to promote the survival and/or growth of populations of neurones, without requiring fulfilment of the full range of criteria for the developmental regulation of neuronal connections as originally suggested in the case of NGF.

There are other differences from the original concept of a full neurotrophic factor that also need to be clarified. First, the issue of selectivity and specificity has become muddied as more and more factors are identified and studied in the CNS. Many neurones respond to a number of different neurotrophic molecules, and one neurotrophic factor can influence several different populations of neurones. For example, whereas cholinergic neurones in the CNS exhibit a relatively pure NGF dependence, the survival and growth of nigral dopamine neurones is promoted both *in vivo* and in culture by a variety of neurotrophic molecules, including GDNF, CNTF, fibroblast growth factor (FGF), neuroptrophin (NT)-3 and NT-4, 5, but not NGF.

Second, the interplay of trophic factors in a given neuronal population may be more dynamic than once supposed. In the adult CNS there is continuous remodelling of synapses as part of the normal representation of learning, memory, and experience. It is probable that this occurs, at least in part, as a consequence of selective afferent inputs activating different neurotrophic molecules, which may also provide a basis in development for the competition of inputs in gaining synaptic space (q.v.). Therefore, neurotrophic molecules may be as important in sculpting synaptic inputs in the mature CNS as in regulating the development of the system embryologically. We will see that neurotrophic factors can be useful in both these respects in promoting the survival and growth of the neural grafts and in providing support to the endogenous postmitotic neurones that have been damaged or are degenerating.

Types of neurotrophic factors

The number of neurotrophic factors is constantly increasing, as are the numbers and types of receptors at which they act (Glass & Yancopoulos, 1993; Patterson & Nawa, 1993). However, the neurotrophic factors can be grouped into various families (see Table 2.2), which have common patterns of action and molecular mechanisms.

These factors act through specific receptors, of which the best characterised are those associated with the neurotrophin family of molecules, comprising the first identified neurotrophic factor, NGF, brain-derived neurotrophic factor (BDNF), and several other structurally related molecules (the neurotrophins NT-3, NT-4/5, etc.). These neurotrophins act through three related receptors on neurones (known as trk A, trk B and trk C) that take the form of tyrosine kinases located in the neuronal cell surface membrane (see Fig. 2.3). For example the septo-hippocampal cholinergic cells are dependent on NGF in development, and their survival can be promoted by both NGF and BDNF. The principal high-affinity receptor for NGF is trk A, and these receptors are located not only on the presynaptic terminals of the axons in the hippocampus but also on the cell bodies in the septum. Each trk receptor has three distinct molecular domains—one domain is found outside the cell membrane and is the extracellular ligand

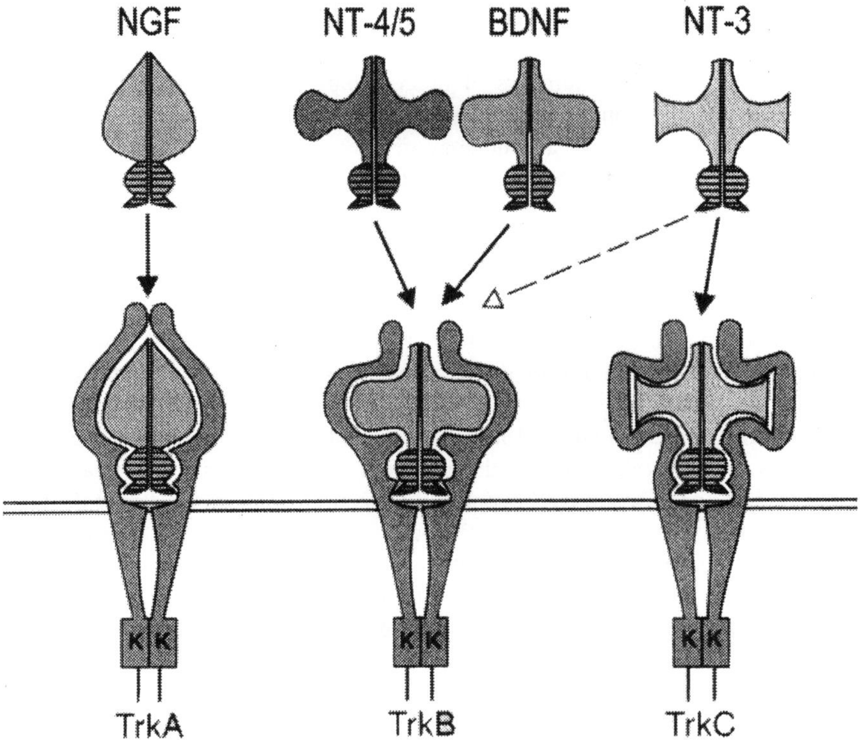

FIG. 2.3. The tyrosine kinase (trk A, trk B, trk C) family of receptors for the neurotrophin (NGF, NT-4/5, BDNF, and NT-3) family of neurotrophic factors (Reproduced from Lindsey et al., 1994, with permission © Elsevier Science.)

binding region, the second domain is a hydrophobic transmembrane region, and the final part is a cytoplasmic region that often contains tyrosine kinase activity (see Fig. 2.3). The activation of the receptor by a neurotrophin molecule leads to a cascade of intracellular proteins, alterations that often involve the adding of phosphate groups to a variety of molecules (i.e. phosphorylation and autophosphorylation). This in turn induces changes within the cell, including alterations in membrane transport and trafficking, cytoskeletal interactions, and gene expression, that together promote the metabolic vitality of the cell.

The importance of these receptors to our discussion is that in order for neurotrophic factors to be effective, the correct receptor with all its component parts must be present. Simple replacement of the neurotrophic input is not in itself sufficient if the receptors are themselves dysfunctional. Whether in areas of damage or regeneration, neurones must be able to bind the neurotrophic ligand and transform it into a response by means of the relevant receptor.

Neurotrophic factors and CNS diseases

The discovery of large numbers of neurotrophic factors within the CNS has stimulated the question of whether some (or even all) neurodegenerative diseases may be the result of a deficiency of one or several of these factors (e.g. Lipton, 1989; Snider & Johnson, 1989). However, this hypothesis has not survived critical examination. First, whilst certain CNS neuronal populations have some selectivity for neurotrophic factors, e.g. cholinergic forebrain neurones and NGF, this is the exception rather than the rule. Second, in contrast to the original notion of lifelong dependence, most CNS neurones appear to have changing patterns of responsiveness to neurotrophic factors over time. Third, it has proved extremely difficult to identify deficiencies in specific neurotrophic factors in specific diseases

Therefore, there remains little evidence that a deficiency of neurotrophic factors is causally related to the development of neurodegenerative conditions. Nevertheless, once we move beyond a pure neurotrophic model, growth factor administration may have a substantial role to play in treatment, by promoting cell survival and regrowth both of intrinsic neurones affected by trauma or disease and of grafted neurones implanted to replace or repair damage.

One of the major problems with considering growth factor administration is that of delivery in the CNS. Whereas their efficacy can be studied in tissue culture models by their simple addition to the culture medium, it turns out that most neurotrophic molecules are rapidly degraded, do not cross the blood–brain barrier, penetrate the brain poorly, and diffuse only short distances within the CNS parenchyma. Consequently, peripheral administration of neurotrophic factors is not effective and the route of delivery becomes a major issue in the development of any effective growth factor therapy. A number of different strategies have been proposed.

The blood–brain barrier can be circumvented by direct infusion into the ventricles or brain parenchyma. This has been the strategy adopted not only in experimental trials of the ability of NGF to protect septal cholinergic cells from axotomy-induced atrophy in rats but also in initial clinical trials of NGF application in Alzheimer's disease and Parkinson's disease in man (Seiger et al., 1993). Typically, in order to sustain prolonged delivery, the infusion cannula is attached to a slow-release pump device carried external to the cranium (see Fig. 2.4).

Although slow-release systems work well for infusions into the ventricles, chronic delivery directly into the parenchyma causes a marked inflammatory reaction. Therefore, in order to reach deep intraparenchymal sites, multiple injections via repeated insertion of an injection cannula via an implanted guide is necessary. This works well in rats, but has not been systematically investigated in man.

Third, perhaps the most promising developments will be to use graft tissues to deliver growth factors directly into the CNS (Dunnett & Mayer, 1992). This

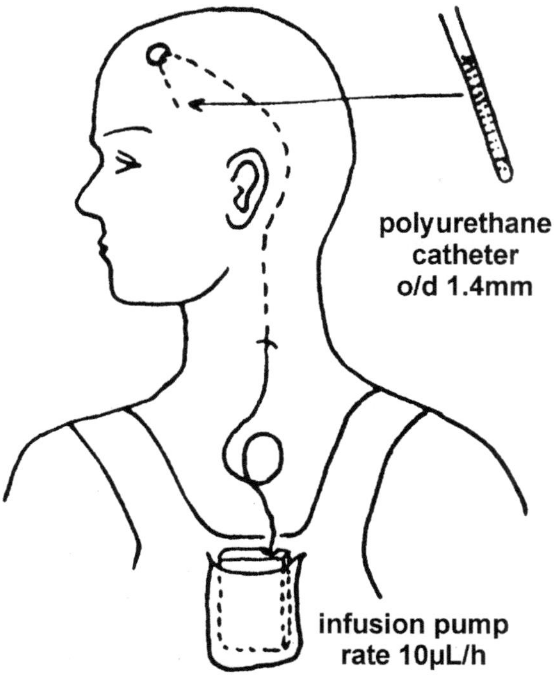

FIG. 2.4. Intracerebral cannula attached to a subcutaneous minipump for intracerebroventricular infusion of NGF in Alzheimer's disease patients. o/d, Outside diameter. (Reproduced from Seiger et al., 1993, with permission © Elsevier Science.)

may involve implantation of a donor tissue that naturally secretes the growth factor molecule, such as a segment of peripheral nerve as a source of NGF, or engineering of neutral cells (such as fibroblasts from the skin of the patients or host animals themselves) to express particular growth factor molecules. These can then be implanted to deliver the neurotrophic molecule at physiological concentrations into selected sites within the brain (see Chapter Nine).

Finally, rapid advances are being made in completely novel delivery technologies for drug targeting into the brain. These include attaching the neurotrophic molecule to either a carrier molecule or an engineered activated T-lymphocyte (Thoenen et al., 1994). In either case the vehicle serves as a Trojan horse to transfer the neurotrophic molecule across the blood–brain barrier and into the CNS. This not only has the advantage that the molecule is delivered to the site where it is needed, but also prevents the neurotrophic molecule from inducing adverse side effects in the periphery.

An associated approach is to engineer an appropriate virus (i.e. one that can infect mature neurones) with the trophic factor gene, and then inject the gene–virus construct into the nervous system (Verma & Somia, 1997). The virus infects the neurones in the vicinity and transfers the trophic gene into the brain. The infected neurones then translate the gene to generate and secrete the encoded molecule. Although classical retroviruses only infect dividing cells (which thereby excludes their use to infect neurones in the adult brain), certain atypical viruses have the capacity to infect postmitotic neurones. These include the herpes simplex virus, adenovirus, and adeno-associated virus. This method of "*in vivo* gene transfer" can provide a powerful alternative strategy to induce cells in the brain to make and secrete increased levels of growth factor that can promote both self-preservation and preservation of other neurones in the vicinity. Nevertheless, the technique is not without problems, not the least being the toxicity of several of the main viruses used. In addition, neurones can switch off expression of transferred genes within 1–2 weeks of infection, and there remain problems with sustained long-term expression with most viral delivery systems and gene promoters.

These new technologies are undergoing intensive investigation with rapid advances being made, and can be expected to develop substantially within the next few years. They will be considered in greater detail in Chapter Nine.

NEURAL TRANSPLANTATION

It remains the case that once neurones are lost in the adult mammalian nervous system they are not replaced. If we are to repair the damaged neural system fully, when all neuroprotective and neurotrophic strategies are exhausted, we have no alternative but to seek ways to replace the missing and damaged cells. The only available strategy, both at present and in the foreseeable future, is by neural transplantation. This is the main topic of the following chapters.

Rationale for transplantation

As already stated, the overall aim of any graft to the CNS is to replace lost cells and restore the damaged part of the CNS. In the ultimate case this is achieved if and when the graft becomes reciprocally connected with host neurones, provides a reconstruction of damaged neural circuits, and restores functional information processes within the host brain. Many conditions need to be fulfilled for full reconstruction to take place. For example, the graft must comprise the correct population of cells at their correct stage of development and be placed at the appropriate CNS site, in the presence of the variety of neurotrophic and neurotropic signals necessary to reproduce accurately the processes of development. Moreover, the graft must be able to stimulate sprouting and re-innervation of the normal afferent inputs and make the appropriate efferent connections. In addition it must display the same physiological and neurochemical processes as the normal host tissue at rest and when challenged.

Inevitably, most grafts fall short of this ideal, and it is debatable whether this level of repair has ever been achieved. Nevertheless, many grafts can go a significant way to achieving the recreation of the local circuitry.

TABLE 2.3
Possible mechanisms of action of grafts

Mechanism	*Description*
Reconstruction	Grafts replace lost cells, extend processes into host brain and form relevant synaptic connections.
Paracrine	Grafts release neurotransmitters in a non-specific fashion to produce (pharmacological) effects on neighbouring cells.
Neuroendocrine	Grafts release neurohormones into local blood vessels, which are then transported to both brain and peripheral targets through the host circulatory system.
Neurotrophic	Grafts exert neurotrophic effects by release of neurotrophic factors from the grafts, indirect stimulation of neurotrophic release from host, or induced release of neurotrophic mediators as a result of an inflammatory cellular infiltrate.
Bridge	Grafts provide a substrate on which host axons may grow and re-innervate distant targets.
Non-specific	Grafts exert their actions as a result of direct damage at the site of implantation, irrespective of the type and state of the graft at that site.

Mechanisms of transplant function

Although the rationale for intracerebral grafting was initially replacement of lost neurones and reconstruction of damaged circuits of the brain, it has become apparent over the past 20 years of research into graft function that functional repair can also be achieved by a variety of additional mechanisms that greatly expand the utility of this technology (see Table 2.3; Dunnett & Björklund, 1987). We have already mentioned transplantation strategies using engineered cells to deliver growth factors into the brain, and it turns out that cellular implants provide a powerful method of delivering a variety of molecules to precise locations in the brain. Although such molecules secreted by the grafts (whether neurotransmitters, neurohormones, or growth factors) will exert a primarily pharmacological influence on the host brain, grafts of living cells may improve on all other pharmacological techniques in that delivery is stable, is self-sustaining over long periods of time, maintains physiological concentrations of the compound at the precise sites where it is required, and affords additional possibilities of engineering regulation of turnover and release.

As a consequence of these diverse modes of action, the potential applications of graft techniques are now considered to be substantially wider than originally conceived when the focus was exclusively on cellular replacement and circuit reconstruction. These different applications will be illustrated in the course of the following chapters.

SUMMARY

In this chapter we have discussed ways of preventing and restoring function to the damaged CNS. In the first instance this involves limiting the extent of damage within the damaged CNS by a variety of pharmacological and neuroprotective strategies. Second, we may seek to stimulate and enhance endogenous repair processes using neurotrophic factors. Third, we may seek to replace lost cells by transplantation.

CHAPTER THREE

Experimental principles of neural transplantation

INTRODUCTION

In this chapter we shall overview the basic principles and techniques that have been developed over the last 25 years for achieving efficient survival of neural transplants in experimental animals, before going on in subsequent chapters to consider applications in particular model systems and human diseases.

Historically, the first published report of an attempt to transplant neural tissue was by Walter Thompson in 1890. He implanted cortical tissue taken from adult cats into the brain of adult dogs and reported surviving cells on post-mortem analysis several weeks later. With the benefits of hindsight, it is unlikely that there were any surviving neurones in these grafts, and the most likely interpretation that can now be placed on his microscopic line drawings is the presence of inflammatory and other glial cells within the graft site, some of which may have been of graft origin, although the techniques were not then available to demonstrate this. Nevertheless, Thompson considered the results sufficiently promising to warrant further investigation, and suggested that neural transplantation techniques would benefit from the attention of those who followed him.

The next landmark was a paper by Elizabeth Dunn in 1917 in which she reported the results of over 50 attempts to transplant cortical tissue from neonatal mice into the brains of adult mice. In what was probably the first instance of successful neural transplantation, she documented surviving graft tissue in two cases. Again with the benefit of hindsight, there were two features of her procedure that led to success where previous studies had failed. First, she used neonatal (rather than more mature) donors, during which period the selected neocortical tissues are still undergoing the final stages of cell division. Neuronal tissues from most subcortical sites are now known to require collection during the embryonic period of development, so her choice of cortical tissue for transplantation was fortuitous. Second, the grafts were implanted into cortical cavities but, in the two cases in which the grafts survived, the cavities were seen to expose the lateral ventricle, so that the graft tissue would have come into contact with the choroid plexus and ependymal cells of the ventricular lining. These two sites in the lateral ventricles have naturally rich and specialised capillary networks. It is now known that graft tissues must be placed in a site that can provide a rich vascular blood supply in order to nourish the implanted tissues in the phase immediately post-transplantation and to allow rapid incorporation into the host vascular network.

The following 50 years saw scattered reports of effective graft survival in the brain and spinal cord. Indeed, several of these reports, such as in the works of Wilfred LeGros Clark (1940, 1942) and Paul Glees (1940, 1955), provided convincing developments in the reliability of survival of neonatal and embryonic tissues implanted in the brain that went well beyond the demonstrations of principle provided by Dunn. However, these studies were largely ignored, in part because the *Zeitgeist* was simply against any consideration of regeneration as a possible event in the mature CNS (central nervous system) (see Chapter One), and partly because the anatomical tools of the day were not sufficient to address the necessary issues of specificity and organisation that were raised.

The turning point came at the end of the 1960s when Raisman (1969) provided the first unequivocal demonstration that regenerative regrowth of axons is possible in the mature nervous system (see Chapter One). This was closely followed by the clear elaboration of the principles that enabled transplantation to be achieved in the brain on a reliable and reproducible basis by several independent research teams under Lars Olson and Åke Seiger (in Stockholm), Anders Björklund and Ulf Stenevi (in Lund), Gopal Das (at Purdue University) and Ray Lund (in Charlottesville).

The critical features, (on which we expand in the following sections) were:

(1) Whereas PNS (peripheral nervous system) tissues may survive transplantation from older donors, CNS donor tissues need to be taken during early development.
(2) Grafted tissue pieces require a rich vascular supply if they are to survive, although the normal capillary network of the brain parenchyma may suffice for direct intraparenchymal injection of very small fragments or dissociated suspensions of cells.
(3) Immunological factors are less critical in the brain than we might expect from consideration of the problems encountered in organ transplantation. At least when grafting between donors and hosts of the same species, poor graft survival is more often related to infection, poor tissue preparation, or traumatic implantation techniques, rather than to rejection.

Definitions

Transplantation is the removal of tissue from one site and insertion of it into another location.

A first distinction relates to the relationship between donor and host. This can involve the removal of one part of the brain or body and placing it at a different site in that same individual, for example as in the case of adrenal medulla grafts to the CNS. These are known as "autografts". Alternatively tissue can be removed from one individual and placed into another of the same species, for example the transplantation of rat foetal nigral or striatal tissue. These are known as "allografts". Finally, tissue can be removed from an individual of one species and placed into a recipient from a different species, for example foetal human nigral cells grafted to the rat striatum, or pig cells into the human brain. These are known as "xenografts".

A second distinction relates to the site where tissue is placed. Cells or tissue placed back into the same site in the brain or body from which they originated (even if from a different individual) are known as "homotopic" (e.g. implanting foetal nigral cells back into the substantia nigra, or striatal cells into the striatum). Cells or tissue placed into a different site are known as "heterotopic" (or "ectopic"). Ectopic grafts include engineered fibroblasts or adrenal medulla grafted anywhere in the brain, or foetal nigral cells grafted into the striatum.

The tissue for transplantation can be prepared in a number of ways. For example, tissues can either be implanted as solid pieces or injected as single cell suspensions, with various levels of dissociation between these extremes (see later). The methods of preparation and implantation will influence the type of grafts that can be performed, and the likely survival and integration of the implanted tissues.

TECHNIQUES OF TRANSPLANTATION

Intraocular grafts

The first successful grafts of this recent period were provided by Olson and Malmfors (1970). They used the new catecholamine fluorescence technique to visualise survival of adrenaline-secreting cells of the adrenal medulla following implantation into the anterior chamber or the eye.

The intraocular graft technique is simplicity in the extreme. A piece (or pieces) of graft tissue is inserted via a fine glass pipette through a small nick in the cornea of the eye to lay on the iris (see Fig. 3.1). In the rat, this operation is rapid, simple, involves a minimum of surgical trauma, and heals quickly.

Although the choices of the adrenal gland as donor tissue and of the anterior eye chamber as transplantation site in that first study by Olson and Malmfors may seem obscure, in fact this model offers one of the simplest and most powerful techniques for experimental investigation of features of graft survival and

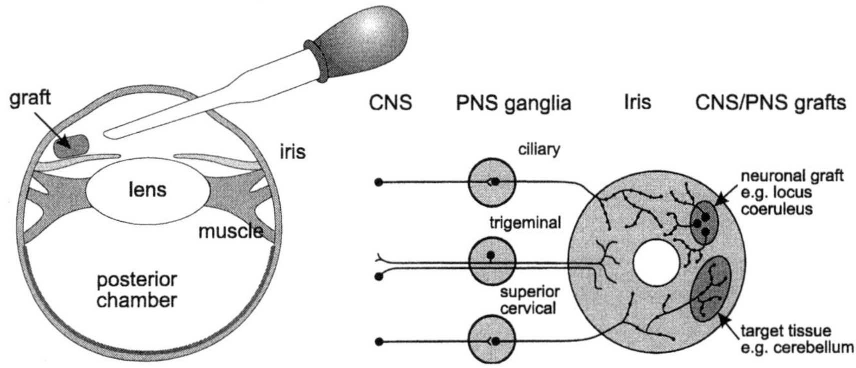

FIG. 3.1. The intraocular graft model. On the left is a schematic diagram of the graft technique, and to the right the host and graft innervations in the iris. (Data from Olson et al., 1983.)

growth in a controlled way. The anterior chamber of the eye is an immunologically protected site like the brain; the iris has a rich vascular supply to nourish the graft; and the survival and growth of the graft can be easily monitored on a day-by-day basis in a non-invasive way by simple inspection through the lens of the eye. The Stockholm group of Olson, Seiger, Strömberg, and colleagues has provided the most systematic comparison of the survival and growth of a wide variety of tissues under different conditions of age, preparation, co-transplantation, and growth factor treatment that provides the experimental basis and parameters for many other more complex techniques. For example, it has been used to provide some of the first demonstrations of both fibre outgrowth from neuronal grafts and the specificity of innervation by different populations of host afferents (see Fig. 3.1).

In spite of its great suitability for addressing a wide range of fundamental parametric and neurobiological questions, the greatest disadvantage of the intraocular model relates to the fact that grafts located in the eye cannot easily be used to model functional impairments following neurodegenerative conditions in the brain.

Intraventricular grafts

The second main grafting strategy is to place graft tissues directly into the brain. Whereas small tissue fragments can often survive when tamped or injected directly into the cortex or cerebellum of neonatal rats, this technique does not work well in adult animals. The critical issue proved to be the identification of a suitable rich vascular site to nourish the graft. The pia of the brain surface, the ependymal lining of the ventricular wall, and the choroid plexus of the ventricular fissures all offer suitable sites, making intraventricular placement of graft tissues a natural choice. As in intraocular grafts the technique is relatively simple. The tissue to be transplanted is drawn up into a fine steel or glass cannula,

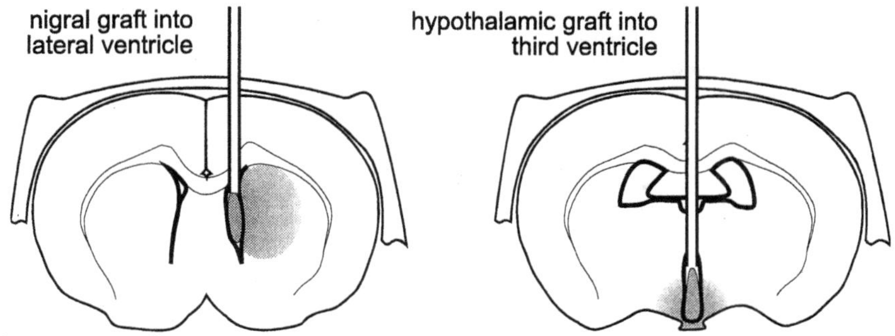

FIG. 3.2. Intraventricular grafts in the lateral and third ventricles.

which is stereotaxically positioned into one ventricle, and the graft tissue is then ejected (see Fig. 3.2).

The intraventricular approach has been used by several groups, most notably Freed and colleagues (1980; Perlow et al., 1979), to insert embryonic nigral tissues into the lateral ventricles in animal models of Parkinson's disease (see Chapters Four and Five). Similar techniques have been used to implant various hypothalamic tissues into the third ventricle (Gash et al., 1980; Kreiger et al., 1982) in order to restore hypothalamic–pituitary control of a variety of neuroendocrine functions. Rosenstein and Brightman have proposed the fourth ventricle for transplantation of peripheral nerve grafts with a poor blood–brain barrier as a route for delivering drugs that do not cross the normal blood–brain barrier from the periphery into the brain.

The main limitation of intraventricular placement is that only a limited range of graft sites is available, and many sites in the depths of the brain are not accessible.

Intracerebral solid grafts

In order to achieve greater flexibility of placement, an alternative approach is to implant solid pieces of tissue into specially prepared cavities of the brain, but then particular attention needs to be paid to providing an adequate vascular supply for the grafted tissues. Three opportunities offer themselves (Stenevi et al., 1976). First, cavities in some cortical sites can expose a natural vascular bed such as the lateral ventricle or choroidal fissure (see Fig. 3.3). Second an artificial vascular bed might be created, for example by co-grafting or manipulating other vascular rich tissues such as choroid plexus, iris, omentum, or muscle, although these procedures are all rather tricky and unreliable. Third, good results can be achieved by undertaking a delayed transplant operation. A small aspiration cavity is made in the cortex, the bleeding is staunched, and the cavity is plugged with gel foam. When the gel foam is carefully removed several weeks later a new pial lining is found to have reformed over the surface of the floor and walls of the cavity. This provides a suitable bed to receive the graft.

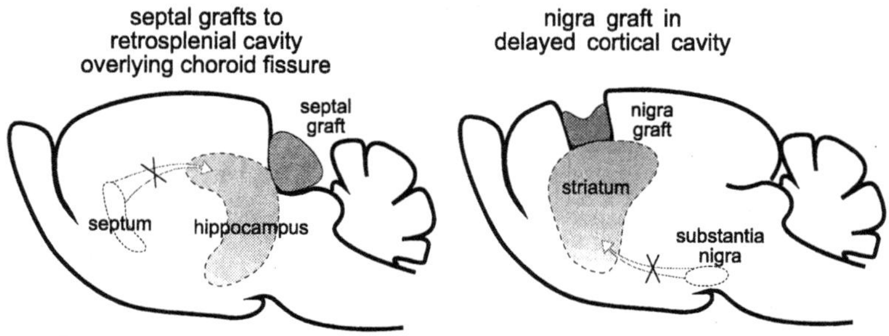

FIG. 3.3. Implantation of solid grafts into cortical cavities by single-stage (septal) and delayed (nigral) graft procedures.

Cavity implants were used in many of the early studies detailing the patterns of innervation provided by alternative tissues implanted into the denervated hippocampus, as well as the functional capacity of embryonic nigral tissues targeted at different neostriatal sites.

One of the main advantages of solid grafts implanted into cavities is that they can be easily identified in a subsequent surgical session. This can be exploited experimentally to allow for the injection of anatomical tracers, implantation of electrodes, or even graft removal as a way to assess the specificity of graft-derived functional recovery from lesion deficits. However, solid grafts suffer from the same major limitation as intraventricular grafts, in that only a limited range of graft sites are available. In addition the cavitation procedures induce greater trauma to the host brain than is involved in other implantation procedures.

Intracerebral cell suspensions

Björklund, Schmidt, and Stenevi (1980b) introduced the cell suspension method for implanting nigral and striatal cells to deep brain sites not immediately accessible from ventricular or cortical cavity placements. The procedure involved a simple adaptation of standard tissue culture procedures used for dissociating embryonic neural tissue. The resulting dense cell suspension is then injected directly into the brain using standard stereotaxic placement techniques (see Fig. 3.4).

The essential stages in graft preparation are as follows:

(1) The tissue is dissected from the embryonic brain under sterile conditions.
(2) The tissue is digested using an enzyme (usually trypsin) that breaks cell–cell adhesion.
(3) The tissue is washed, the enzyme is inactivated (with a trypsin inhibitor), and DNase added to prevent cell clumping.

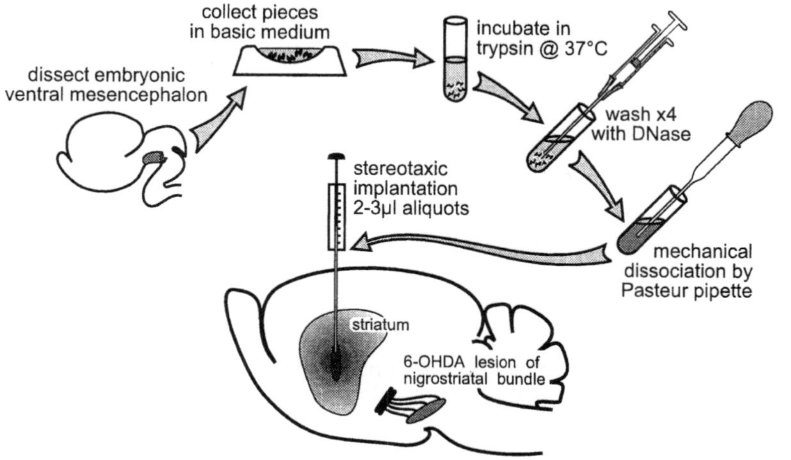

FIG. 3.4. Techniques for preparing and implanting dissociated cell suspensions in the adult brain. (Based on Björklund et al., 1983a.)

(4) The tissue is dissociated into suspension by mechanical aspiration and dispersion through a fine glass Pasteur pipette.
(5) The density of the cell suspension is counted and cell viability assessed with a "vital" stain that distinguishes live from dead cells.
(6) Finally, the cell suspension is drawn up into a fine-calibre syringe and aliquots are implanted by stereotaxic injection into a single or multiple sites in the host brain, using standard surgical procedures.

The particular advantage of the suspension method is that the apposition between the dissociated cells and the fine capillary network intrinsic to the brain parenchyma is sufficiently close that the grafts appear to survive injection directly into any site within the brain without the need for any additional steps to ensure a special vascularisation of the transplants. Consequently, grafts can be placed into deep brain sites with little additional trauma, almost at will, and there are few limitations on making multiple injections to increase the area of graft influence or to make co-grafts of different cell types. The injection of dissociated cell suspensions, as compared to other transplantation methods, allows the greatest ingrowth and outgrowth of host afferent and graft efferent fibres, respectively. In addition, the ability to assess the number and viability of cells in a suspension and to draw a large number of aliquots from a single preparation from multiple donors facilitates the design of properly counter-balanced experiments with carefully matched groups.

There remain, however, a number of situations where solid grafts are favoured. First, the dissociation procedure itself inevitably causes a greater degree of trauma than is involved in other techniques of graft preparation, so that this method may be less suitable for particularly sensitive cells. Second, the cell suspension technique favours grafting multiple hosts with a cell suspension prepared from multiple donors, and it is difficult working with the very small volumes that would be required to make a cell suspension from a single embryo. This becomes a problem when only single donors are available, as when identifying embryos with a particular genetic mutation or chromosomal abnormality (see Chapter Seven), or where individual embryos need to be genetically typed on an embryo-by-embryo basis for correlation with features of graft function. Third, there are occasions when it is necessary to expose the graft for manipulation under visual guidance, as in the implantation of electrodes or the injection of anatomical tracers. This can only be done based on stereotaxic placement in a suspension graft, which can be inaccurate if there is any migration of cells or dynamic change in the topography of the underlying lesion, as indeed occurs in the case of striatal grafts in animal models of Huntington's disease (see Chapter Six).

Nevertheless, for most purposes the cell suspension is the method of choice in both experimental and clinical situations. In the 15 years since its introduction, the dissociated cell suspension procedure has been found to be the most reliable and flexible of all transplantation procedures, and has been widely used to study many different cell types and model systems in the nervous system, as will be illustrated repeatedly through this volume. Similar implantation procedures are used for implanting cultured and engineered cells as well as cell lines of different neuronal, glial, and precursor phenotypes (see Chapter Nine).

SOURCES OF CELLS FOR TRANSPLANTATION

CNS tissues

The early studies of this century identified the need to use embryonic or neonatal donors if CNS tissue is to survive transplantation in the brain. This has been investigated most systematically by Olson and colleagues in the anterior eye chamber. For example, they have grafted noradrenergic cells of the brainstem locus coeruleus from embryonic, neonatal, and young adult donors, and measured the survival and volume of growth of the grafts. As shown in Fig. 3.5, the grafts showed the greatest growth when the tissues were dissected from the younger embryos, had declining viability with increasing foetal age, and were effectively not viable once the donor had reached a postnatal age.

It turns out that the same principle applies to all CNS tissues of interest (with the possible exception of the olfactory bulb). However, it is not simply the case that the younger the better; neither is the optimal donor age the same for all cell groups in the CNS. Rather, Olson and colleagues (1983) have emphasised that the optimal donor age for harvesting a particular group of neuronal cells correlates closely with the date at which the cells are undergoing their genetically determined final cell division. At this time they then commence a period of

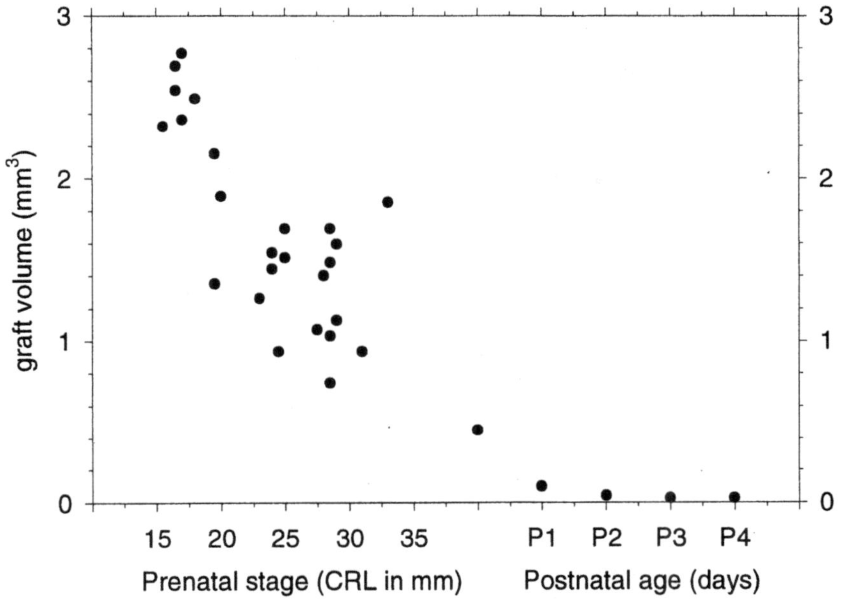

FIG. 3.5. The age of embryonic donor tissues is critical for viability of transplants. Illustrated for intraocular grafts of embryonic locus coeruleus from donors of different embryonic or postnatal ages. (Data from Olson et al., 1983.)

vigorous neurite outgrowth directed towards appropriate targets in the developing brain. Even when isolated from their normal site and transplanted into an adult environment, embryonic neurones continue to express these genetic programmes, grow, and seek out appropriate targets for connection in the host brain. Olson et al. (1983) provide tables of optimal donor ages for different populations of CNS neurones, based on systematic empirical investigation in the anterior eye chamber model. The same ranges have been found to apply in other transplantation paradigms in the CNS. Indeed, it appears to be the case that the time window may be even narrower for cell suspension grafts, with an earlier upper limit to the effective time window. This may be because the cells are already differentiated and first exhibiting neurite outgrowth by this time, and so are particularly sensitive to the increased trauma involved in dissociating the cells in this procedure.

PNS tissues

The tight restriction to a particular developmental time window does not appear to apply to PNS tissues, whether we are considering the Schwann cells in peripheral nerve grafts or the neuroendocrine and autonomic neurones of peripheral ganglia. This relates, of course, to the fact that these cells (unlike CNS neurones) continue to have the capacity to divide and regenerate throughout life.

So as a consequence, adrenal medulla, enteric ganglia, and sympathetic ganglia can be grafted even from adult donors. There has therefore been considerable interest in whether PNS ganglia may provide an alternative to CNS tissues for neural transplantation into the brain and spinal cord. Although such grafts are inevitably heterotopic and may not exhibit the same phenotypes as central neurones, nevertheless they may have several advantages.

(1) They may be more readily available than foetal tissues. PNS tissues may be easier to dissect, available in larger amounts, and (in the case of human tissues) without the ethical complications surrounding foetal or embryonic donors.
(2) They offer the possibility of autografts. If graft tissue comes from the patient him- or herself, then there are fewer ethical problems of informed consent. Moreover, notwithstanding the relative immunological privilege of the brain (see later), any immunological problems associated with transplantation between unrelated individuals are abolished at a stroke.

Cells and cell lines

The last decade has seen increasing attention to selecting, manipulating, and engineering cells in culture prior to transplantation. The technique for implantation of cultured cells is straightforward: stereotaxic injection following the same procedures as are employed for grafting dissociated primary cell suspensions.

Glial cells can be readily expanded in culture, and cultured glial cells survive transplantation well. Indeed, a period of growth *in vitro* with specific culture media is the general method for exclusion of neurones and selecting particular populations of glia for subsequent experimentation whether by transplantation or further *in vitro* analysis. By contrast, primary neurones appear to have a declining efficacy when maintained in culture. Several studies have found that nigral, septal, or striatal neurones grown in culture for 2 days to 1 week yield lower numbers of surviving cells when subsequently implanted than if the grafts had been implanted directly upon initial dissociation. In order to overcome the limited survival of grafts derived from primary neuronal cultures, several basic strategies have been investigated.

Cell lines. The first approach is to identify and maintain cell lines that express particular neuronal properties of interest. The source of neuronal cells that will proliferate in culture has traditionally been isolation from nervous system tumours, such as neuroblastomas, glioblastomas, and phaeochromocytomas. Their malignant properties *in vivo* are recruited to enable them to divide and grow over long periods *in vitro*. Whereas this has proved extremely powerful in experimental studies of factors regulating cell differentiation *in vitro*, the very properties that enable these cells to be grown in culture render them extremely problematic for use as an alternative source of cells for transplantation. Most studies have found that when untreated cell lines are implanted they give rise to aggressively invasive tumours. Alternatively, if the cells are treated with antimitotic drugs or X-irradiation sufficient to block their continuing proliferation, then the cells do not survive well long-term.

Immortalised cells. The second approach is to seek to "immortalise" neurones so that they will continue to divide in culture, in a manner such that proliferation can be terminated and differentiation induced when the cells are subsequently harvested for transplantation. After various strategies were tried, immortalisation has been achieved by inserting the Sv40 T temperature-sensitive oncogene into primary neurones. This gene induces the cells to proliferate at 33°C, the temperature at which they are cultured, but to differentiate into post-mitotic neurones at 37–39°C after transplantation into the mammalian brain. Shihabuddin and colleagues (1995, 1996) have demonstrated that immortalised neurones adopt a phenotype appropriate to the site of implantation when subsequently transplanted into the adult rat hippocampus.

Neurospheres. The third strategy is to culture cells under conditions where the differentiated neurones in fact all die off, but a small population of stem and precursor cells survive. Reynolds and Weiss (1992) first identified the conditions for proliferating neuronal stem cells in culture by treatment with high concentrations of epidermal and fibroblast growth factors (EGF and FGF). The proliferating balls of cells, called "neurospheres" by Reynolds and Weiss, can then be expanded exponentially through multiple passages over many weeks. Under these conditions the expanded populations of cells appear to retain a "multipotential" capacity to develop down different precursor, neuronal, or glia lineages when subsequently differentiated under different culture conditions. This procedure then may offer a powerful strategy for generating large numbers of embryonic neurones for transplantation, although the techniques to ensure good post-transplant survival and differentiation *in vivo* into appropriate populations of neurones relevant to particular neurological deficits is still not well resolved (Svendsen et al., 1996).

We will return to a more detailed consideration of these alternative sources of cells for transplantation in Chapter Nine, after we have developed the models for their analysis in the intervening chapters.

Cell preservation

Foetal neuronal tissues need to be implanted within hours of tissue donation if they are to maintain their viability. Therefore, in addition to the search for alternative sources of neuronal cells for transplantation, there has also been an extensive investigation of alternative techniques for preserving suitable embryonic cells and tissues to prolong their viability.

Cell culture. One strategy is of course to grow or maintain the cells *in vitro*, which, as described in the previous section, compromises the viability of the cells, at least with presently available techniques.

Cryopreservation. A second approach is cryopreservation. Adopting the conditions and media first developed for cryopreservation of organs and other cells, it is certainly possible to freeze neuronal tissues for thawing and transplantation on a subsequent occasion that may be months later (Jensen et al., 1987; Redmond et al., 1988). However, as in tissue culture, all attempts at transplanting cryopreserved cells have yielded substantially poorer survival compared to the use of fresh embryonic neurones.

Hibernation. A third approach is to keep the pieces of dissected embryonic tissue in a chilled hibernation medium that has a low calcium/low magnesium composition and slows down cell metabolism dramatically. It has been found that embryonic neuronal tissues can survive hibernation for up to 4–5 days with no loss of viability for subsequent transplantation (Sauer & Brundin, 1991). This technique may therefore introduce considerable flexibility in allowing a separation of the timing of tissue donation and implantation surgery, in particular in situations where multiple or rare tissues are required for a particular experimental or clinical application.

IMMUNOLOGICAL FACTORS IN GRAFT SURVIVAL

Immune privilege in the brain

The CNS has often been regarded as an immunologically privileged site. Thus, it was known even before the present era of neural transplantation that tumour cells from unrelated donors would survive transplantation into the brain whereas similar grafts placed elsewhere in the body would be rapidly rejected. This is equally true for grafts of embryonic neurones which readily survive intracerebral grafting between animals of the same species. Thus, experimental studies based on outbred colonies of mice, rats, or monkeys have all encountered very few problems of rejection, even though a skin or organ graft between the same donors and hosts would be rapidly rejected.

The immunological privilege is based on several features.

Low immunogenicity of neuronal tissues. Neurones express few histocompatibility antigens—the molecules on the cell surface that enable immune cells to distinguish "self" from "non-self". Consequently, neurones have a relatively low capacity to induce an immune response, even when implanted outside the nervous system. However, glial cells do express more histocompatibility antigens, and this increases further in response to injury or inflammation.

The blood–brain barrier is protective. The blood–brain barrier is effective in screening brain tissue from circulating cells of the immune system. Consequently, at least in the resting state, circulating lymphocytes would not routinely encounter foreign antigens in the brain. However, this restriction is not absolute; if the immune system is primed, peripherally activated lymphocytes can penetrate the blood–brain barrier. Moreover, standard graft implantation procedures themselves all involve surgical trauma that, however mild, will still be expected to open the blood–brain barrier. Such damage will heal rapidly, typically within a couple of weeks, but acute treatment with immunosuppressive drugs may be warranted over a brief period before and after surgery, even if prolonged treatment is not necessary.

Lymphatic drainage is absent in the brain. The specialised lymphatic drainage system found throughout the body is very poorly developed in the brain so that the potential transport and immune activation that follows the recognition of an antigen as foreign is greatly reduced.

It should, nevertheless, be appreciated that the immunological protection in the CNS is only partial, not complete. Whereas allografts of neuronal tissue generally survive well within a species (unless donor and host differ substantially in both minor and major histocompatibility antigens, which can occur with very divergent strains, Mason et al., 1986), rejection can be induced if a host response is primed by a skin graft across the same boundaries. This suggests that even if the brain is relatively protected against recognising foreign tissues, an activated immune system can produce a response in the brain that is quite as efficient as any in the periphery. Once donor and host differ across species boundaries, a vigorous and efficient rejection is the norm rather than the exception.

Immune protection in the brain

In situations where immunological reactions can be expected, a number of strategies for immune protection are available (Lund & Bannerjee, 1992).

First, a variety of immunosuppression drugs have been developed in recent years. Cyclosporin A has been repeatedly demonstrated to be effective for protecting neural xenografts in experimental rats and monkeys, and there is a limited but accumulating literature that this drug, either alone or in a "triple therapy" with azathioprine and prednisolone, is also effective in humans. It is still a matter of debate, as will be elaborated in Chapter Five, whether immunosuppression should be used in human allografts on the prophylactic principle that we still understand little about immune responses in the human CNS and an active rejection process in a patient might have devastating consequences.

A second strategy, promoted by Bartlett and colleagues (1990), is to sort a mixed cell population to remove the more antigenic cells prior to transplantation. What showed the feasibility of this strategy was the demonstration that purified neuronal populations after removal of glial cells survived xenotransplantation in much greater numbers than did unsorted grafts of mixed neurones and glia.

Finally, Lund and colleagues have shown that xenografts show much better survival when implanted into the brains of neonatal animals, owing to the fact that the implanted cells are already established in the host brain at the time when the immature immune system is still in the process of learning to distinguish "self" from "non-self" (Lund & Bannerjee, 1992). Although this can provide a powerful technique for studying developmental neurobiological issues in experimental animals, it is unlikely to prove a useful therapeutic strategy, at least in adults.

In summary, the immunological response of the animal to a graft is an important consideration in both experimental and clinical transplantation studies. Autografts of course have no direct immunological consequences. Allografts, in practice, provide few problems associated with adverse immunological reactions, although a modest acute protection may be warranted in critical or particularly adverse combinations. Xenografts, by contrast, will show minimal survival unless appropriate steps are taken to protect the grafted tissues against immunological rejection.

PRACTICAL ASPECTS OF CELL SURVIVAL

The preparation of tissue in an appropriate state for implantation is one of the key issues to be addressed in any experiment or practical therapy, especially when selective subpopulations are required, e.g. the dopaminergic nigral neurones in suspensions of ventral mesencephalic tissue (Barker et al., 1994). It is therefore a topic that will appear repeatedly throughout this book. We will therefore only summarise the major issues, and leave their discussion for later.

Graft preparation

In the standard cell suspension procedures, large numbers of cells are lost in the preparation process (Fawcett et al., 1995). This means that the transplantation process is generally inefficient. This can have important repercussions in the clinical arena, where the availability of foetal tissue is particularly limited. Strategies to enhance the viability of cells for transplantation by improvements in the preparative techniques is therefore an area of active investigation (Barker et al., 1994; Fricker et al., 1996).

Foetal age

The use of foetal tissue of the appropriate donor age is critical. Different populations of CNS neurones develop at different times embryologically, and grafts of such tissue are maximally effective when the tissue is harvested at the time of this development. This therefore means that foetal tissue of a given gestational age should be used, and that this gestational age needs to be known accurately (Dunnett & Björklund, 1992; Olson et al., 1983). Most populations of human foetal neurones for clinical application will need to be collected during the first trimester of pregnancy.

Graft placement

The number and location of grafts within the CNS need to induce maximal innervation and integration. This can create major logistical problems in terms of obtaining sufficient quantities of tissue that can be transplanted into a number of appropriate sites, in particular when donor tissue is scarce or the target structure is large, as can be expected to apply in many clinical situations.

Transplant environment

The site of transplantation immediately after grafting is probably not favourable for the grafted cells by virtue of the complex host tissue reaction induced by the implantation procedure itself. This will include oedema, local tissue damage, oxidative stress, and a variety of other molecular and ionic changes. Indeed, the highest level of cell death in neuronal grafts occurs within the first 24 hours of implantation (Fawcett et al., 1995). Consequently, a variety of growth factor, antioxidant and other neuroprotective treatments can reduce the susceptibility of cells to toxic changes in the host environment, enhance their survival and promote neurite outgrowth and connectivity of the cells once transplanted. In Chapter Five we see how the developments in this area provide a major strategy for enhancing the viability of grafts in the clinical context.

Glial reactions

The glial reaction to the graft may induce some loss of cells in the graft and/or reduce its re-innervation potential. The trauma of implantation will induce a glial response, which in theory may adversely affect the graft, although the balance between the adverse and reparative consequences of glial (and in particular astrocytic) reactions in and around grafts is only now becoming a topic of active investigation.

Therefore, a number of factors are important in determining the ultimate success of a graft. Although all of these factors have only briefly been discussed here, they represent an important area of transplantation technology and as such will resurface a number of times in later chapters of this book. At this stage it is sufficient to be aware of the large number of possible factors that govern the success or failure of a transplant in the host brain, whether in an experimental animal or a human patient.

SUMMARY

In the adult mammalian brain, lost neurones are not spontaneously replaced. Consequently, the only viable strategy for replacing critical neuronal populations lost through damage or disease is by explicit surgical replacement, i.e. by cell transplantation. Transplantation offers not only a way of replacing lost cells but also a means of providing support for surviving cells within the damaged CNS. In this chapter we have discussed the basic techniques, rationale, and aims of intracerebral grafting, as well as highlighting some of the major technical problems that have to be addressed in any transplantation programme.

The main emphasis of our discussion in the following chapters will be on the use of grafts to replace neurones lost through damage in identified CNS systems or particular neurodegenerative diseases. In each case the fundamental principles, procedures, and difficulties will be addressed experimentally, in studies involving normal development, cell culture, and experimental animals, before the clinical arena is entered. However, certain problems will only ever be answered by undertaking controlled clinical trials with patients. We shall, therefore, now turn our attention to Parkinson's disease, a disease in which clinical trials of neural transplants are under way, as a prototypical case of a neurodegenerative disease that can be treated and possibly cured by intracerebral grafts.

CHAPTER FOUR

Nigral grafts in animal models of Parkinson's disease

PARKINSON'S DISEASE (PD)

Parkinson's disease (PD) is a common neurodegenerative disorder that usually presents in middle age or early old age. It is found everywhere throughout the world, with an estimated prevalence of between 30 and 330 per 100,000 population (reviewed in Tanner & Goldman, 1996). The disease is characterised clinically by a picture of tremor, difficulty initiating movement (bradykinesia), and rigidity, which is due to an underlying degeneration of the pigmented dopaminergic cells of the substantia nigra (SN), the pathological appearance of Lewy bodies in the SN and elsewhere, and a severe biochemical decline in dopamine in the nigrostriatal pathway (Agid, 1991; Forno, 1990) (Fig. 4.1). The clinical picture of parkinsonism is a feature of many CNS (central nervous system) diseases involving the basal ganglia in the brain and as a result misdiagnosis of idiopathic PD is not uncommon (Hughes et al., 1992). This is important because the ability accurately to diagnose true idiopathic PD is not only critical for an understanding of the aetiology of this condition, but will also be central to any transplantation programme.

The cause of idiopathic Parkinson's disease is unknown, but there is accumulating evidence that its pathogenesis may in some way be related to a reduced ability of the cell to deal with metabolic stresses. Dopaminergic neurones of the SN generate large numbers of toxic free radicals in response to metabolic stresses, which is compounded by their reduced ability to deal with them (Jenner & Olanow, 1996). The first protein of the mitochondrial respiratory chain, complex I (NADH coenzyme Q), is selectively deficient in nigral dopaminergic neurones in patients with idiopathic PD relative to controls. This enzyme can

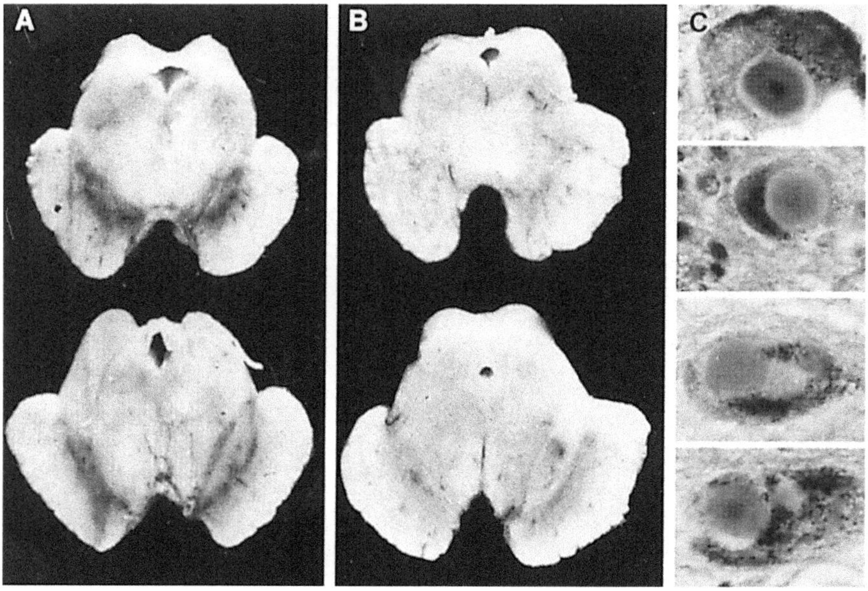

FIG. 4.1. Neuropathology of Parkinson's disease. (A) Normal pigmented dopamine neurones of the substantia nigra. (B) Loss of pigmented neurones from the substantia nigra in Parkinson's disease. (C) Four examples of Lewy bodies in neurones of the parkinsonian substantia nigra, the classical pathological hallmarks of the disease. This brainstem pathology and cell loss results in degeneration of the nigrostriatal pathway, leading in turn to dopamine depletion in the basal ganglia. (Reproduced from Forno, 1990, with permission © Chapman and Hall.)

also be inhibited by a variety of neurotoxins, most notably MPP+ (1-methyl-4-phenylpyridium ion), the active metabolite of the selective neurotoxin 1-methyl-4-phenyl-1,2,3,6-tetrahydropyridine (MPTP, Burns, 1991). The consequence of a deficiency in this enzyme's activity is that oxidative phosphorylation (which generates the energy of a cell) is inhibited, which in turn leads to reduced levels of adenosine triphosphate (ATP) and ultimately cell death (Schapira, 1992). Furthermore, there is increasing evidence that there is an elevated state of oxidative or metabolic stress within the SN in PD, which will also contribute to the selective death of these neurones.

The importance of this theory to our discussion is that if PD is due to an intrinsic defect in the patient's own dopaminergic nigral neurones, rather than an environmental agent (Rajput, 1993), then there is no reason to believe that the grafted neurones will die in the same way as the patient's own original population of dopaminergic nigral neurones. Of course, there is the potential that the donor embryo would have developed PD, but as the disease typically does not present until 40–50 years of age this seems more of a theoretical than a real risk and, as we shall see in Chapter Five, has not turned out to be a substantive problem in the first clinical trials.

Although the classical biochemical deficit in PD results from the loss of the dopaminergic nigrostriatal neurones, the disease is by no means confined to this one anatomical or biochemical system. Pathology is often found outside the SN (Forno, 1990) and is associated with extensive changes in multiple transmitters within the CNS, including the acetylcholine and noradrenaline systems of the forebrain (Agid et al., 1989). This may be reflected in the diversity of cognitive and other non-motor features in this disease (Gibb, 1989), some of which are relatively unresponsive to dopaminergic replacement therapy. This therefore means that grafts specifically designed to replace striatal dopamine deficiencies will only ever treat the core pathology of this disease, although this may nevertheless be sufficient to alleviate the most disabling components of PD.

ANIMAL MODELS OF PD

Anatomical organisation of forebrain dopamine systems

Animal models of PD typically rely on the use of selective dopaminergic toxins. In order, however, to understand the effects of these neurotoxic lesions a brief summary of the pharmacological anatomy of the basal ganglia is required (see Fig. 4.2).

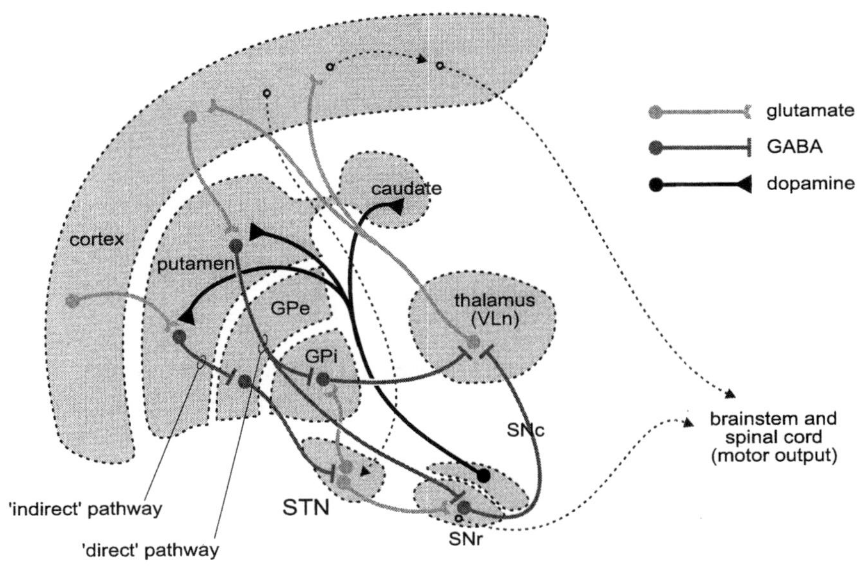

FIG. 4.2. Chemical neuroanatomy of the basal ganglia, showing the main nuclei and the transmitters that mediate their interconnections. GPe, GPi, external and internal segments of the globus pallidus; SNc, SNr, pars compacta and pars reticulata of the substantia nigra; STN, subthalamic nucleus; VLn, ventrolateral nucleus of the thalamus. (Based on Henderson & Dunnett, 1998.)

The basal ganglia are made up of several major nuclei, including the substantia nigra (SN), globus pallidus (or "pallidum"), subthalamic nucleus, and striatum. This latter structure has a large dorsal part (called the "neostriatum") made up of the caudate nucleus and putamen and a ventral part (called the "ventral striatum") made up of the nucleus accumbens and olfactory tubercle. Both the dorsal and the ventral striatum receive a dense dopaminergic innervation which originates in the SN and adjacent ventral tegmental area (VTA) of the brainstem. In this book we shall be concentrating on the dorsal parts, and any reference to the "striatum" will imply the dorsal neostriatum; when the ventral striatum is being discussed, this will explicitly be made clear.

The dopaminergic innervation of the dorsal striatum is important in modulating the other striatal inputs from the cortex and thalamus, which is then coded for in the output from the dorsal striatum to the pallidum and SN, which in turn relay information to the thalamus and from there to the premotor areas of the cortex (see Fig. 4.2). The subthalamic nucleus serves to modulate both the pallidal and nigral output to the thalamus. In PD, therefore, there is a loss of the dopaminergic input to the dorsal striatum, which ultimately leads to increased inhibition within the thalamus from the basal ganglia outflow nuclei.

The dopaminergic neurones of the SNc (the pars compacta part of the SN) receive a major feedback input from the striatum. This striatonigral projection contains a number of different neurotransmitters, some of which might coexist together, including GABA (γ-amino butyric acid), substance P, dynorphin and enkephalin. This striatonigral pathway originates from a different cell population than those directed to the globus pallidum, and, although the predominant termination is to the pars reticulata part of the SN (SNr), the long dendrites of the dopaminergic cells in the SNc mean that these neurones are influenced by descending striatal projections (Beckstead & Cruz, 1986). The other afferent inputs to the SN include a glutaminergic input from the cortex and a serotonergic input from the raphé nuclei, as well as a host of lesser inputs from other brainstem sites (reviewed in Condé, 1992).

Development of forebrain dopamine systems

The SN, containing the dopamine neurones that project to the striatum, is located in the ventral mesencephalon, which develops as part of the midbrain. On gross inspection, this nucleus consists of two major parts, the predominantly GABAergic SNr and the dopaminergic SNc (see Fig. 4.2). In the adult rat, the SNc contains 21,000 dopaminergic neurones (Björklund & Lindvall, 1986; German & Manaye, 1993), which together with 22,000 dopaminergic neurones in the ventral tegmental and other adjacent areas make up the midbrain dopaminergic system. These dopaminergic neurones have relatively large cell bodies with numerous very long dendrites (frequently over 500μm). The dendrites themselves contain and release dopamine (DA) and may be subserving some local neuromodulatory function on other neuronal populations, such as the GABAergic output neurones of the SNr (Chéramy et al., 1981). However, the major site of action for the DA contained in these neurones is in their axonal terminal fields that project to the neo- and ventral striatum.

Developmentally, the dopaminergic neurones of the SNc and VTA arise from the ventricular zone along the central aqueduct between 12 and 15 days of embryonic age (E12–E15) in the rat (Lauder & Bloom, 1974; Reisert et al., 1990). These cells migrate to the ventral surface of the developing midbrain (Shults et al., 1990), during which period they attain the large cell bodies and ramified dendrites that are characteristic of mature DA neurones. In the developing embryo, precursor cells first start to differentiate into neurones at E12, and by E15 the majority of the dopaminergic neuronal precursor cells have undergone their final division. By E18 all of the nigral precursor neurones have completed their migration from the subventricular zone to the developing SNc (Shults et al., 1990). However, from E14 onwards, long before this period of cell formation is completed, the first-born cells start to extend axons rostrally towards their targets, reaching the striatum between E16 and E21. The axons are distributed in the striatum in a topographic pattern that lasts throughout life (Voorn et al., 1988).

Perinatally, there is a decrease in activity within this dopaminergic pathway (Santana et al., 1992), which is followed by two periods of naturally occurring cell death within the SN at postnatal days 2 and 14 (Janec & Burke, 1993). The size and nature of this postnatal cell death is unclear, but the scale of the loss is estimated at between 20–80% of all the cells of the SN, although the proportion of these that are dopaminergic neurones is unknown. The final adult pattern of dopaminergic innervation of the striatum is not achieved until 21 days of age, about the stage when the developing rat pup is weaned.

The mature dopaminergic nigrostriatal tract projects onto the ipsilateral striatum in an orderly topographic manner (medial nigra to medial striatum, lateral to lateral, rostral to rostral, and caudal to caudal, but with dorsal and ventral tiers inverted), with only relatively minor projections to other areas (Björklund & Lindvall, 1986; Moore & Bloom, 1978).

The relevance of this developmental and anatomical account of the SNc is that it highlights the main limitations of placing grafts of embryonic ventral mesencephalic tissue from different-aged donor animals into the ectopic environment of the striatum. In the first instance it points to the period when the neurones to be grafted should ideally be harvested, and second, it highlights the complex connectivity of the system one is attempting to recreate with grafts.

Neurotoxic lesions of forebrain dopamine systems

Animal models attempt to mimic clinical PD first and foremost by making selective lesions of the dopaminergic nigrostriatal pathway. A variety of neurotoxins are available for this purpose, of which the two most widely used are

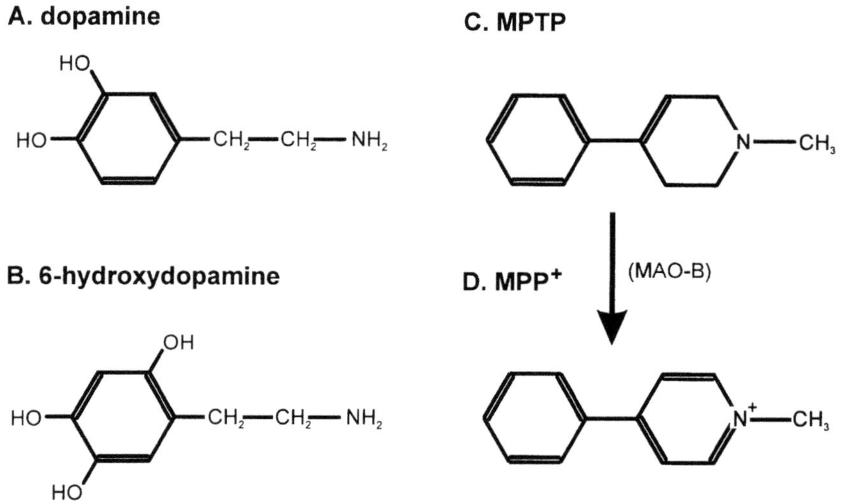

FIG. 4.3. Dopamine neurotoxins. (A) Structure of dopamine itself. (B) 6-OHDA, with the extra OH group on the carbon ring. (C, D) MPTP, which is converted by monoamine oxidase to the active toxic ion, MPP^+.

6-hydroxydopamine (6-OHDA) and 1-methyl-4-phenyl-1,2,3,6-tetrahydropyridine (MPTP) (Fig. 4.3). These two toxins act in different ways, and thus produce slightly different patterns of neuronal and neurotransmitter loss in different species. They each reproduce many of the anatomical, biochemical, and behavioural features of the human disease, and so provide useful models to evaluate new therapeutic strategies such as cell transplantation. Nevertheless, it should be remembered from the outset that in neither case is the precise pattern of cell loss or functional deficit identical in all respects to that seen in idiopathic Parkinson's disease in man.

6-OHDA is a locally acting specific toxin against catecholamine neurones. It does not cross the blood–brain barrier, and so must be injected by stereotaxic infusion via a fine cannula placed either in the lateral ventricle or (more accurately) directly into the nigrostriatal pathway, on one or both sides of the brain. 6-OHDA is structurally similar to the endogenous transmitter and so is concentrated in dopamine neurones by active uptake mechanisms, but is then metabolised intraneuronally to produce a number of toxic free radical compounds (including hydrogen peroxide) that kill the cell from within. Injection of 6-OHDA into the midbrain produces a rapid irreversible destruction of dopaminergic neurones in the SN and VTA, leading to a loss of dopamine inputs to both the dorsal and ventral striatum, depending on the precise placement of the injection cannula (see Fig. 4.4). Alternatively, injection into the lateral ventricles of the brain induces a widespread bilateral depletion of dopamine (and of the other major catecholamine, noradrenaline) throughout the forebrain, which results in

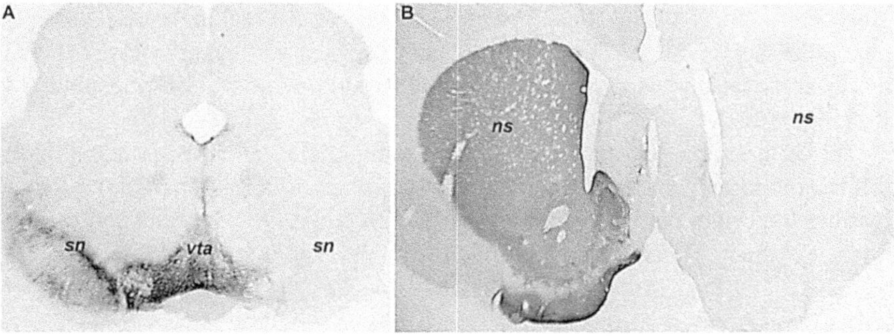

FIG. 4.4. Unilateral 6-OHDA lesions of the nigrostriatal pathway in rats, visualised with tyrosine hydroxylase immunohistochemistry. (A) The brainstem at the level of the substantia nigra, showing the intact substantia nigra (sn) and ventral tegmental area (vta) on the intact left side of the brain but almost total loss of dopamine cells on the right, the side of the 6-OHDA injection. (B) The 6-OHDA lesion results in total loss of nigrostriatal terminal staining in the neostriatum (ns) on the side of the lesion. (Original sections courtesy of Lucy Annett and Eduardo Torres.)

an extremely sick animal (of which, see more later). 6-OHDA is an efficient and safe toxin for experimental use to target dopamine neurones in all mammalian species studied, including rats, mice, and monkeys.

MPTP on the other hand is a far more risky compound. Ingestion of MPTP will produce parkinsonism in humans (Langston et al., 1983) and thus it may be a better toxin for mimicking PD in animal models (Gerlach et al., 1991; Pifl et al., 1991). It has the particular advantage that it can be given systemically, and so does not require special stereotaxic surgery for delivery into precise locations in the depths of the brain. Ingestion or peripheral injection of MPTP will produce bilateral lesions of forebrain dopamine systems, which can kill the animals if they are not maintained with intensive nursing care. However, this problem can be partially overcome by a modified technique in which the toxin is administered by unilateral infusions into the carotid artery in the neck on just one side to produce a predominantly unilateral lesion on the injected side in the brain (Bankiewicz et al., 1986).

In spite of its simplicity and face validity, problems with MPTP relative to 6-OHDA still exist. MPTP is known to be an effective neurotoxin in monkeys, mice, cats, and even goldfish but its lack of effects in rats has greatly hampered its use as an experimental tool (Gerlach et al., 1991). Moreover, its efficacy as a neurotoxin is both age- and species-dependent (Gerlach et al., 1991), and even within species there is great individual variation in the response to the toxin (Burns, 1991). MPTP is more effective as a neurotoxin in these species when the animal is aged. This is possibly as a result of the increasing activity of the MAO (Monoamine oxidase) type B enzyme, which converts MPTP to its active metabolite MPP+, with age (Gerlach et al., 1991). Furthermore, the deficits induced by this toxin, unlike those induced by 6-OHDA, are often transient (Burns,

1991; Russ et al., 1991). This appears to be due to the induction of compensatory processes involving host fibre sprouting, which can occur with MPTP by virtue of its selective sparing of the ventral striatum (Burns, 1991; Schneider & Rothblat, 1991).

The different modes of action of MPTP and 6-OHDA along with their slightly different topographical profiles of catecholamine (especially dopamine) terminal loss are important considerations in the interpretation of the results and mechanisms by which grafts may work under different lesioning paradigms.

Behavioural deficits associated with forebrain dopamine lesions

As already mentioned, bilateral lesions of forebrain dopamine systems produce an extremely debilitated animal. As first characterised in detail by Zigmond and Stricker (1972), the animals exhibit a profound aphagia (not eating), adipsia (not drinking) and akinesia (not moving), akin to the classic lateral hypothalamic syndrome. The animals will die unless maintained by regular tube feeding. Indeed, the deficit is not simply a failure of general regulatory systems: the animals exhibit a profound akinesia and do not engage in any voluntary goal-directed activity. If kept alive by gastric intubation and intensive nursing care the animals will eventually recover the ability to eat, drink, and maintain body weight, and the mechanisms of plasticity and recovery have been a major topic for investigation in their own right (Marshall et al., 1974; Zigmond et al., 1984). Nevertheless, this may take a period of months to achieve, and the level of debilitation exhibited by the bilateral nigrostriatal rat does not offer an ideal model for experimental analysis of transplantation strategies for repair.

The restrictions of the bilateral lesion model have largely been resolved by using a unilateral lesion model. Unilateral injections of 6-OHDA or intracarotid infusions of MPTP induce a marked motor asymmetry in rats, involving motor and sensory deficits on the opposite ("contralateral") side of the body to the lesion. The fact that the nigrostriatal system remains intact on one side of the brain is sufficient to maintain normal ingestive and regulatory functions. Furthermore, this allows for each animal to act as its own control in terms of evaluating the nature and extent of functional deficits (and their recovery) on the side of the body contralateral to the lesion with reference to performance on the ipsilateral side.

The lateralised deficits of a unilateral 6-OHDA lesioned rat are apparent in a variety of simple and more complex motor tests. Rats have a weakness of grasp when climbing a grid and a failure in tactile placing with the contralateral forepaw; they exhibit a postural bias towards the ipsilateral side of the body and a neglect of stimuli presented in the contralateral half of space in all modalities (visual, olfactory, and tactile). Marshall and colleagues (1974) have characterised this syndrome in some detail and shown that the deficit is not a failure of

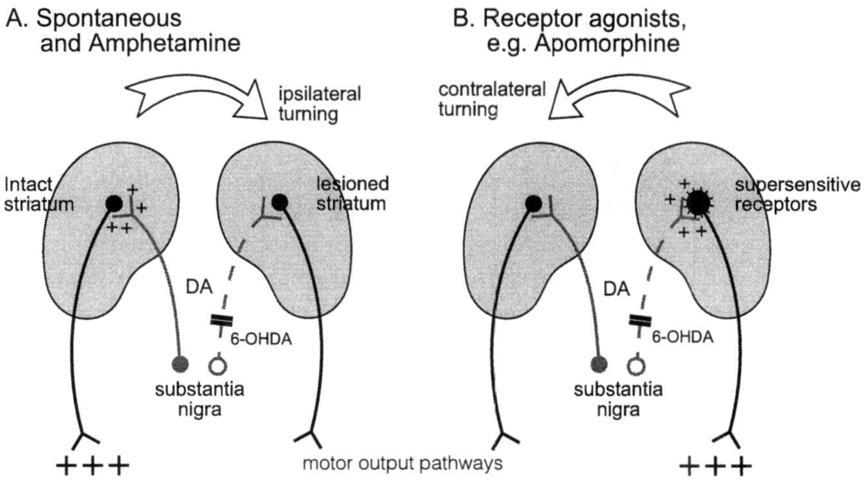

FIG. 4.5. Rotation after nigrostriatal lesion in rats. (A) After unilateral lesion of the right nigrostriatal pathway, animals have a postural bias to the right (ipsilateral) side, which becomes a strong ipsilateral rotation after peripheral injection of the stimulant drug, amphetamine. (B) Unilateral lesions result in the development of supersensitivity of the dopamine receptors on postsynaptic neurones. Peripheral injection of dopamine receptor agonists such as apomorphine activate supersensitive receptors and striatal outputs on the lesion side at doses subthreshold for influence of normal receptors on the intact side, driving rotation to the left (contralateral) side.

sensation *per se*, but a failure of the rat's ability to co-ordinate lateralised responses to a contralateral stimulus, a deficit that they describe as essentially "sensorimotor" in nature. Further analysis, in particular using a lateralised choice reaction time task, has shown that the deficit involves a failure in the animal's ability to initiate rather than to execute voluntary goal-directed responses on the contralateral side (Brown & Robbins, 1989; Carli et al., 1985).

The most dramatic symptoms are seen when the unilateral lesioned rat is aroused by activating stimuli. This may be achieved by stressing a rat with loud noise, pinching the tail, or placing it on an ice-cold surface. These stimuli increase general locomotion, which, when combined with the rat's postural bias, results in a head-to-tail turning phenomenon known as "rotation" (Ungerstedt, 1971a). The turning is in the ipsilateral direction, i.e. towards the side of the lesion (see Fig. 4.5). Even more dramatic and consistent rotation is produced if the animals are activated pharmacologically. Thus, the presynaptic stimulant drug amphetamine induces increased dopaminergic release and prolonged receptor activation on the intact side but has no effect on the lesion side, increasing the functional asymmetry of striatal outputs on the intact side, and resulting in prolonged rotation at a rate of 10–20 turns per minute lasting for the 3–4 hour duration of drug action (Fig. 4.5).

One of the advantages of rotation as an experimental measure of behavioural deficits following lesion is that it is easy to quantify and easy to automate.

Ungerstedt and Arbuthnott (1970) first described a simple "rotometer" apparatus in which a rat is placed in a circular bowl and connected via a harness and wire tether to an overhead cam and pivot that would register (then electromechanically, nowadays on a microcomputer) the turning rates in either direction over time, simply and efficiently. Rotation turns out to be a highly stable and reliable measure of asymmetry in individual animals and yields consistent dose–response curves for different levels of activation. Moreover, the rate of turning between animals yields highly consistent correlations with independent indices of the size of the lesion, such as post-mortem measurements of striatal dopamine loss. Whereas most behavioural effects studied in physiological psychology are variable and dependent on statistical tests based on groups of animals to reveal clear lesion effects, amphetamine rotation correlates closely with the levels of dopamine depletion ($r = 9$), so that an accurate estimate can be made on an animal-by-animal basis of the completeness of the individual lesion (Dunnett et al., 1988b; Ungerstedt, 1971a). This allows selection of carefully matched groups for analysis of graft effects, and any resulting recovery to be monitored quantitatively over time.

The rotation test revealed another unexpected consequence of nigrostriatal lesions. Whereas amphetamine and related stimulant compounds induced strong ipsilateral rotation, the dopamine receptor agonist apomorphine induces strong rotation in the contralateral direction, i.e. away from the lesion side (Ungerstedt, 1971b). This was the first evidence for receptor "supersensitivity', originally proposed to account for this behavioural observation and subsequently demonstrated in receptor binding assays as both an increase in the numbers and the affinity of dopamine receptors on striatal neurones as a compensatory response to the loss of their synaptic inputs. Consequently, a low dose of a receptor agonist will stimulate supersensitive receptors on postsynaptic neurones, inducing rotation away from the lesion side, at doses below the threshold of any detectable effects on intact receptors (Fig. 4.5).

NIGRAL GRAFTS IN ANIMAL MODELS OF PD

Preliminary studies

Transplantation of embryonic nigral tissue in the dopamine-depleted striatum was the first model system in which the behavioural effects of neural transplants were investigated. The first studies were reported simultaneously in 1979 by two laboratories: Perlow, Freed, and colleagues in the USA and Stockholm, Sweden, and Björklund and Stenevi from Lund, Sweden. Both groups employed dopamine-rich tissue of the developing SN dissected from the ventral mesencephalon of the embryonic brainstem and implanted as solid pieces into adult rats with unilateral 6-OHDA lesions. Perlow et al. (1979) placed the graft into the lateral ventricle, whilst Björklund and Stenevi (1979) placed the tissue into a dorsal cortical cavity, as shown in Figs. 3.2 and 3.3 respectively. Catecholamine fluorescence was used in both cases to show that the grafts had survived and contained healthy-appearing dopaminergic neurones, and subsequent studies by both groups provided more detailed descriptions of the anatomical appearance of the grafts and demonstration of dopaminergic fibre outgrowth from the graft into the host striatum (Björklund et al., 1980a; Freed et al., 1980). Finally, both groups showed compensation by the grafts on simple rotation tests of the motor asymmetry, using reduction in apomorphine-induced rotation in the case of the intraventricular grafts (Freed et al., 1980; Perlow et al., 1979) and of both amphetamine- and apomorphine-induced rotation in the case of the cavity grafts (Björklund & Stenevi, 1979; Björklund et al., 1980a; Dunnett et al., 1981a).

The first studies of transplant function suggested that although good compensation could be observed on simple rotation tests, the range of deficits on which the animals showed recovery was rather limited. Thus for example, no recovery was seen on other deficits characteristic of unilateral lesions, such as the marked contralateral sensory neglect (Björklund et al., 1980a; Dunnett et al., 1981a). This has turned out to be due, at least in part, to the limited extent of fibre outgrowth and re-innervation derived from solid grafts in dorsal cavities and in the lateral ventricle. Sensorimotor functions appear to be mediated by the lateral striatum, i.e. by areas not reached from either of those initial graft placements, and so when grafts were positioned in a lateral cortical cavity some recovery was demonstrated (Dunnett et al., 1981b). This study provided the first clue that both the topography and extent of graft re-innervation are critical factors determining the functional efficacy of the implants. However, solid graft techniques are intrinsically limited in the flexibility of their placement, and it was only with the advent of the cell suspension method that the experimental analysis of functional nigrostriatal repair really took off.

Following the procedures outlined in Chapter Three (Fig 3.4), Björklund et al. (1980b) first used the 6-OHDA lesion model to demonstrate the survival of dopamine-rich nigral cell suspension grafts in the rat brain. Nigral suspension grafts survive transplantation into the denervated striatum, where hundreds (or occasionally thousands) of dopamine cells are seen to survive in the aggregated deposit of graft tissue at the injection site in the depths of the striatum, surrounded by a halo of graft-derived dopaminergic fibres growing into the host brain (Fig. 4.6).

Cell suspension grafts are particularly powerful because of their flexibility for placement singly or in combination into multiple sites in the depths of the brain almost at will. This was used early on to explore issues of functional topography (Dunnett et al., 1983a). Thus, a cell suspension graft into the dorsal striatum will ameliorate deficits in amphetamine, apomorphine, and spontaneous rotation but not the contralateral neglect associated with unilateral nigrostriatal lesions. Conversely, lateral grafts alleviate the neglect but not the rotation deficits. Moreover, multiple grafts can yield an additive pattern of recovery on a range of tests sensitive to the individual graft placements.

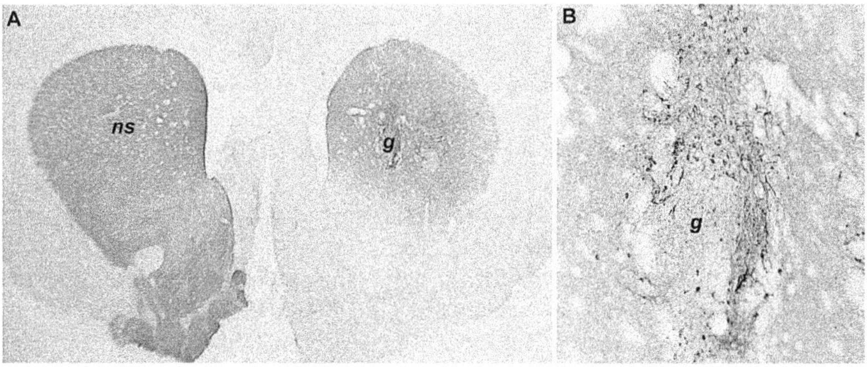

FIG. 4.6. Photomicrographs of dopamine-rich nigral graft in the dopamine-depleted neostriatum of the unilateral 6-OHDA lesioned rat brain, as visualised by immunohistochemical staining with antibodies against the dopamine-synthesising enzyme tyrosine hydroxylase. (A) Low magnification of graft with halo of fibre re-innervation into host striatum. (B) High magnification of dopamine cells in the graft itself. g, graft; ns, neostriatum (Original sections courtesy of Lucy Annett and Eduardo Torres.)

The anatomy and connectivity of foetal nigral grafts

In the intervening years since those first studies, considerably more has been learned about the connections and integration of nigral grafts into the host brain and the limits and mechanisms of functional recovery.

The dopamine cells of nigral grafts develop morphologically to exhibit the large cell bodies, ramified dendritic branches, and long axons characteristic of normal nigral neurones. Since the implants are composed of mixed ventral mesencephalic neurones and precursors rather than pure populations of dopaminergic cells, not surprisingly the grafts are seen to include many other cell types, including CCK (cholecystokinin), GABA, enkephalin, substance P, and serotonin-containing neurones (Mahalik & Clayton, 1991; Schultzberg et al., 1984). Indeed probably only 0.1–2% of the cells in the graft are actually dopaminergic (Brundin et al., 1985, Herman & Abrous, 1994), reflecting the proportion of these target cells within the normal ventral mesencephalon. Nevertheless, the dopamine and non-dopamine neurones together can occasionally be seen to organise themselves into a SNc–SNr like arrangement within the grafts (Björklund et al., 1980a).

Dopamine axons grow out into the host striatum, producing a terminal density up to 50% of the normal level close to the grafts but declining at progressively greater distances (Doucet et al., 1990). When examined in the electron microscope, the outgrowing dopamine fibres establish synaptic connections onto target neurones in the host striatum. In particular, asymmetric synapses are made onto the necks of spines and shafts of dendrites of the medium spiny neurones, which is the morphologically appropriate form and correct target for a normal nigrostriatal innervation (Freund et al., 1985; Mendez et al., 1991). Nevertheless, some other contacts have also been seen which are not found normally, for example onto the cell bodies of giant cholinergic neurones, which are not a normal target. Although the grafts contain many different types of cells, the dopamine neurones are the predominant source of outgrowth, and systematic retrograde labelling suggests that the serotonin neurones that occur in varying numbers in nigral grafts (depending on how caudal the embryonic dissection extends into the brainstem) appear to be the only other source of (in this case non-dopamine) neurones innervating the host brain (Mahalik & Clayton, 1991).

Conversely, the grafts receive a range of inputs from the host brain. On the one hand, the host cortex and serotonin fibres from the host raphé as well as local connections from host striatal neurones all appear to give rise to fibre ingrowth into nigral grafts (Doucet et al., 1989; Mahalik et al., 1985). In addition, the grafts probably also receive collateral connections from striatal interneurones as well as output medium spiny neurones (Clarke et al., 1988a). Thus, at least anatomically, implanted nigral cells become reciprocally connected with the host brain. However, whereas the existence of afferent inputs to the graft is not in doubt, the detailed patterns of their innervation are most probably far from normal. As we shall see, whether and how the inputs regulate activity in the dopaminergic outputs and control release of dopamine in the host striatum is a more difficult issue to resolve.

Electrophysiology and neurochemistry of intrastriatal nigral grafts

The functional activity of grafted nigral neurones is very similar to that found within the normal intact nigra, although some of the neurones seem to retain a more immature pattern of firing whilst others clearly have a firing pattern characteristic of non-dopaminergic components of the grafted brainstem (Fisher et al., 1991a). The mature dopaminergic nigral neurones have a relatively high resting rate of discharge, which the grafted and developing nigral neurones take time to acquire (Fisher & Gage, 1993). Furthermore, the dopaminergic nigral neurones not only display the firing rates and waveforms of dopaminergic neurones *in situ*, irrespective of location, they also respond to the local application of dopamine agonists and antagonists in a similar fashion (Arbuthnott et al., 1985; Wuerthele et al., 1981). These neurones not only have similar intrinsic discharge patterns but, in agreement with the anatomical studies, they also have been found to respond appropriately to stimulation of the host cortex, raphé, locus coeruleus, and striatum (Arbuthnott et al., 1985; Fisher et al., 1991a). Thus, nigral grafts appear to recreate some of the local circuit relays of the nigrostriatal loop, and can normalise the firing rates of striatal neurones over time (Fisher et al., 1991a; Strömberg et al., 1991).

Biochemically grafted nigral neurones synthesise and release dopamine in a similar manner to that of the intact nigrostriatal neurones. The levels of dopamine are clearly greatest in the graft and fall off as one moves away from it, giving a mean figure for dopamine levels in the grafted striatum of around 10–30% of normal (Freed et al., 1981; Schmidt et al., 1983). Furthermore, the grafted dopaminergic cells spontaneously release dopamine, the amount of which is increased by amphetamine and decreased by apomorphine (Strecker et al., 1987; Zetterström et al., 1986). This re-innervation of the host striatum and the associated release of dopamine from nigral transplants results in a normalisation of dopaminergic receptor sensitivity (Dawson et al., 1991a,b; Mendez et al., 1993; Mennicken et al., 1995; Rioux et al., 1991). Furthermore, there is some evidence that cortical glutaminergic afferents can control the release of dopamine from the graft via a non-NMDA (N-methyl-D-aspartic acid) receptor (Kondoh & Low, 1994). Thus the normalisation of dopamine release in response to stimulant drugs and the stabilisation of receptor sensitivity in the lesioned striatum re-establish the symmetry between the two striata underpinning the reversal of amphetamine- and apomorphine-induced rotation observed behaviourally.

Beyond the postsynaptic receptor, the restored dopamine inputs to the striatum derived from the grafted cells restore normal levels of metabolic and synthetic processing by the postsynaptic neurones. Activation of the normal dopaminergic input to the striatum induces an activation of "immediate early genes" such as c-*fos* that provides a rapid marker of cellular activation. This signalling mechanism is markedly reduced after a nigrostriatal lesion but restored by grafts (Abrous et al., 1992; Cenci et al., 1992). Indeed the level of cellular activation reflects not only the rate of rotation, but also the direction of rotation in animals in which recovery is "overcompensated"—a phenomenon in which the graft paradoxically induces rotation away from the grafted side in response to an amphetamine challenge (see later for a more detailed discussion; Abrous et al., 1992). Moreover, lesion-induced changes in the synthesis by striatal neurones of their primary neurotransmitters can also be restored by grafts. For example, glutamic acid decarboxylase and preproenkephalin mRNAs are increased in striatal neurones following 6-OHDA lesions, and both are restored to normal levels in the grafted striatum (Segovia et al., 1991; Sirinathsinghji & Dunnett, 1991).

Promoting graft survival and integration

Following the demonstration that nigral grafts can and do survive and connect with the host brain, one issue that has become of increasing importance as the techniques develop to clinical application is how to optimise graft survival. In particular, whereas the grafted neurones clearly survive, connect, and function, the actual yields turn out to be rather poor when subjected to systematic quantitation. As mentioned before, there are approximately 45,000 dopaminergic neurones in the ventral mesencephalon (SN and VTA together) in the normal rat brainstem. By contrast, the nigral grafts derived from the equivalent of one brainstem-worth of embryonic ventral mesencephalon typically contain several hundred or at most 1000–2000 dopamine neurones as stained by catecholamine fluorescence or tyrosine hydroxylase histochemistry. This implies that the average nigral graft prepared by the standard method contains only 1–5% of surviving dopamine neurones. Although it is possible to pool tissue from multiple donors when we are considering experimental studies in rats, the efficiency of present nigral grafting techniques has become an increasingly critical issue as the procedures develop to clinical application (see Chapter Five), not least because of the much more precious nature of tissues derived from human embryonic/foetal donors. Consequently, the last decade has seen an increasing attention to alternative ways to improve the viability and survival of nigral tissues both at the stage of preparation and following transplantation into the host brain.

Improvements in preparation conditions. It is sensible to start out by considering the methods for cell preparation—perhaps the high levels of cell death are simply due to the trauma involved in their dissection, handling, dissociation, and implantation. In fact, detailed parametric studies on the media used and the mechanisms for handling and preparing the cells yield only very small improvements in graft viability (Barker et al., 1995). Moreover, when cells are prepared in the same way but grown in three-dimensional tissue culture very much higher yields are obtained, so their death following implantation must be related to later events rather than to the methods of their harvesting and preparation *per se* (Fawcett et al., 1995).

Growth factors. We know that the fate of all neurones during their development is controlled and regulated by a variety of growth factors (see Chapter Two). Consequently, it may be possible to promote the survival of embryonic neurones developing in grafts by providing or supplementing them with the same growth factor molecules on which they are dependent during normal development *in situ*. Fibroblast growth factor is a general, rather broad-acting, survival factor in tissue culture that has a modest effect in promoting the survival of dopamine neurones in nigral grafts when injected into the graft site in the host striatum over 10–20 days following implantation (Mayer et al., 1992). Several other factors have subsequently been shown to have similar, rather modest effects, including PDGF (platelet-derived growth factor), BDNF (brain-derived neurotrophic factor) and NT (neurotrophin)-4/5 (Haque et al., 1996; Nikkhah et al., 1992; Yurek et al., 1996), but by far the most potent effect has so far been achieved with glial cell line-derived neurotrophic factor (GDNF, Apostolides et al., 1998; Sinclair et al., 1996, Rosenblad et al., 1997). Although GDNF will have a small effect when the nigral tissue is simply incubated in it prior to implantation, better effects are obtained when it is infused chronically into the graft site over several weeks following transplantation (Fig 4.7).

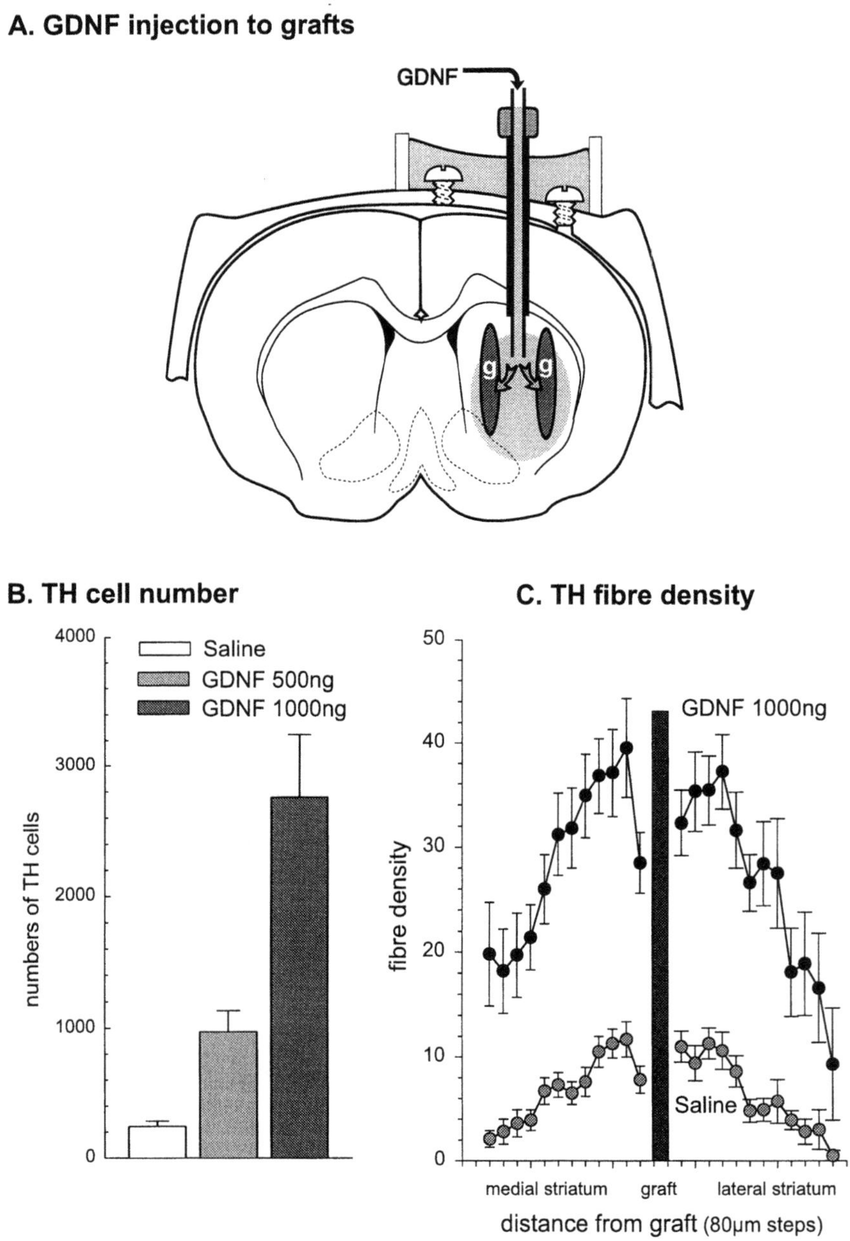

FIG. 4.7. Infusions of the trophic factor GDNF promotes the survival and fibre outgrowth of nigral grafts. (A) Technique for local infusion of GDNF into the graft site. (B) Enhanced survival of DA neurones in the grafts. (C) Enhanced density of dopamine fibre outgrowth into the host brain. TH, tyrosine hydroxylase. g, graft. (Data from Sinclair et al., 1997.)

Antioxidants and excitotoxicity. A third strategy to promote the yields of implanted dopaminergic nigral neurones is to seek to protect them from the various toxic processes involved in active cell death. Nigral dopamine neurones are known to be particularly sensitive to free radical damage—indeed we have seen that this may be one of the primary mechanisms of cell death in Parkinson's disease. Brundin and colleagues have demonstrated that enhancing the free radical scavenging capacity of graft tissues or the host striatum can enhance the survival of dopamine cells both *in vitro* and in nigral grafts (Barkats et al., 1997; Grasbon-Frodl et al., 1997), and a number of antioxidant molecules, including lazaroids, n-acetyl cysteine, and vitamin E are under active investigation for their capacity to promote graft survival with clearly significant (even if so far incomplete) success (Nakao et al., 1994).

Cryopreservation and hibernation. An alternative approach to the difficulties in co-ordinating the availability and timing of foetal tissues for transplantation following the poor yields obtained from individual donors is the possibility of storing and of pooling tissues to be made available at a subsequent time. Early attempts to cryopreserve tissues for long-term deep-frozen storage has led to only moderate success—it is certainly possible to freeze, thaw, and implant tissues, and get surviving dopamine neurones in the grafts, but the yields are consistently even lower than that obtained with fresh tissues (Collier et al., 1993; Sautter et al., 1996). Similarly, cells can be maintained and grown in culture, but again the trauma of lifting off and dissociating cultured cells results in poorer survival than in the baseline case (Brundin et al., 1985). However, an intermediate strategy, involving cool storage of tissue pieces in a "hibernation" medium that is non-physiological and slows down cellular metabolism can maintain cells for survival over several days with no loss of efficacy (Sauer & Brundin, 1991), opening the way for a variety of growth factor treatments, labelling of cells, or a variety of other manipulations with a greater flexibility than was hitherto possible.

Notwithstanding these specific strategies for promoting survival of dopamine-rich embryonic nigral grafts, there is now an increasing interest in moving completely away from the dependence on availability of primary embryonic CNS neurones to the search for alternative sources of peripheral cells, cell lines, engineered cells, and even completely non-cellular strategies for molecular replacement and repair. However, none of these strategies is close to application. We will return to this topic, after considering what is possible today, to look at developing future options in Chapter Nine. Having seen that nigral grafts can survive and integrate in the host striatum, however imperfectly, let us return first to the experimental analysis of trying to understand their function better.

FUNCTIONAL ANALYSIS OF NIGRAL GRAFTS

Functional specificity of intrastriatal nigral grafts

The structural, chemical, and electrophysiological reorganisation provided by a nigral graft can account for many aspects of the behavioural recovery observed in transplanted rats (Herman & Abrous, 1994), in particular with regard to the alleviation of asymmetry in simple motor tests such as drug-induced rotation in unilateral lesioned rats or akinesia in animals with bilateral lesions. In addition, the behavioural phenomena can provide additional information on the ways in which the grafts work, and the critical features of the transplantation methodology necessary to achieve good functional effect.

The specificity of nigral graft effects is illustrated in a study of alternative control procedures (Dunnett et al., 1988b). This study brought together three different lines of evidence to suggest that the functional effects of the grafts are critically dependent upon dopamine replacement by grafted neurones. First, only grafts derived from embryonic nigra ameliorated the rotation deficit; neither embryonic raphé rich in another group of brainstem monoamine neurones (i.e. serotonin), nor embryonic striatum (i.e. a population of cells relevant to the target area) had any functional effect (Fig. 4.8A). Secondly, the removal of the dopamine cells within the implanted nigral tissue by injecting 6-OHDA into the vicinity of the grafts led to an immediate restoration of the initial lesion-induced level of rotation (Fig. 4.8B). This is just one of several studies in which grafts have been removed and the initial deficits reinstated—by lesion, by

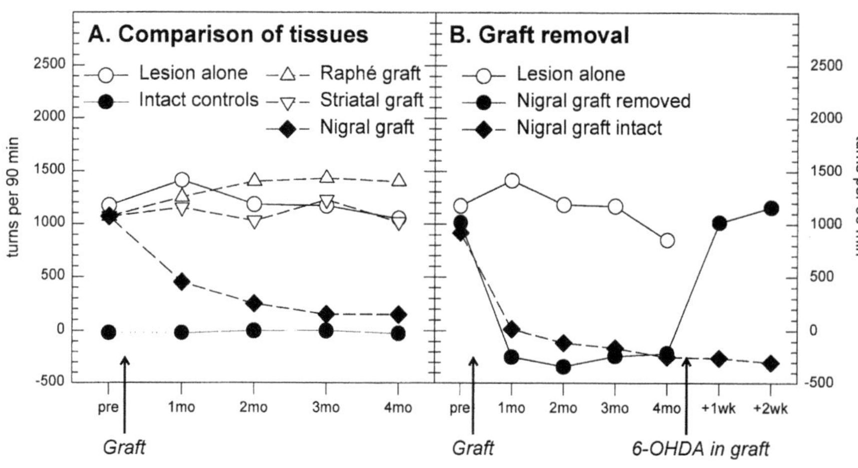

FIG. 4.8. Specificity of graft-derived recovery on dopamine replacement in rats with unilateral nigrostriatal lesions. (A) Ipsilateral rotation induced by amphetamine is long-lasting in rats with lesions, alleviated over 1–2 months in rats with nigral grafts, but unaffected in rats with control striatal or raphé grafts. (B) Removal of dopamine neurones from nigral grafts by local injection of 6-OHDA reinstates the initial rotation deficit. (Data from Dunnett et al., 1988b.)

aspiration, or by immunological rejection (Björklund et al., 1980a; Brundin et al., 1986)—as the basis for demonstrating that the recovery is dependent on the continued survival of the grafted cells and not, for example, due to a non-specific effect of the surgery or a trophic stimulation of recovery processes in the host brain (LeVere & LeVere, 1985). Third, when the animals were brought to post mortem, there were clear and highly significant correlations on the one hand between the rate of turning and the extent of dopamine depletions induced by nigrostriatal lesions (in the lesion rats) and on the other hand between the recovery of turning and the extent of dopamine replacement provided by the nigral grafts (in the transplanted rats) (Dunnett et al., 1988b).

Limits of functional recovery

The ability of embryonic nigral grafts to reverse many of the behavioural deficits induced by experimental lesions of the nigrostriatal tract is well documented and summarised in Table 4.1.

Although there are some problems with the sensitivity of the standard rotational model, it is a useful screening test for the efficacy of these grafts (Brundin et al., 1985). Indeed, embryonic nigral grafts appear not only to reduce drug-induced rotation (e.g. Perlow et al., 1979) but also actually to induce a seemingly paradoxical contralateral rotational response to amphetamine. In response to amphetamine challenges, some grafted animals not only fully recover but also actually rotate away from the grafted side (e.g. Björklund et al., 1980a; Herman et al., 1985; see also Fig. 4.4). The basis of this rotational "overcompensation" is

TABLE 4.1
Profiles of recovery in rats with nigrostriatal 6-OHDA lesions and standard nigral grafts

Unilateral lesions/grafts	*Bilateral lesions/grafts*
Tests that show recovery with nigral grafts	
Amphetamine rotation	Spontaneous akinesia
Apomorphine rotation	Amphetamine hypoactivity
Spontaneous rotation	Apomorphine hyperkinesia
Conditioned rotation	Bilateral neglect
Contralateral neglect	
"Sticky labels" test	
T-maze bias	
Intracranial self-stimulation	
Placing, stepping, and support reflexes	
Grip strength	
Tests that do not recover with nigral grafts	
Skilled paw reaching	Aphagia and adipsia
Disengagement behaviour	Hoarding*

* Ventral tegmental area lesion; Herman et al. (1986)

unclear, as the levels of dopamine in the grafted striatum are not higher than those found on the control side, and neither is the functional status of the postsynaptic dopamine receptors. It may be related to the abnormal synaptic relationship between the outgrowing dopaminergic fibres from the graft and the host striatal neurones, and is reflected in increased activity of striatal output neurones on the lesioned side as identified by an increase in their expression of the immediate early gene c-*fos* (Abrous et al., 1992). It therefore seems probable that the "overcompensation" observed with these embryonic nigral grafts reflects an abnormal postsynaptic event between the innervating dopaminergic fibre and the host striatal neurones.

Recovery is not simply dependent upon pharmacological activation, as the heavy focus on rotation tests in the literature might suggest. Recovery can be equally apparent in the undrugged animal in tests of other forms of lateralised turning bias: spontaneous turning in rotometer bowls, exploratory turning in a T-maze, and conditioned turning in which the animals are trained for water reward to turn in the direction contralateral to the lesion.

Similarly, as described earlier, recovery can be seen on a variety of sensorimotor tests provided the grafts are positioned laterally in the striatum. This applies not only to the classic neurological tests of neglect as first developed by John Marshall but also on a range of other tests such as reflexive placing and stepping with the forepaws when the rat is held and displaced manually (Olsson et al., 1995), the speed with which they will remove sticky labels (L. Annett, unpublished data), and a rigid disturbance in grip strength when the animals hold onto and are pulled away from a holding bar (Dunnett et al., 1998).

Lastly, recovery can be seen in tests of learning, even in unilaterally lesioned rats, both in the lateralised conditioned turning task already mentioned (Dunnett et al., 1986), and also in providing a substrate for intracranial self-stimulation reward to reinforce learning in a conventional operant lever press test (Fray et al., 1983).

All of these tests would suggest that nigral grafts can provide a rather dramatic and extensive profile of recovery. However, recovery is not complete, and animals that show good or even complete recovery on some tests may remain profoundly affected on others. For example, rats showing good recovery on both rotation and contralateral neglect remain completely impaired on test of skilled forelimb reaching (Dunnett et al., 1987; Montoya et al., 1990). Whereas rats with nigral lesions can show good recovery of their ability to detect single contralateral stimuli, they are unable to "disengage" from an ongoing task when actively engaged in another goal-directed activity (Mandel et al., 1990). Similarly, rats with bilateral lesions that exhibit good recovery in symptoms of akinesia and bilateral neglect fail to recover from the profound regulatory deficits in eating and drinking (Dunnett et al., 1983b) and in the deficits in food hoarding exhibited by rats with ventrally positioned lesions (Herman et al., 1986). In each of these cases it is not as if the grafts have a partial effect across the board—

rather some classes of deficit are completely unaffected by the grafts, whereas others can exhibit dramatic or complete recovery. It therefore becomes an important issue: What are the key factors that differentiate those behaviours (or functions) that recover from those that do not?

In the first instance it is not simply a matter of complexity of stimuli or of the controlling response. Presumably the response and its controlling conditions are as complex in the case of several of the conditioning tasks (intracranial self-stimulation, ICSS, conditioned rotation) as they are in reaching, hoarding, or basic consuming of food.

A more extensively studied hypothesis is that the issue of placement is important. We have seen that placement is critical; and perhaps for these non-recovered tasks the critical target fields are not reached, notwithstanding extensive re-innervation elsewhere. This is hypothetically plausible, and certainly accounts for many of the early dissociations (Dunnett et al., 1981a,b, 1983a). However, it cannot readily account for many of the remaining deficits. Thus, several studies have implicated the lateral striatum in particular in the control of skilled paw reaching, yet nigral grafts placed here are no more effective than anywhere else, whereas a striatal graft into the same site can restore reaching in rats with lesions of intrinsic striatal neurones (Fricker et al., 1997; Montoya et al., 1990). Moreover, in the case of the regulatory deficits, animals with bilateral lesions have been prepared with large numbers of graft placements, throughout the forebrain not just in the striatum, without alleviation of the aphagia and adipsia (Dunnett et al., 1983b).

An alternative hypothesis is that the incomplete recovery relates to the ectopic placement of the graft in the striatum. The dopamine neurones are lost from the SN, not the striatum. If the grafts are placed back into the homotopic site, i.e. back into the SN, the dopamine cells survive well but the axons growing out from the grafts penetrate only a few hundred microns into the host brain. In the adult host brain, the embryonic axons do not have a capacity to grow long distances to reform connections with the appropriate distant striatal targets, and such grafts are without functional benefit on virtually all tests (Dunnett et al., 1983a). We have therefore proposed that the reason rats do not recover on tests such as skilled paw reaching is that these tests measure functions that are dependent on the relay of patterned information via the nigrostriatal pathway, which is not restored by standard ectopic graft procedures (Dunnett et al., 1987, 1989b). Conversely, in view of the relatively diffuse regulatory function of ascending dopamine systems, many tests primarily reflect functional dopaminergic activation of the neostriatum, and it is these that are alleviated by a nigral graft. Added plausibility is given to this hypothesis by the demonstration that whereas nigral grafts are unable to restore skilled reaching in rats with nigrostriatal lesions, striatal grafts do restore performance on the same test after implantation into animals with excitotoxic striatal lesions (Fricker et al., 1997; Montoya et al., 1990). Although the striatal lesions induce more extensive damage, the grafts in the two models differ in that the former is ectopic and does not restore nigrostriatal connectivity, whereas the latter is homotopic and striatal grafts do re-establish cortico-striato-pallidal connections (see Chapter Six).

Nigrostriatal bridge grafts

A clear test for the ectopic hypothesis would be if it were possible to reconstruct the nigrostriatal projection and then demonstrate recovery on tests such as skilled paw reaching. The experimental requirement is to replace nigral cells in the nigra in combination with a treatment that would overcome the inhibitory nature of the CNS environment to allow the axons to grow back to their appropriate striatal targets. This was first attempted using bridges of peripheral nerve tissue. Aguayo and colleagues applied the techniques first developed for bridging spinal cord injury (as described in Chapter One, see Fig 1.6) by implanting a segment of peripheral nerve as a bridge over the top of the brain to connect a solid nigral graft placed over the midbrain with distant targets in the striatum (see Fig. 4.9A). They were able to show extensive growth of fluorescent dopamine fibres from the nigral grafts through the bridge to re-innervate the host striatal targets. Thus, bridge grafts to enable long-distance axon regrowth and guidance to their appropriate targets are certainly possible in the adult forebrain, although the ectopic nigral graft used here did not favour functional evaluations.

We introduced an alternative bridge grafting strategy which involved laying down a track of a suitable cellular substrate in a series of injections made via an oblique cannula along the nigrostriatal pathway (Dunnett et al., 1989b). That study explored a number of alternative cellular and matrix bridges and found a clear stimulation of long-distance axon growth using target-relevant striatal cells. Dopamine fibres grew the full length of the grafts to re-innervate the striatum in several cases, and rotation was alleviated in just those cases in which such regrowth was seen. A similar pattern of long-distance growth has been reported using both laminin tracks (Zhou & Azmitia, 1988) and pathways of endogenous glia made reactive by an injection of an excitotoxin (Zhou & Chiang, 1995). However, the clearest results to date have been achieved by Brecknell et al. (1996) using tracks of Schwann cells that had been engineered to secrete a variety of growth factors including FGF and GDNF (see Fig. 4.9B). Again the grafts were shown to reconnect over long distances, the striatal innervation was demonstrated to be derived from the nigral grafts by retrograde tracing, and functional recovery in a test of rotation correlated on an animal-by-animal basis with the numbers of fibres regenerating back to the striatum and the numbers of back-labelled dopamine neurones in the grafts.

However, none of these studies has yet achieved a reliability and extent of re-innervation necessary to test out the initial hypothesis that tests such as skilled paw reaching as well as tests of rotation will reveal recovery if, but only if, we can achieve extensive repair of the degenerated nigrostriatal circuitry itself.

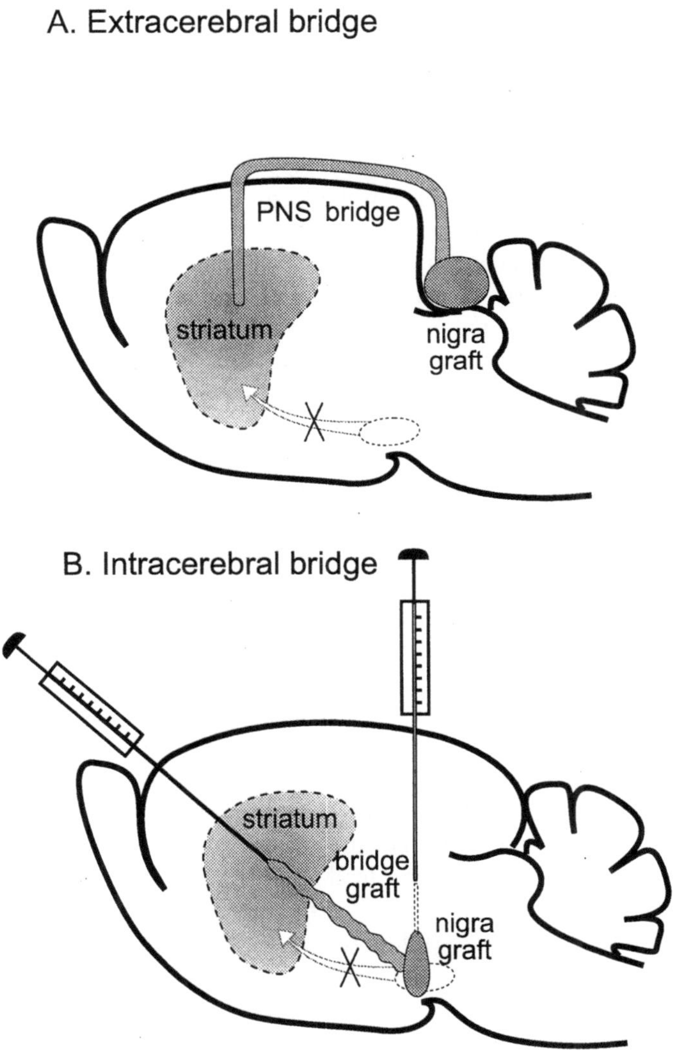

FIG. 4.9. Bridge grafts in the nigrostriatal system. (A) Extracerebral peripheral nervous system (sciatic nerve) bridge linking a nigral graft implanted over the tectum to the denervated striatum (Aguayo et al., 1984). (B) Intracerebral Schwann cell graft linking a nigral graft implanted in the substantia nigra with the denervated striatum (Brecknell et al., 1996.)

L-dopa and the nigral dopaminergic neurones

There has been a considerable debate about whether grafted nigral neurones interact positively or negatively with concurrent pharmacological treatment. This issue has important clinical implications as well as raising important questions about the mechanisms by which nigral grafts exert their functional effects. We need to establish whether the nigral neurones are adversely affected by drugs used in the treatment of PD such as the dopamine precursor drug, L-dopa. One of the long-running controversies in the treatment of PD is whether treatment with L-dopa should be started early or late in the disease. This arose because some early clinical studies suggested that whereas L-dopa may alleviate the symptoms of PD it may be detrimental to the underlying survival of stressed neurones, resulting in more rapid progression of the disease (reviewed in Factor & Weiner, 1993). This issue has obvious implications that carry over to the use of nigral grafts in PD, and the subsequent pharmacological treatment of patients who have received grafts.

A recent *in vitro* study has shown that L-dopa does appear to be toxic to the dopaminergic nigral neurones in culture at concentrations similar to that found in the serum of patients with PD (Mena et al., 1993). Although other workers report similar findings, serious doubts as to the relevance of studies using high doses of L-dopa must be raised even though in the grafted situation the blood–brain barrier may be compromised (but see Geist et al., 1991) and thus higher concentrations of L-dopa may be present at the grafted site. However, a more significant factor may be the presence of glial cells, as *in vivo* studies have largely failed to substantiate a toxic action for L-dopa, at least in the partially lesioned rat brain or normal human brain (Murer et al., 1998; Quinn et al., 1986). Indeed some recent studies suggest that L-dopa may actually have a trophic action on the nigral dopaminergic neurones (discussed in Agid, 1998). These observations may help explain the discordant results reported for the effects of L-dopa on embryonic nigral graft survival and functional effects. Blunt, and more recently Adams, have demonstrated that long-term treatment of rats with L-dopa and carbidopa did not prove detrimental to either the survival or functional effectiveness of the ventral mesencephalon graft (Adams et al., 1994; Blunt et al., 1991, 1992). In contrast, Steece-Collier and colleagues have reported that chronic L-dopa treatment does impair the behavioural recovery of animals with nigral grafts, possibly by affecting the degree to which the neurones can grow axons out into the host striatum (Steece-Collier et al., 1990, 1995; Yurek et al., 1991). In these two groups of studies the concentrations and preparations of L-dopa were different, and this may well account for the difference in their results.

The extent to which L-dopa is detrimental to grafted nigral neurones is therefore at present unresolved. Although receptors for dopamine are found on these neurones (Robertson, 1992), chronic stimulation does not adversely affect their survival in culture (Van Muiswinkel et al., 1992, 1995). The most parsimonious interpretation is that at clinically relevant concentrations L-dopa is without effect on the normal healthy nigral dopaminergic neurone, but that in abnormal situations it may adversely affect their ability to develop neurite outgrowth. Unfortunately, from a clinical point of view there is no evidence to support or refute this theory, as all patients tend to be on oral L-dopa post-grafting.

SUMMARY

Embryonic nigral grafts can survive long-term in the CNS of rodents and primates. They receive and form synapses from the host striatum and can release dopamine tonically as well as in response to electrophysiological and pharmacological stimuli. However the synaptic relationship between the graft and host is not fully normal and is limited in terms of the extent of re-innervation, which may in part explain the ability of grafts placed in different parts of the striatum to have differential effects on the recovery of behavioural deficits. The poor survival of transplanted dopaminergic nigral neurones coupled to the ectopic placement of the graft has meant that not all of the behavioural deficits that result from lesions of the dopaminergic nigrostriatal tract can be reversed by these grafts. Various strategies have been employed to try to improve on the synaptic relationship between the graft and host either by grafting to the host nigra or by increasing the number of surviving dopaminergic neurones within the graft by the use of neurotrophic factors. To date these approaches have met with only modest success.

CHAPTER FIVE

First clinical trials: Neural grafts in Parkinson's disease

INTRODUCTION

Parkinson's disease (PD) is a neurodegenerative condition of unknown aetiology, for which there is a treatment but no cure. As discussed in the Chapter Four the core pathology in PD is the loss of the dopaminergic nigrostriatal pathway, and thus the mainstay of current therapy is in pharmacologically restoring this network. The main drugs that are commonly used in PD are L-dopa, which is converted into dopamine by the remaining dopaminergic neurones of the nigrostriatal tract, and dopamine agonists (e.g. bromocriptine, pergolide, lisuride, apomorphine, and ropinirole), which directly activate dopamine receptors within the CNS (central nervous system). These agents are effective early on in the disease but, with time, complications of therapy start to appear and these initially consist of wearing off phenomena and unpredictable changes in the patient's motor state from one of relative normality ("on") to one of relative immobility ("off"). Furthermore, the drugs induce a range of unwanted movements, "dyskinesias", which the patient can find especially disabling. As a result, 5–10 years after first developing symptoms, patients with PD often have major problems in the control of their disease despite taking complex regimes of medication (reviewed in Stocchi et al., 1997).

As a consequence of these problems with pharmacological approaches, a number of surgical alternatives have been developed for application in advanced PD. These include making strategic lesions in the outflow pathways of the basal ganglia—pallidotomy, subthalamotomy, and thalamotomy (Obeso et al., 1997; see Fig. 5.1). Both the internal part of the globus pallidus and the subthalamic nucleus are overactive in PD (Hutchison et al., 1994), so that their lesion should

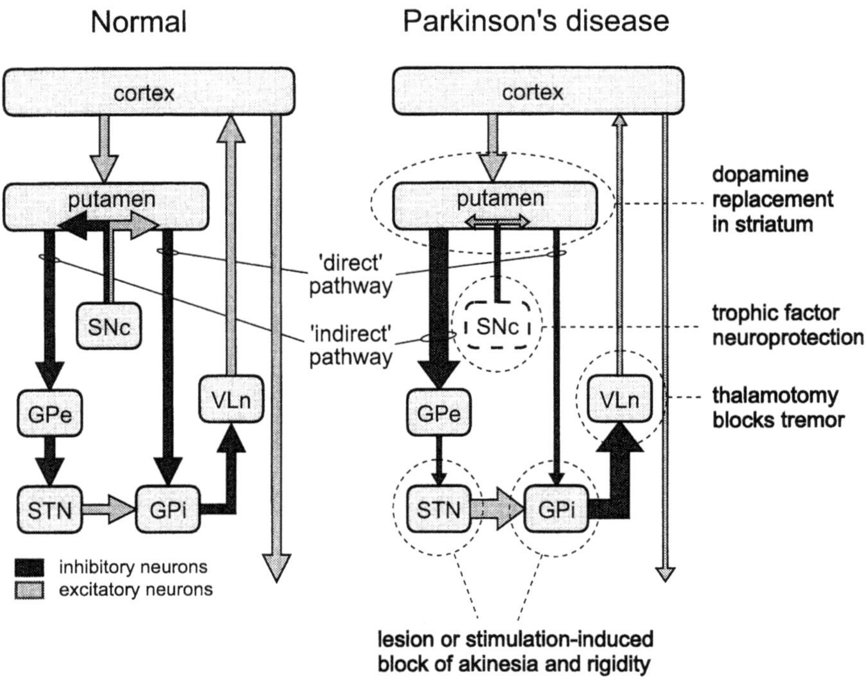

FIG. 5.1. Schematic figure of the basal ganglia in normal state and in PD, indicating the sites for surgical intervention. GPe, GPi, external and internal segments of the globus pallidus; SNc, pars compacta of the substantia nigra; STN, subthalamic nucleus; VLn, ventrolateral nucleus of the thalamus. See Fig. 4.2. for further details of the anatomical organisation of these systems.

(at least theoretically) release the thalamus from its excessive inhibition by basal ganglia output nuclei that occurs in PD. To date these lesions appear particularly effective in ameliorating drug-induced dyskinesias but seem to provide less clear-cut benefit on the underlying motor deficits of PD (Olanow, 1996). Thalamotomy on the other hand appears specifically to help the tremor but has little effect on other aspects of the disease (Fox et al., 1991).

An alternative approach to the use of destructive surgical lesions is the use of electrical stimulators. High-frequency stimulation can induce a conduction block at their site of implantation, and stimulating electrodes have therefore been implanted in the same sites as those used for lesioning. These stimulators appear to have a clear effect in modulating some of the symptoms of PD, especially in subthalamic targets (Krack et al., 1998).

Whilst these surgical approaches can be effective in controlling the symptoms and as such are an important aid to patient management, they cannot halt, repair, or cure the underlying disease process. Transplantation, on the other hand, strives to restore the dopaminergic loss of PD by replacing dopaminergic cells lost from the diseased basal ganglia, with the goal of achieving lasting survival and explicit repair of the underlying degeneration. The extent to which this is achieved in part depends on the type of tissue that is transplanted. At the simplest level this may take the form of dopamine-secreting cells to provide the missing neurotransmitter in a rather non-specific fashion. At the other end of the spectrum is the use of embryonic nigral cells, which try to recreate the host dopaminergic network, both anatomically and functionally.

In this chapter our discussion begins with adrenal medulla grafts, which were the first to be applied clinically in PD, based on the hypothesis that they could provide an active replacement source of dopamine in the parkinsonian striatum. However, it soon became clear that any functional effect they had could be mediated via a variety of different possible mechanisms. As a result of the complications and inconsistency of this approach coupled to the increasing experimental data on embryonic ventral mesencephalic tissue (see Chapter Four), the use of human embryonic nigral tissue as the donor source in patients with PD rapidly developed as the alternative, preferred, transplant option. This will form the second half of our discussion in this chapter.

ADRENAL MEDULLA TRANSPLANTS

The adrenal medulla (AM) lies at the core of the adrenal gland, of which there are two, with each one being located above each kidney. It was the first tissue to be transplanted into the CNS in patients with PD, and although it has been used extensively in this disorder, there have been instances in which it has been used for other conditions, most notably to relieve severe pain (see Chapter Eight). However, before discussing the clinical results of such transplants, we should first review the experimental data and rationale behind the use of this tissue in patients with PD.

Rationale for AM grafts

The original reason for using the AM as a donor tissue in PD relates to the fact that it is rich in catecholamines. It is this gland that secretes adrenaline into the blood stream under conditions of stress and arousal. Adrenaline is synthesised within the cell by metabolism of tyrosine in a series of enzyme-regulated steps into adrenaline via dopa, dopamine, and noradrenaline. Consequently, the cells make dopamine and noradrenaline as steps in the synthesis of adrenaline, and *in vitro* low levels of these intervening catecholamines can be measured, albeit at much lower levels than the primary hormone adrenaline. Two additional qualities of the cells of the AM made them an attractive donor tissue. First, they demonstrate a marked postnatal plasticity under the regulation of certain growth factors and steroids, which in turn has effects on their profile of catecholamine synthesis and release. Second, the patient can provide his own donor tissue and by so doing we may avoid many of the immunological, practical, and ethical problems inherent in the use of embryonic human nigral tissue.

It was therefore hypothesised that AM grafts might continue to secrete catecholamines, and in particular serve as a replacement source of dopamine (DA), after transplantation into the lesioned brain. Indeed, under the right conditions, they may even be induced to adopt a neuronal phenotype with axonal outgrowth and synaptic interactions with the host brain, in an analogous fashion to the foetal nigral grafts. Although this was a useful starting point from which to investigate the AM graft, it has proved to be a misleading view of its mode of action. Indeed the mechanisms by which AM grafts work are largely unresolved, and may indeed be different under different transplant conditions (reviewed in Barker & Dunnett, 1993).

AM development and anatomy

The adrenal gland consists of a cortex and medulla, with the former secreting steroid hormones, whilst the medulla, which developmentally is related to the sympathetic nervous system, secretes predominantly catecholamines (see Fig. 5.2).

Developmentally, the catecholamine-secreting chromaffin cells of the AM are, like other cells of the sympathetic nervous system, derived from the neural crest (Anderson, 1993). The trigger that switches the sympathoadrenal precursor to a chromaffin cell type probably involves glucocorticoids (GCs) produced by the developing adrenal cortex and FGF (fibroblast growth factor). The continued presence of GCs (as occurs in the adrenal gland) ensures that the cell develops along the chromaffin cell lineage. On the other hand, the development of sympathetic neurones from the same neural crest precursor cells relies on the absence of GC and the presence of FGF and NGF (nerve growth factor) (Doupé et al., 1985a).

This interconversion between these cell types can to some extent continue in postnatal life in the rat—NGF promotes the development of the sympathetic neuronal phenotype in mature chromaffin cells *in vitro*, whereas dexamethasone (an exogenous GC) maintains these cells in the chromaffin cell phenotype even when NGF is present (Doupé et al., 1985a; Unsicker et al., 1978). However, the situation is made more complex when one starts to consider both the age of the chromaffin cell and species. In the rat, the chromaffin cells display a reduced ability to respond to NGF with age (Tischler et al., 1982; Unsicker, 1986), whilst human chromaffin cells appear to be responsive irrespective of age (Silani et al., 1990) and bovine chromaffin cells never respond postnatally to NGF with neurite outgrowth (Naujoks et al., 1982). This plasticity of the isolated chromaffin cell has been exploited in the transplantation of this tissue both experimentally and clinically.

The chromaffin cells are the major, but not the only, cell type of the AM and, as one would expect from their developmental origin, they receive a preganglionic cholinergic input from the spinal cord, the cells themselves being specialised

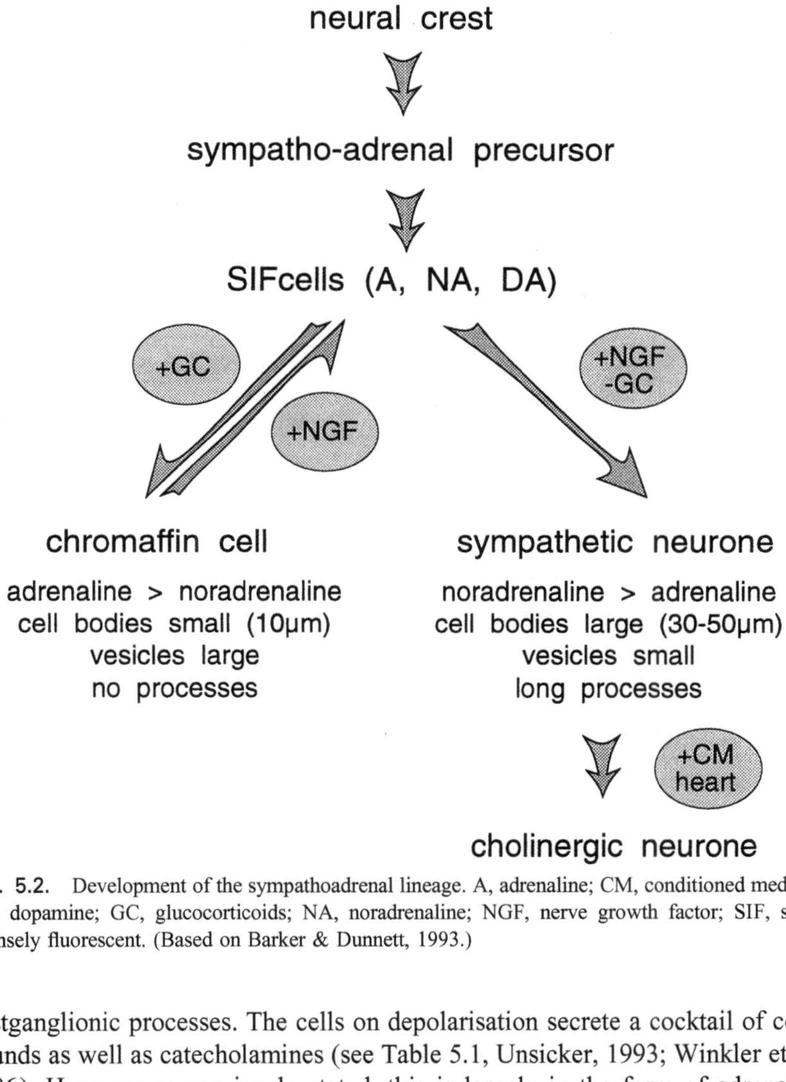

FIG. 5.2. Development of the sympathoadrenal lineage. A, adrenaline; CM, conditioned medium; DA, dopamine; GC, glucocorticoids; NA, noradrenaline; NGF, nerve growth factor; SIF, small intensely fluorescent. (Based on Barker & Dunnett, 1993.)

postganglionic processes. The cells on depolarisation secrete a cocktail of compounds as well as catecholamines (see Table 5.1, Unsicker, 1993; Winkler et al., 1986). However as previously stated, this is largely in the form of adrenaline (A) and noradrenaline (NA) rather than dopamine (DA). In the rat, for example, DA represents less than 0.1% of the total catecholamine content of the adrenal gland (Verhofstad et al., 1985), which is of obvious relevance to the use of this tissue as a donor source for transplantation in PD. However, a different situation is seen when chromaffin cells are cultured *in vitro* or intracerebrally transplanted (Freed, 1983; Freed et al., 1983; Müller and Unsicker, 1981; Tischler et al., 1982). Under these conditions there is an increase in DA relative to NA and A by an unknown mechanism. This encourages the view that although the chromaffin cells secrete very low levels of DA in their normal adrenal environment,

TABLE 5.1
Cell types and contents of chromaffin cells

Types of cell found in adrenal medulla	*Components of the chromaffin cell*
Chromaffin cells	Catecholamines
	Calcium
	Ascorbic acid
	Chromogranins
	Enkephalin-like peptides
	Variety of neurotrophic factors
Adrenocortical cells	
Small intensely fluorescent (SIF) cells	
Ganglion cells	
Vascular endothelial cells	
Smooth muscle cells	
Fibroblasts	
Schwann cells	

their capacity to release DA may be enhanced substantially in the very different environment of an intracerebral AM graft.

It is therefore important to realise that a grafted piece of AM does not represent a pure dopaminergic transplant for several reasons:

(1) It mainly contains catecholamines other than DA.
(2) It co-releases many non-catecholaminergic compounds on depolarisation.
(3) It contains large numbers of non-catecholaminergic cells, and this includes cells from the adrenal cortex.

Consequently, dissection of the functional effects of AM transplants is not straightforward.

AM grafts in animal models of PD

The original work on AM transplantation was pioneered by Olson and colleagues. They used an intraocular implantation site to demonstrate that chromaffin cells could survive transplantation, extend axons and innervate deafferented iris or cografted brain tissue (see Chapter Three; Olson & Malmfors, 1970; Olson et al., 1980; Strömberg et al., 1985a; Unsicker, 1985). Furthermore, NGF produced a permanent phenotypic transformation of transplanted rat chromaffin cells into a primarily neuronal phenotype, irrespective of age (Strömberg et al., 1985a).

The first implantations of AM into the brain were undertaken by Perlow and colleagues using the model already developed for implanting solid nigral grafts into the lateral ventricle (Freed et al., 1980; Perlow et al., 1979). Thus, Perlow

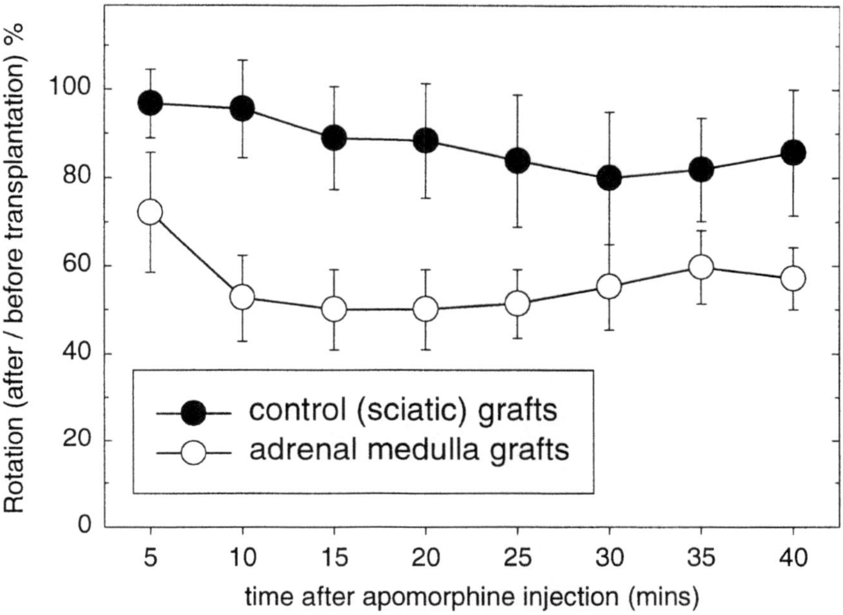

FIG. 5.3. Rotational behaviour of 6-OHDA lesioned rats receiving intraventricular grafts of adult adrenal medulla tissue (Data from Freed et al., 1981, reprinted with permission from *Nature*, © Macmillan Magazines Limited.)

et al. (1980) first grafted bovine adrenal chromaffin cells into the cerebral ventricles of rats and demonstrated modest survival for at least 2 months after transplantation.

A more detailed and extended study then reported the first functional and histological study on intracerebral AM allografts (Freed et al., 1981). In this second study, AM pieces derived from rat donors were grafted into the lateral ventricle of adult rats, resulting in a significant reduction in turning 8 weeks later in the apomorphine rotation test (see Fig. 5.3). The degree of reversal of rotation appeared to correlate well with the number of cells seen on tyrosine hydroxylase (TH) staining, except in one case where over 5000 cells survived without any significant effect on rotational behaviour. This lack of effect was attributed to the presence of adrenal cortical tissue within the graft. This in turn may have led to reduced levels of DA in the transplanted chromaffin cells, which have been demonstrated to contain substantial (if somewhat variable) quantities of DA 5 months after grafting (Freed et al., 1983).

Unfortunately, in these early studies there was no correlation made between the levels of different catecholamines, the number of TH-positive cells, and the behavioural effects of the graft. However, the hypothesis that high levels of catecholamines and the presence of some surviving chromaffin cells are critical to the functional success of the grafts was supported by the studies of Strömberg

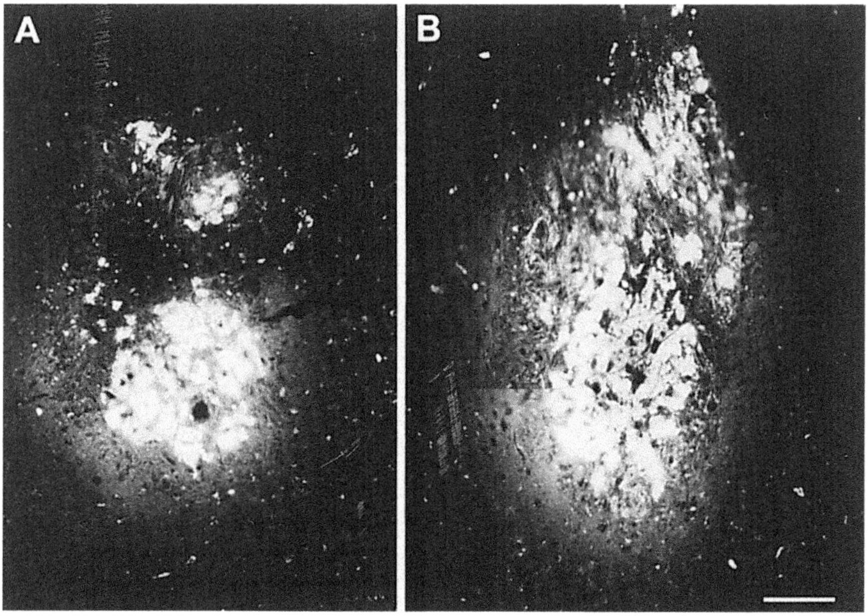

FIG. 5.4. Histology of adrenal medulla grafts in rats, (A) treated with and (B) without NGF following implantation. Tissue sections are stained by catecholamine fluorescence in order to visualise adrenal chromaffin cells surviving in the striatum of the host brain. (Reproduced from Strömberg et al., 1985a, with permission © Springer-Verlag.)

and colleagues. These investigators demonstrated, first of all, that in the acute stages after transplantation there is a dramatic release and then loss of catecholamines as the cells die and that the spontaneous rotational behaviour seen after grafting is mediated via DA (Herrera-Marschitz et al., 1984; Strömberg et al., 1984, 1985a). Survival of these grafts was dramatically improved if NGF was given either intermittently or for a continuous period after grafting (Strömberg et al., 1985b). In this latter study, donor tissue was taken from adult rat adrenal medulla and if NGF was given continuously via an implanted osmotic minipump for 14–28 days after grafting the recipients were observed to have functional benefits that lasted at least 18 months. After 18 months the animals were killed, and histology at this time revealed that a significant number of chromaffin cells had survived and many had undergone differentiation with process outgrowth; but none of these processes appeared to make synapses with the host CNS (see Fig. 5.4). The decreases in apomorphine-induced rotational behaviour after grafting correlated well with the histological findings.

These studies of Strömberg and colleagues (1984, 1985a) involved placing pieces of AM into the neostriatum as opposed to the lateral ventricle. Attempts at using stereotaxically injected suspensions of chromaffin cells, in contrast to the situation with foetal nigral tissue, have overall been disappointing with poor cell survival and therefore limited functional recovery (Brown & Dunnett, 1989; Freed et al., 1986a; Morihisa et al., 1984; Patel-Vaidya et al., 1985). This has led some investigators to propose that AM grafts are only effective if placed into the lateral ventricle of the recipient (Freed et al., 1990), although other studies do not necessarily support this view (Bing et al., 1988; Nishino et al., 1988). For example, Nishino et al. (1988) reported that neonatal AM cells could transmute into dopaminergic neurones when injected into the lesioned striatum and that these neurones did form synapses with the host caudate.

Mechanisms of AM graft function

Overall, these studies tend to imply that the AM graft may be working by releasing DA, irrespective of the phenotypic endpoint of the transplanted cell. This possible role for DA as at least *a* factor responsible for some of the benefits of the graft is reinforced by two further observations. First, Hargraves and Freed (1987) and later Becker et al. (1990) have demonstrated that direct intrastriatal infusion of DA can reverse to some extent apomorphine-induced rotational behaviour in 6-OHDA (6-hydroxydopamine)-lesioned rats. Second, AM grafts that are behaviourally and anatomically effective cause an increase in DA turnover, amphetamine-stimulated striatal DA release, and DA concentration in the blood *without* producing an increase in CSF (cerebrospinal fluid) or striatal extracellular concentrations of DA (Becker & Freed, 1988). This led Becker and Freed (1988; Becker et al., 1990) to propose that the graft may be acting by releasing catecholamines, especially DA, into local blood vessels and that these catecholamines are then transported through the circulatory system into the host brain where they produce their effect.

This latter hypothesis has its origins in the observed differences in the vascularisation of different types of grafts. Solid AM grafts contain the fenestrated capillary endothelium of the donor tissue, which produces a local defect of the blood–brain barrier (BBB), so that the effects may extend outside the site of the graft (Pappas & Sagen, 1988; Rosenstein, 1987). In contrast, the vasculature of cell suspension grafts, the predominant form in which embryonic neural tissue is transplanted, is host-derived, and so does not contain graft-derived endothelial cells (Pappas & Sagen, 1988). In this respect Curran and Becker (1991) have recently shown that changes in BBB permeability are associated with some of the behavioural and neurochemical indices of recovery in 6-OHDA-lesioned rats receiving intraventricular AM.

In 1987, Martha Bohn and colleagues (1987) proposed an alternative mechanism of action to the DA replacement hypothesis for AM grafts. They observed that in MPTP (1-methyl-4-phenyl-1,2,3,6-tetrahydropyridine)-treated mice the AM graft promoted sprouting of the host striatal dopaminergic fibres (see Fig. 5.5). This observation has since been corroborated both in monkeys (Bankiewicz et al., 1988; Plunkett et al., 1990) and in two human post mortems (Hirsch et al.,

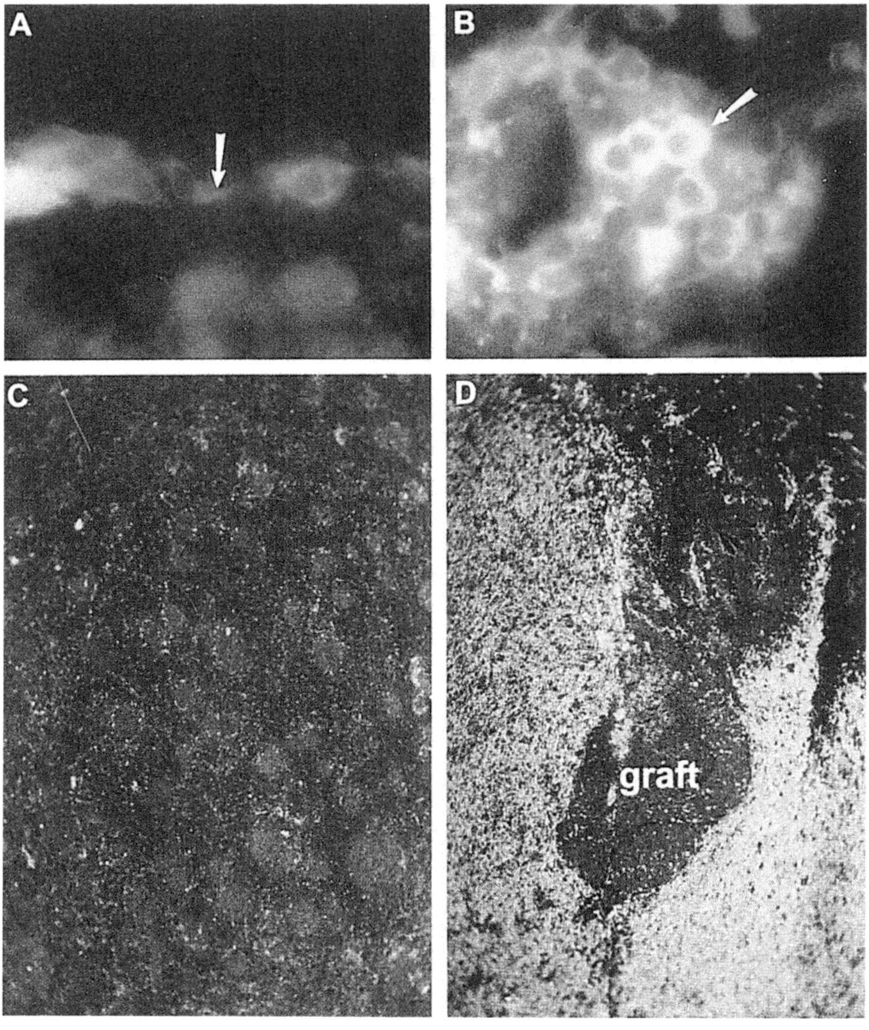

FIG. 5.5. Histology of adrenal medulla grafts in the MPTP-lesioned mouse brain showing host fibre sprouting. (A) Tyrosine hydroxylase stain of catecholamine-producing adrenal cells surviving in the grafts. (B) Adrenal cells also stain for the enzyme, phenylethanolamine-N-methyltransferase (PNMT) that converts noradrenaline into adrenaline. (C) The striatum of a control mouse with MPTP lesion alone, showing almost complete loss of TH-stained fibres in the dorsal striatum. (D) The striatum of a grafted mouse showing massive increase in TH fibre staining in the grafted striatum. These fibres appear to originate not from the grafts but by sprouting from more ventral parts of the host striatum. (Reproduced from Bohn et al., 1987, with permission © American Association for the Advancement of Science.)

1990; Kordower et al., 1991). This suggested an alternative mechanism of graft function, *viz*. that the graft was acting by releasing a humoral neurotrophic agent into the adjacent neostriatum and CSF that stimulated sprouting of host DA fibres spared by the lesions. This alternative hypothesis would also help explain the bilateral improvements seen in some of the unilaterally transplanted parkinsonian patients (see later). It should also be noted that the sprouting response induced by AM grafts is only seen when the host animals have partial lesions, as for example induced by MPTP in these studies (Bankiewicz et al., 1988; Bohn et al., 1987), whereas after relatively complete lesions of the host system, as induced by 6-OHDA in rats, no similar sprouting response can be observed (Brown & Dunnett, 1989).

There are several possible candidates for the neurotrophic stimulus mediating AM-induced sprouting. A variety of neurotrophic factors are found within and released by chromaffin cells of the AM, including bFGF (basic FGF), NGF, chromogranin A, a ciliary neurotrophic-like factor, and possibly other cytokines and neuropeptides (Unsicker, 1993; see Table 5.1). Although none of these factors has been measured in experimental AM grafts in animals, in a series of AM transplants in humans no significant changes were found in either bFGF or chromogranin A levels in the CSF following transplantation (Shults et al., 1991). However, few of their patients showed any significant improvement following grafting, so this negative biochemical result may simply be attributable to poor graft survival in this series.

A third explanation as to how AM grafts may function is that they may provide a nidus for the release of host-derived trophic factors. Evidence for this relates to the observation that the AM graft *does not* necessarily have to survive in order for it to produce an effect in MPTP-treated mice and primates (Bohn & Kanuicki, 1990; Fiandaca et al., 1988; Hansen et al., 1988). Date and colleagues (1990), in agreement with the earlier work of the Rochester team (Bohn et al., 1987; Bohn & Kanuicki, 1990), demonstrated that degenerating AM grafts in mice were associated with a substantial sprouting response in young animals, but one which was markedly reduced for older animals. Furthermore, Fiandaca and colleagues (1988; Hansen et al., 1988) demonstrated that grafted cells in *Cebus* monkeys rapidly degenerated and that the transplantation of non-neural tissue in MPTP-treated monkeys produced host TH fibre sprouting and some behavioural recovery, an observation confirmed in the MPTP-treated *Rhesus* monkey (Bankiewicz et al., 1991; Plunkett et al., 1990). This, coupled to a study in which the use of non-neural tissue and NGF was as effective as AM grafts (Pezzoli et al., 1988), led to the suggestion that the benefits of AM grafts may be either directly due to the release of neurotrophic factors from the damaged striatum, or indirectly, through providing a nidus for an inflammatory infiltrate and the release of cytokines, many of which can have a neurotrophic action.

Evidence in support of this first interpretation came with the demonstration that insertion of a graft does directly damage the neostriatum, with the release of host neurotrophic factors (Nieto-Sampedro et al., 1983, 1984). These factors, however, can only have a trophic effect when some host fibres are still present, as occurs in the MPTP, as opposed to the 6-OHDA, lesioned animal by virtue of the fact that the toxin spares to some extent the ventral striatum. Support for the alternative second explanation is to be found in the fact that grafts do induce an inflammatory response with the release of inflammatory mediators, such as interleukin-1, which have a known neurotrophic action (Riopelle, 1988; Wang et al., 1991). In this respect the transplantation of both cytokine-producing cells and interleukin-secreting pellets has been associated with a reduction in amphetamine-induced rotation in rats with partially lesioned nigrostriatal tracts. This reduction in rotation appears to be associated with a host TH fibre sprouting response (Ewing et al., 1992; Wang et al., 1991). However, the prolonged benefits of some grafts in the absence of an inflammatory response does argue against this being the only mechanism by which AM grafts act.

In view of the studies demonstrating that NGF enhances chromaffin cell and AM graft survival (Doupé et al., 1985; Strömberg et al., 1985b), interest has turned to the use of cografts in which the AM is co-transplanted with an NGF-rich tissue such as peripheral nerve (Doering, 1992; Hansen et al., 1990; Kordower et al., 1990; Watts et al., 1990), amitotic C6 glioma cells (Bing et al., 1990; Unsicker et al., 1984) and astrocytes transfected to produce NGF (Cunningham et al., 1991, 1994). These studies have demonstrated that cell survival is improved in these grafts, which is reflected functionally in their ability to reduce the animal's rotational response to apomorphine, and to a lesser extent amphetamine.

Summary of adrenal medulla grafts in animals

It is clear that the mechanisms outlined above are simplistic models of effect. Indeed, it is probable that AM grafts will exert their effects via a variety of different mechanisms in different situations. Apart from the possible role of DA as the effector system of AM grafts under certain circumstances, several other conclusions can be drawn from these animal studies.

(1) In the first instance AM grafts do survive transplantation but their long-term survival may be limited, although this can be prolonged with trophic agents including NGF.
(2) The number of surviving TH-positive cells resulting from transplantation appears to relate to functional recovery irrespective of the phenotypic morphology of the transplanted cells, although graft survival is not an absolute prerequisite for a reduction in rotation. This raises doubts as to the role of DA in mediating the effect of AM grafts. Indeed the variable results with different types of AM grafts in different animals with different lesions mean that it is probable that AM grafts act by a *variety* of actions.

(3) Only in animals with partial lesions (e.g. MPTP) can grafts appear to be capable of exerting a trophic influence on surviving host dopaminergic neurones. This sprouting response seen under these conditions relates in part to the release of host neurotrophic molecules at the time of surgery; in part to the release of inflammatory mediators which have neurotrophic actions; and in part to trophic molecules secreted by grafted cells.

CLINICAL TRIALS OF ADRENAL MEDULLA TRANSPLANTS

It is on the background of these experimental animal studies, to some extent, that the first clinical trials of AM transplants were undertaken in patients with PD (Parkinson's disease). However, it must be stressed that many of the experimental data discussed above actually post-date the first clinical trials. This highlights the need for caution and patience in any experimental procedure such as this, as the premature introduction of a poorly researched approach can have detrimental effects both clinically and in terms of scientific credibility.

General principles

As one would expect, the first PD patients chosen for AM transplantation had entered the final stages of the disease process where control by conventional medical treatment was becoming increasingly difficult, if not impossible. By this stage, many parkinsonian patients have significant cognitive difficulties as well as depression, especially in the more elderly cases (Cummings, 1992; Marder et al., 1995). However, in order to be suitable for transplantation, patients in general had to be free of such cognitive and affective abnormalities whilst displaying marked motor difficulties, and so, as a result, most patients in the initial trials were relatively young. Thus the population that received the AM transplants (as is true for *all* clinical transplant programmes to date) are highly selected and unrepresentative of most patients with idiopathic PD.

A second consideration that cannot be over-stressed at the outset is that the loss of dopaminergic neurones within the SN (substantia nigra) in idiopathic PD is only part of a much wider spectrum of neuronal loss within the nervous system, and these other losses are associated with widespread alterations in a spectrum of neurotransmitters (Agid et al., 1989; Fearnley & Lees, 1996). The significance of these additional changes to the aetiology and natural history of the disease is unknown, but may be an important factor in limiting the success of any graft designed simply to replace the dopaminergic deficiencies of the disease alone.

The PD process is not localised to the CNS alone. Of some significance is the fact that the adrenal glands themselves appear also to be involved. At post mortem, the adrenal medulla derived from PD patients contains less than normal levels of catecholamines (Carmichael et al., 1988; Cervera et al., 1988; Stoddard et al., 1989a, b). Consequently, if the patients' own adrenal glands are used for autotransplantation (which is the primary advantage of AM grafts and thus typically the case) then not only may any disease-related abnormality be transferred with the transplant into the brain, but also the whole rationale of replacement with catecholamine-secreting cells may be compromised from this source.

These problems, coupled to the heterogeneous nature of the disease, make interpretation of any clinical study of AM transplants difficult. However, this difficulty has been compounded by the use of different transplantation procedures, measures of disability, and medical treatment. Each of these factors is extremely important and may help explain some of the differences between studies. For example, if maximal L-dopa treatment is withheld prior to surgery, and then optimal dosing strategies are only subsequently introduced after transplantation, we can get a very distorted perspective of the apparent effectiveness of the transplantation procedure. Stable baseline measures of a number of variables need to be established prior to any grafting procedure and then continued post-grafting, and for ease of comparison, medical treatment should, if possible, be left unchanged.

This unfortunately still does not help to establish whether the underlying disease process will influence the survival and growth of grafted cells, nor whether the continued use of L-dopa therapy after transplantation will in itself be harmful to the graft (see Chapter Four). However, in the case of the AM there is no evidence of toxicity with L-dopa, but the presence of DA receptors on the AM chromaffin cells could theoretically affect the release of catecholamines in the transplant.

It is on this background that the clinical transplant programmes were started and must be interpreted. It is therefore not surprising that dramatic claims and counterclaims have been made in this field.

The clinical trials

The first clinical trial of AM transplants was undertaken in Sweden in the early 1980s by Backlund and colleagues. They stereotaxically transplanted AM tissue into the neostriatum; the caudate nucleus in the first two patients (Backlund et al., 1985) and the putamen in the next two (Lindvall et al., 1987). It was only this latter site which produced any demonstrable recovery, although the benefit was only moderate in degree and short-lasting in duration (see Fig. 5.6).

At about the same time, in Mexico, Madrazo et al. undertook an open surgical approach and, in contrast to the Swedish series, reported apparently dramatic results. Their approach was more invasive, involving direct visualisation of the transplant site in the head of the caudate nucleus, and creating a cavity in the ventricular wall of the caudate into which the auto-grafted AM tissue was anchored. In their original paper, Madrazo et al. (1987) reported persistent improvements in the first two patients, which was then followed by a second report of 11 patients all of whom had dramatic improvements in motor and cognitive

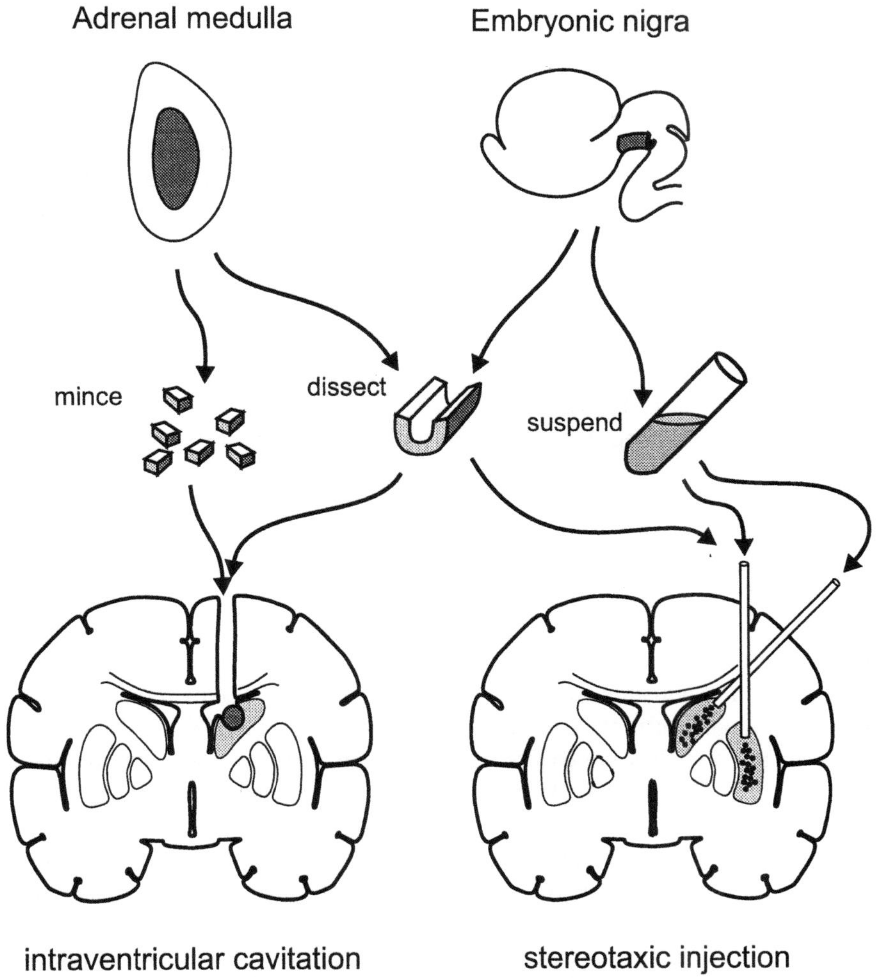

FIG. 5.6. Basic techniques for clinical intracerebral transplantation in Parkinson's disease. Tissue for implantation may be harvested from the patient's own adrenal medulla or from the substantia nigra of a donor embryo. The tissue may be transplanted as solid pieces, minced pieces, or as a dissociated cell suspension. Tissue is then transplanted as solid or minced pieces into a cavity made in the ventricular wall of the head of the caudate nucleus or as pieces or dissociated cells by stereotaxic injection into the depths of the basal ganglia.

function (Drucker-Colin et al., 1988; Ostrosky-Solis et al., 1988). These improvements were bilateral even though the grafts were unilateral, were apparent immediately after surgery, and occurred whilst reducing or even stopping the antiparkinsonian medication.

Following such apparently dramatic success, a host of further operations were performed world-wide, but especially in the USA (Goetz et al., 1991), even though some caution was expressed at the time about the strength of the initial results. This scepticism was based on the fact that the original patients of Madrazo et al. were highly atypical, being very young with rapidly progressive disease, and with one having an affected relative. Furthermore, the possibility could not be excluded that their apparent improvement was not so much due to the actual effect of the graft *per se* but to the way this effect was scored (see W.J. Freed et al., 1990 for further discussion on this). This is best illustrated by the fact that although one of their patients improved on their scoring system from grade 1 to 5 following transplantation, this improvement was not seen by other neurologists several months after surgery, nor by the family several weeks after the operation. Moreover, this patient had an element of dementia which made assessment difficult, and at post mortem he was found to have a necrotic, non-surviving graft (Peterson et al., 1989).

Nevertheless, among the subsequent trials using a similar surgical protocol, many were undertaken within a more rigorous experimental context, enabling systematic evaluation of safety and outcome. In particular two major multicentre collaborations were established in North America, the first co-ordinated by the American Association of Neurological Surgeons (Bakay et al., 1990) to collate information on surgical procedures, safety, and complications of surgery, and the second co-ordinated by the United Parkinson Foundation to provide a registry of trials in the USA and Canada, along with establishing standards for assessment and collation of outcome data (Goetz et al., 1990). A summary of published reports of trials and individual cases is shown in Table 5.2.

From these studies we can see that although none supported the dramatic improvements claimed by Madrazo et al., many did find that the majority of patients gain some detectable benefit from the procedure and that in a few patients improvement can be striking. Overall, patients with AM grafts have a mean increase of "on" time from 47.6% to 75%, with an increase in "on" time without abnormal movements (especially chorea) from 27% to 59%. In most cases, however, the improvement has not been a permanent one, with significant benefits at 6 months generally dissipating by 18 months (Goetz et al., 1989, 1990; Olanow et al., 1990), in contrast to the patients receiving foetal nigral grafts, where the converse is true (see later).

To be offset against this apparent benefit, however, is the fact that the surgical procedure is not benign. The undertaking of an open neurosurgical approach into the caudate nucleus, in conjunction with an abdominal operation to harvest one adrenal gland, in a patient with advanced PD, who is thus frail, is fraught with difficulty, as these transplant studies have shown. Peri-operative morbidity from this procedure is relatively high, particularly in older patients (Drucker-Colin et al., 1988; Goetz et al., 1991). For example, Allen et al. demonstrated that four of their six elderly patients experienced prolonged alterations in mental state (Allen et al., 1989), and overall over 78% of operated patients experienced some adverse side effects from the procedure, such as haemorrhage and

TABLE 5.2
Summary of major clinical studies on AM grafts in humans with idiopathic PD

Author	*Number of patients*	*Operation*	*Improvements*[1]	*Side effects*[2]	*Deaths*
Ahlskog et al.	8	CN/open	4	6	0
Allen et al.	18	CN/open	4	9	0
Apuzzo et al.	10	CN/stereo	4	1	0
Backlund et al.	2	CN/stereo	1	1	0
Bakay et al.	12	CN/open	9	12	0
Broggi et al.	4	CN/open	2	2	0
Broseta et al.	1	CN/open	0	1	1
Cahill & Olanow	6	CN/open	5	14	1
Choi et al.	8	CN/open	5	6	0
Chung et al.	5	CN/stereo	5	0	0
Fazzini et al.	4	CN+Put/stereo	4	2	1*
Flores et al.	24	CN/open	14	14	2
Gildenberg et al.	12	CN/stereo	11	5	0
Hitchcock et al.	1	CN/stereo	1	0	0
Jankovic et al.	3	CN/open	3	2	0
Jiao et al.	4	CN/stereo	4	0	0
Koller et al.	6	CN/open	3	17	0
Liebermann et al.	9	CN/open	6	9	0
Lindvall et al.	2	Put/stereo	0	0	0
Lopez-Lozano et al.	20	CN/open	17	17	3
Machado-Salas et al.	9	CN/open	3	4	1
Madrazo et al.	22	CN/open	18	0	4
Petruk et al.	5	CN/open	3	5	0
Pezzoli et al.	3	2CN/stereo	2	2	0
		1CN/open	0	1	0
Rush Research Group	7	CN/open	7	11	0
Schvarcz et al.	2	CN+Put/stereo	2	0	0
Takeuchi et al.	1	Put/stereo	1	0	0
Velasco et al.	10	CN/open	5	8	2
Zhang	24	CN/open	17	0	2
Total	190	Open : 145 Stereo : 45	159	156	16

Open, open surgical approach; Stereo, stereotaxic implantation of graft; CN, caudate nucleus; Put, putamen.

[1] Improvement at 6 months post grafting. [2] Any complication per patient is classified as a single side effect.

* In the study of Fazzini et al. one patient had a graft placed accidentally in the medial thalamus and one patient developed a glioma thought to be unrelated to the graft procedure.

infarctions, with postoperative psychiatric disturbances being particularly common. A review by Quinn (1990) of studies published within the first 5 years of the operation indicated at least 17 deaths of various cause out of 231 operations, many of which could be attributed to some aspect of the surgical procedure, a rate approaching 10%.

The collation of these reviews has led to a consensus among most parties that the high level of morbidity and mortality associated with the procedure, combined with the poor survival of the grafts (see later), outweighs the modest and transient improvements that the AM graft offers the patient. Consequently, continuation of AM transplantation is no longer justified, at least when based on the standard protocols that have hitherto been employed. That does not of course preclude experimental developments that make it plausible that improved techniques may be developed. However, this will require the following measures:

(1) Improved surgical procedures that reduce morbidity and mortality.
(2) Improved graft survival, including survival of the chromaffin cells.
(3) Demonstration of sustained dopamine replacement.
(4) Improved collection or alternative sources of adrenal chromaffin cells (e.g. cross-species) that eliminate the requirement of additional surgery for autograft harvesting.
(5) Clarity about the mechanism of graft function, including the demonstration that simple dopamine secretion is sufficient to yield functional recovery.

Mechanism of action for adrenal medulla transplants in humans

The disparate results of this procedure have meant that any mechanism of action for the benefits seen with these AM grafts is controversial. However, it is still important to understand the mechanism of action in those adrenal grafts that yielded at least some benefits. Only then can we rationally design the next step forward.

The most obvious interpretation is that the clinical effects of AM grafts are mediated through their acting as a source of catecholamines, especially DA, in the depleted striatum. Evidence to support this is that while levels of the DA metabolite homovanillic acid (HVA) in the CSF are increased after surgery in those patients who improve, there is no increase in the concentration of DA (Ahlskog et al., 1990; Fazzini et al., 1991; Jankovic et al., 1989; Penn et al., 1990; Watts et al., 1989).

This is confirmed by the lack of any consistent increase in the intrastriatal uptake of the dopamine reuptake ligand [^{18}F]-fluorodopa when patients with autologous AM grafts are given PET (position emission tomography) scans (Guttman et al., 1989; Sawle & Myers, 1993). Whilst this does not exclude a small local increase in DA release from either the graft or host striatum, it is possible that some other factor from the AM graft is being released, especially given the bilateral effects of unilateral grafts in the original Mexican series.

Schults et al. studied the ventricular fluid of transplanted patients for chromogranin A and bFGF (basic FGF), both of which are found in chromaffin cells and are considered to have neurotrophic actions. They found no significant differences, although none of their patients reported any benefit from AM transplantation (Shults et al., 1991). On the other hand, one of the most consistent changes seen in the CSF of these patients is an elevation in levels of endorphin, a peptide that can be reduced in idiopathic PD (Nappi et al., 1985). It is conceivable, therefore, that this is the humoral agent of successful AM grafts; but it seems more likely that it is responsible for the hypersomnolent state and the surprising lack of pain experienced by many patients postoperatively (Goetz et al., 1991; Jankovic et al., 1989; Shults et al., 1991). Indeed, these results point the way to a possible useful application of adrenal grafts in the treatment of pain itself (see Chapter Eight).

In addition one cannot exclude the possibility that the improvement seen in patients with AM grafts is simply the result of surgery to the neostriatum and/or disruption of the BBB, which in turn may allow for a more consistent and better delivery of drug therapy to the CNS. However, there are several reasons for doubting that this is the main mechanism of graft efficacy. First, there is no improvement in patients with idiopathic PD who have a caudate nucleus (CN) biopsy (Motti et al., 1988). Second, there appears to be little long-term alteration in BBB permeability despite some long-term improvements in function (Ahlskog et al., 1989). Finally, the accidental placement of an AM graft outside the striatum is without benefit (Fazzini et al., 1991).

The difficulty of studying the functional state of AM grafts in the living patient has meant that greater emphasis has had to be placed on the information gained at post mortem. Several cases have now come to post mortem. Surprisingly, these reveal that in the majority of cases few, if any, TH-positive adrenal medulla cells survive (Table 5.3). Although the agonal state causing death coupled to the delay in performing the post mortem may lead to apparent graft death in life, this seems unlikely given the consistency of the post-mortem results with AM grafts and the contrast with findings under similar circumstances with nigral grafts (see later).

One of the best-documented post-mortem accounts of an intracerebral adrenal graft in a patient with PD comes from Kordower et al., who reported on a case in which the patient had 18 months benefit after his graft, following which he slowly returned to his pre-operative status. At 30 months he suddenly died and at post mortem he had a few TH-positive cells present in the graft surrounded by a dense network of TH-positive terminals and processes that appeared to be of host origin (see Fig. 5.7, Kordower et al., 1991). This sprouting response of host TH fibres in the presence of only a few chromaffin cells is similar to the findings that had been reported by Hirsch et al. (1990), although in this case no surviving

TABLE 5.3
Post-mortem studies in patients with Parkinson's disease who have received an adrenal medulla graft

Author	*Time of PM after grafting (months)*	*Surviving TH cells in graft*	*Host response as assessed by TH fibre sprouting in vicinity of graft*
Allen et al., 1989	3	None	?
Dohan et al., 1988	4	None	None
Fazzini et al., 1991	12	None	None
Forno et al., 1989	12	None	None
Hirsch et al., 1990	4	None	Yes
Hurtig et al., 1989	4	Few	None
Jankovic et al., 1989	8	None	None
Kordower et al., 1991	30	Few	Yes
Lieberman et al., 1990a	2	None	?
Lieberman et al., 1990b	4	None	?
Peterson et al., 1989	4	None	None
Velasco et al., 1991	1	None	None
Velasco et al., 1991	2	None	None
Waters et al., 1990	1.5	None	None

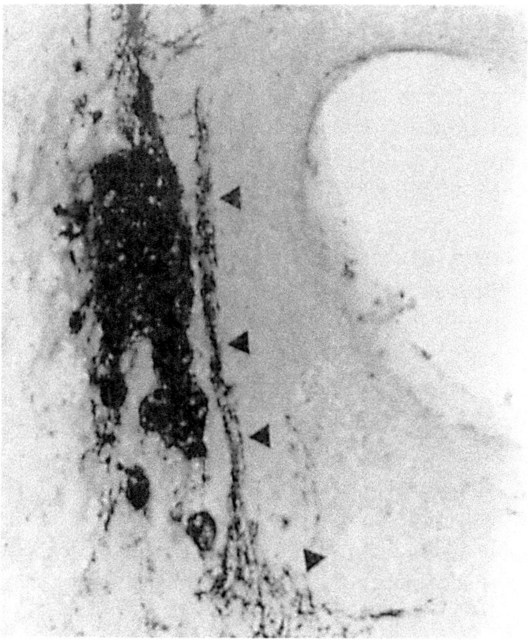

FIG. 5.7. Histology of degenerating AM graft in a patient with Parkinson's disease, visualised by tyrosine hydroxylase staining in the post-mortem brain. A few surviving cells and some host fibre sprouting can be seen. (Reproduced from Kordower et al., 1991, with permission © Lippincott, Williams & Wilkins.)

chromaffin cells were identified. This parallels some of the histological findings seen with MPTP-lesioned animals with AM grafts that failed to survive (see Fig. 5.5). Thus transplanted chromaffin cells can survive for prolonged periods of time within the human CNS although the number doing so is small. They can probably induce a sprouting response of host dopaminergic fibres even in the absence of surviving chromaffin cells, and indeed the degeneration of the graft may actually be a prerequisite for this sprouting response. However, it is unclear whether the few surviving transplanted cells or the host TH fibre sprouting mediate the functional benefits of grafts.

Modified adrenal graft protocols

As a result of the poor survival of AM grafts and their limited clinical success, a number of investigators have tried a variety of modifications to the basic surgical approach. Petruk et al. have modified the original technique by performing a two-stage transplantation procedure in which a cavity in the CN is made first, followed by placing graft tissue into the preformed cavity 7–10 days later (Petruk et al., 1990). This allows for the reabsorption of blood, the removal of post-traumatic neurotoxic agents (e.g. excitatory amino acids), the liberation of trophic factors from the damaged striatum (Nieto-Sampedro et al., 1983, 1984), and the development of new blood vessels locally around the cavity (post-cavitation angiogenesis), which is maximal at 10 days (Nieto-Sampedro et al., 1983), all of which are thought to promote graft survival. Preliminary results reveal improvement in limited numbers of patients.

Alternatively Lopez-Lozano et al. have modified the basic transplantation procedure by perfusing the adrenal gland prior to implantation. In the 20 patients who have been operated on using this approach, 17 have improved bilaterally in all parameters (Lopez-Lozano et al., 1991), although a significant number of these patients experienced transient psychiatric disorders postoperatively and three died. No patient reported in this study had been followed up for more than 7 months and no post-mortem information is available.

The possibility of supporting the graft with neurotrophic factors, especially NGF, has been assessed both by the use of direct infusions and co-grafts of tissue-rich NGF. Olson et al. undertook a study in which patients received an intraputamenal infusion of NGF for a month following an AM autograft for idiopathic PD (IPD) (Olson et al., 1991, 1992). They report that there is some improvement in their cases. This technique closely parallels the earlier work in rats by Strömberg et al. (1985b) and presumably is effective by a similar mechanism (see Chapter Four), as NGF is known to promote neurite outgrowth in aged parkinsonian adrenal medulla cells (Silani et al., 1990). An alternative source of NGF for the AM graft is the sectioned peripheral nerve, which has been used with some success as a co-graft in animals (see previous discussion). This procedure using autologous AM and intercostal nerve co-grafts has been undertaken in a few patients with IPD and the preliminary results are encouraging (Date et al., 1994; Watts et al., 1992, 1997).

Finally, some groups have used foetal adrenal tissue. The initial report on the use of this approach in a single patient demonstrated a poor outcome (Madrazo et al., 1988). This may have related to the gestational age of the donor adrenal gland (13 weeks), as at this time the gland is poorly developed and it is therefore not clear what is being transplanted (Dwork et al., 1988; Silani et al., 1992a). However, these same investigators have recently treated 3 PD patients with foetal AM grafts of this same gestational age, and on this occasion reported some improvement of rigidity and bradykinesia although the improvement was not as great as in those who had received foetal nigral grafts (Madrazo et al., 1990). The reason for these discordant results with the same procedure is not clear.

These new approaches offer hope for improving the efficacy of AM transplants, although the results from animal experiments and trials on human patients suggest that considerable progress will have to be made before they can be considered an effective treatment for PD.

Conclusions on adrenal medulla transplants in humans

It is clear that the dramatic improvement reported by Madrazo et al. for AM grafts in PD patients has not been consistently replicated by others. Many patients do derive some benefit from the procedure, but this benefit is moderate and appears to decline with time. The reported benefit is mainly one of a reduction in "off" periods and an increase in "on" time of improved quality (Goetz et al., 1991). In addition, there appears to be some evidence that the AM grafts may slow down or even halt the disease process. Whether this relates to the graft providing a protective factor or simply reflects the advanced stage of the disease at the time of surgery is unclear. It does, however, highlight the problems in studying a group of patients in whom the natural history of the advanced treated disease is largely unknown.

The modest benefits of the grafts are not gained without an appreciable perioperative morbidity, especially in the older patient (see Table 5.2). Theoretically, not having to use immunosuppression for autologous grafts such as these does mean that the procedure in the long term is safer than operations that employ foetal nigral grafts, or indeed any other tissues between unrelated individuals and/or species. On balance, however, the morbidity of the operation coupled with its limited long-term therapeutic effects makes it extremely difficult to recommend in its current form.

Until research is successful in finding ways to make AM grafts survive and function long-term in experimental models (especially primates), and to make surgical delivery safer, it seems appropriate to postpone use of this procedure in human patients.

EMBRYONIC NIGRAL TRANSPLANTS IN HUMANS

In contrast to AM grafts in humans, the advent of clinical transplants with nigral tissues did not occur for a decade after the first basic experiments in animals had been completed. A large number of such transplants have now been undertaken over the past 10 years, estimated in a recent review at over 200 (Lindvall, 1997). Although they have been exclusively targeted for PD, diagnostic difficulties have meant that occasionally patients with other diseases may have received transplants (see later). In three cases the patients have had MPTP-induced parkinsonism; in the remainder of cases their parkinsonism is idiopathic, i.e. the cause is unknown.

Ethical issues

The decision to use human foetal tissue for clinical transplantation arose out of the failure of alternative sources of the adrenal medulla autografts to provide effective catecholamine-secreting cells in PD. The animal models clearly indicate that it is possible to alleviate Parkinson-like symptoms that result from explicit dopamine loss by dopamine cell replacement. Moreover, the efficacy of the grafts is critically dependent on a combination of factors, not least being the source of cells used for implantation. The available data clearly indicate that using the correct population of cells at the correct stage of developmental growth is by far the most effective for functional repair. In the case of degeneration of the nigrostriatal dopamine system, this is most effectively achieved using foetal nigral neurones at the time of their initial development. Moreover, these cells are best derived from foetuses of the same species, as the move to other species for donor tissue (xenotransplants) creates severe immunological problems. The biology therefore clearly suggests that the most effective source of cells for clinical transplantation in PD is likely to be human foetal nigral neurones of the appropriate developmental age.

There are substantial practical and ethical concerns to be addressed if we are to use human foetal tissues for transplantation. Such tissues might become available through either spontaneous abortion or elective termination of pregnancies, although both of these approaches encounter some strong emotional, moral, and religious sensitivities.

In some countries there is a legal ban on all medical abortions, which would make spontaneous abortions the only source for obtaining foetal tissues (which have been used for transplantation in Mexico and Spain). Notwithstanding the ethical acceptability of this, there are serious practical concerns about the use of this tissue, as spontaneous abortions have a very high incidence of genetic and developmental abnormalities that would make this tissue unsuitable or unsafe for transplantation into a patient.

In other countries, abortion is legal and usually under the control of tight legislation and carefully regulated circumstances; a situation that applies to much of northern Europe and North America. In these circumstances a consideration of the legal and ethical use of human foetal tissues derived from elective abortions needs to be undertaken. Although there has been a long-standing acceptance of using post-mortem foetal tissues for research (e.g. in studies on developmental human anatomy), the issues have become more controversial with concern about the sanctity of life and the rights of the foetus if it is manipulated in early life, whether by *in vitro* fertilisation, stem cell expansion, or growth of embryos in culture.

However, the opinion of the various ethical review commissions that have considered the issues at national and international level is that, if the termination of pregnancy is itself legal, then the subsequent use of resulting tissues for research or therapy is ethical *provided* that there is no influence on the decision of whether, when, and how the abortion is undertaken; that appropriate consent is obtained; and that the tissues are treated with appropriate respect. An example of one such set of guidelines adopted by NECTAR, the network of clinical and research teams in Europe, is shown in Table 5.4 (Boer, 1994). These were derived from an initial consideration by the Swedish Society of Medicine, and subsequently, similar sets of guidelines have been drawn up by many other countries, which are broadly similar in principle even though they may differ in their details. Of course, as well as seeking a consensus position for regulating what is, and is not, permitted or approved within each society, it is also necessary that the individual scientist and clinician confronts and abides by his or her own personal ethical and religious standards.

Development of the human nigrostriatal system

Experimental studies in the rat, marmoset, and other species have shown that the best time to harvest nigral dopaminergic neurones for transplantation is the time when they are first developing. This has been well described in the rat nigrostriatal system (see Chapter Four), and recently Freeman and colleagues (1991, 1995b) have performed similar studies in the developing human nigrostriatal system. These studies have shown that the dopaminergic neurones of the ventral mesencephalon are first detectable in developing human embryos at 6.5 weeks post-gestation. By 8 weeks, they have extended neurites towards the developing striatum and by 11 weeks they have stopped dividing and their subsequent development is in terms of increased innervation of their target structures (Freeman et al., 1991; Silani et al., 1992a).

In a subsequent transplant study, Freeman et al. (1995b) have shown that the best human nigral suspension grafts are obtained from tissue 37–56 days post-ovulation, whilst solid grafts are best harvested 45–65 days post-ovulation.

TABLE 5.4
NECTAR* ethical guidelines for the retrieval and use of human embryonic or foetal donor tissue for experimental and clinical neurotransplantation and research

Clinical and experimental groups or institutions that are members of NECTAR will obey the present ethical guidelines, irrespective of the fact that national legislation may permit them to deviate from these guidelines and provided national legislation allows them to follow these guidelines.

(1) Tissue for transplantation or research may be obtained from dead embryos or foetuses, their death resulting from legally induced or spontaneous abortion. Death of an intact embryo or foetus is defined as absence of respiration and heart beats.
(2) It is not allowed to keep intact embryos or foetuses alive artificially for the purpose of removing usable material.
(3) The decision to terminate pregnancy must under no circumstances be influenced by the possible or desired subsequent use of the embryo or foetus and must therefore precede any introduction of the possible use of the embryonic or fetal tissue. There should be no link between the donor and the recipient, nor designation of the recipient by the donor.
(4) The procedure of abortion, or the timing, must not be influenced by the requirements of the transplantation activity when this would be in conflict with the woman's interests or would increase embryonic or foetal distress.
(5) No material can be used without informed consent of the woman involved. This informed consent should, whenever possible, be obtained prior to abortion.
(6) Screening of the woman for transmissible diseases requires informed consent.
(7) Nervous tissue may be used for transplantation as suspended cell preparations or tissue fragments.
(8) All members of the hospital or research staff directly involved in any of the procedures must be fully informed.
(9) The procurement of embryos, foetuses, or their tissue must not involve profit or remuneration.
(10) Every transplantation or research project involving the use of embryonic or fetal tissue must be approved by the local ethical committee.

* Network for European CNS Transplantation and Restoration

It is therefore clear that the optimal age of donor tissues for human foetal nigral allografts is between 5 and 9 weeks post-gestation. This has proved to be important in explaining some of the disparate results between centres, as older donors are likely to produce grafts with fewer surviving DA neurones.

Clinical results of embryonic nigral transplants in humans

The undertaking of a clinical transplant programme, despite the wealth of animal data to support its use, is still an experimental procedure. As a result, some aspects of the transplantation programme may change with successive patients as some of the problems and technical possibilities in humans, as opposed to animals, become better understood. This has meant that even within one transplantation centre the procedure varies between patients, making comparative studies difficult. Indeed, despite the large number of patients who have received foetal nigral transplants only a minority of these have been fully reported in the detail set out in the CAPIT-PD protocol (Core Assessment Protocol for Intracerebral Transplantation in Parkinson's Disease, see Chapter One). A reluctance by some centres to adopt the recommended consensus protocol for assessment has meant that comparisons between their results and those of other centres is often impossible. It is for this reason that we shall concentrate on only a few centres that have undertaken clinical trials within the format of a scientifically rigorous and objective assessment of patient progress.

The first patients to receive foetal nigral grafts were two PD sufferers in Sweden and one in Mexico at the end of 1987 (Lindvall et al., 1988; Madrazo et al., 1988). Since then a large number of other groups have undertaken clinical transplant programmes with human foetal tissue (see Table 5.5). However, we shall use the large series from Sweden as the focus of our discussion and elaborate with the results from other studies where relevant.

The group in Sweden, co-ordinated by the neurologist Olle Lindvall with Sten Rehncrona as the surgeon, has reported on nigral transplants in 16 PD patients over the past 10 years. Full experimental details have been published on the first 10 cases, although summary data are now available on them all (Widner, 1998). The details of these patients are summarised in Table 5.6.

The first two patients recruited for foetal transplantation were both young and had suffered with PD for about 14 years. Therefore, as with AM grafts, the patients were not representative of the majority of patients suffering from PD. These two patients each received unilateral grafts into the caudate and putamen with tissue from four embryos that were approximately 7–8 weeks old (Lindvall et al., 1989). Both patients were immunosuppressed following the procedure with drugs that are routinely used in kidney transplant programmes (i.e. a "triple therapy" of cyclosporin A, azathioprine, and prednisolone), and maintained on it for 2 years.

In neither case was there a dramatic improvement, although there was an improved response in the effectiveness but not duration of a single dose of L-dopa, a modest increase in the "on" time was observed in one patient, and in both cases there was a transient gait improvement and increase in the motor readiness potentials measured electrophysiologically. However, there was little significant clinical improvement in either patient, which was matched by little evidence of any changes in fluorodopa binding in the PET scans, suggesting rather poor graft survival (Lindvall et al., 1989). Overall then, these patients gained minimal clinical benefit from their transplants. This led to the conclusion that the implantation procedures may have been suboptimal in comparison to what had been achieved in experimental animals, and led to a re-evaluation of the grafting technique in terms of the mode and speed of foetal tissue preparation and the method of implantation. As a result, modifications were made in the implantation procedure, including the design of smaller implantation cannulae

TABLE 5.5
Published studies of human foetal dopamine grafts involving patients with PD

Author	*Numbers of patients*	*Improvement*	*Age of embryo (weeks)*	*Site of graft**	*Time from abortion to grafting*
Swedish group					
Lindvall et al., 1989	2	0	8–10	C+P	5–6hrs
Lindvall et al., 1990/94	2	2	6–7	PUT	2.5–4hrs
Wenning et al., 1997	4	6, but 2 only minor	6–8	2 PUT 2 C+P	<4 hrs
Widner et al., 1992	2 (MPTP)	2	6–8	C+P (bilat)	<4hrs
Widner, 1998	6 (1 MPTP)	6	6–8	1 PUT (bilat) 5 C+P (bilat)	<4hrs
USA group					
Freed et al., 1994	13	13	6–8	2 C+P 11 PUT (bilat)	?
Spencer et al., 1992	4	3	7–11	CN	**
Liebermann et al., 1994a	6	4	?	?	?
Freeman et al., 1995a	4	4	6.5–9	PUT (bilat)	***
Kopyov et al., 1996	22	18	6–10	9 C+P 3 C+P (bilat) 10 PUT (bilat)	<48hrs
UK group					
Henderson et al., 1991	12	3	12–19	CN	5–12hrs
Others					
Madrazo et al., 1990	4	4	12–14	CN	<4hrs
Peschanski et al., 1994	5	4	6–9	C+P	?
Subrt et al., 1991	3	3	?	CN	<3hrs
Zabek et al., 1994	3	3	11–12	CN	?
Molina et al., 1992, 1994	30	30	6–12	CN	45mins
	22	22	8–13	C+P	2.75hrs
Shabalov et al., 1994	4	0	6–9	CN or PUT	?
Lopez-Lozano et al., 1994	10	10	6–8 (8) 15 (2)	CN	?
Total	126	107			

* Unilateral unless otherwise stated with + symbol; ** Tissue was cryopreserved; *** Tissue was stored in hibernation medium prior to grafting.

CN, caudate nucleus; PUT, putamen; C+P, both caudate and putamen; bilat, bilateral; ? Not stated

TABLE 5.6
Details of 16 patients receiving foetal nigral grafts in Sweden

Patient	*Sex*	*Age*	*Diagnosis*	*Graft site 1*	*Graft site 2*
1	F	48	IPD	L CN/Put	–
2	F	55	IPD	R CN/Put	–
3	M	48	IPD	L Put	R Put
4	M	58	IPD	R Put	–
5	M	43	MPTP	R CN/Put	L CN/Put
6	F	30	MPTP	R CN/Put	L Put
7	M	49	IPD	L Put	R Put
8	M	43	IPD/MSA	L CN/Put	R CN/Put
9	M	52	?IPD	L Put	L Put
10	M	43	IPD	R CN/Put	L CN/Put
11	F	25	MPTP	L Put	R Put
12	M	54	IPD	L CN/Put	R CN/Put
13	M	48	IPD	R CN/Put	R CN/Put
14	M	42	IPD	R CN/Put	L CN/Put
15	M	54	IPD	R CN/Put	L CN/Put
16	M	68	IPD	R CN/Put	L CN/Put

IPD, idiopathic Parkinson's disease; MSA, multi-system atrophy; Put, putamen; CN, caudate nucleus

and the use of more physiological media for the dissection process, which was done more quickly (Brundin, 1992).

The next two patients with PD were then recruited and grafted again unilaterally with tissue from four embryos of 6–7 weeks gestational age. In these cases, however, the tissue was placed in the putamen, as this is the site of greatest DA loss in PD (Kish et al., 1988). This site has also been favoured by other centres, for example the group in South Florida (Freeman et al., 1995a). In contrast to their first two patients, the second series of patients from Sweden showed a significant beneficial response that was apparent from approximately 6 months after grafting. On these encouraging results, further series of patients were recruited and transplanted both in Sweden and elsewhere (see Table 5.5). There are now many well-documented cases in which there is clear improvement in clinical state combined with clear evidence of good graft. These have been assessed in several different ways:

Efficacy of L-dopa

The effects of grafts initially develop in the context of concurrent L-dopa treatment. Consequently, it is necessary to assess both the changes in the patients' responses to their drugs due to transplantation, and changes in function during defined periods of their drug therapy, most commonly first thing in the day before they have taken any medication. One of the most noticeable effects in

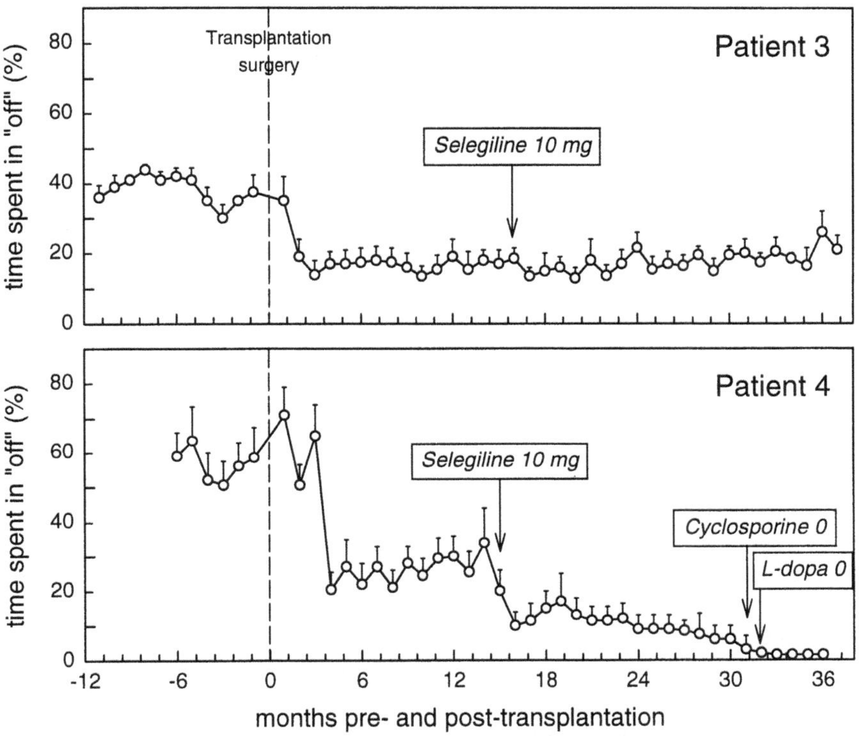

FIG. 5.8. Amount of time spent in the "off" state for two Parkinson's disease patients, numbers 3 and 4 from the Swedish series of grafted patients. Prior to operation, each patient was in an "off" state for approximately 50% of each waking day, even with optimal L-dopa therapy. Both patients showed a dramatic improvement in "on" time following transplantation, which was sustained even when other drug therapy was eventually removed, as in patient 4. (Redrawn from Lindvall et al., 1994, 1997, with permission © Lippincott, Williams & Wilkins.)

patients with effective transplants is an improvement in drug efficacy. Most patients are of course selected at a stage in the disease when they are suffering severe complications in pharmacotherapy, with prolonged periods in the "off" state and severe dyskinetic side effects when they are "on".

The improved response is illustrated in Fig. 5.8 for patient 4 in the Swedish series (Lindvall et al., 1994). This patient was in the "off" state for approximately 60% of each day pre-operatively, but this decreased to 30% by approximately 4 months after transplantation, and to 15% by 16 months. Indeed, from about 3 years after transplantation this patient was in the "on" state all the time, and there was with a progressive reduction and eventual elimination of the need for additional L-dopa therapy. Although this represents a "best case" scenario, many other patients have been seen to exhibit a substantial increase in "on" time during the day, frequently with a progressive reduction in the required doses of L-dopa. Most patients also exhibit a reduction in the major dyskinetic side effect of L-dopa therapy, although whether this is due directly to the grafts or indirectly to the fact that the grafts allow the patient to take lower doses of L-dopa to maintain an effective "on" state is not clear.

The effectiveness of L-dopa itself can be assessed using a single dose after a defined period when the patient has been drug-free, typically for 12 hours overnight. In this situation, the effect of a graft on the drug response can be precisely quantified, and in many patients the grafts not only prolong the duration of an individual "on" period but also reduce peak dose side effects (Lindvall et al., 1990, 1994), enabling a reduction in the frequency of drug taking during the day.

Neurological tests

The neurological deficits exhibited by parkinsonian patients are markedly affected by their drug therapy, and so in order to obtain meaningful data on their neurological status, tests need to be undertaken both in defined "off" (e.g. after overnight drug withdrawal) as well as during "on" states at defined times following L-dopa administration. A variety of neurological tests have been developed for testing the motor capacities of patients, ranging from a variety of simple motor tests, such as the time to complete defined sequences (e.g. walking test or finger tapping), to automated computerised tests of hand and foot tapping that the patients can undertake in their own homes (C.R. Freed et al., 1992).

The CAPIT protocol defines a series of defined movement tests that are now utilised by many centres. An example is where the time to undertake 20 pronation–supination movements of the arm is individually recorded for each hand in the "off" period and thereafter at regular intervals after taking L-dopa. Several studies have indicated a dramatic improvement in the speed with which PD patients can perform this test, in particular during the "off" state, following transplantation. This is illustrated for patient 3 in the Swedish series in Fig. 5.9 (Lindvall et al., 1994). A normal adult subject takes approximately 8 seconds to complete the 20 movements. Pre-operatively, the patient took about 14 seconds using his less affected left side, and about 25 seconds on the more affected right side. These scores were stable over 12 months of baseline testing. The patient then received a unilateral transplant in the right striatum contralateral to the more impaired side, following which the speed of responding returned to almost normal levels within 6 months after transplantation; and that improvement has been maintained since. In addition there was a modest improvement in the ipsilateral side, but not to the same extent; consequently, the performance is now faster on the previously more impaired but transplanted side.

Nigral grafts are capable of restoring performance deficits to normal on a variety of tasks during defined "off" periods, in particular the speed of walking and the speed and dexterity for using the hands. Rigidity is also markedly alleviated in many patients. Nevertheless, even in the best-recovered patients deficits remain. In particular, the tremor has been relatively unaffected in most

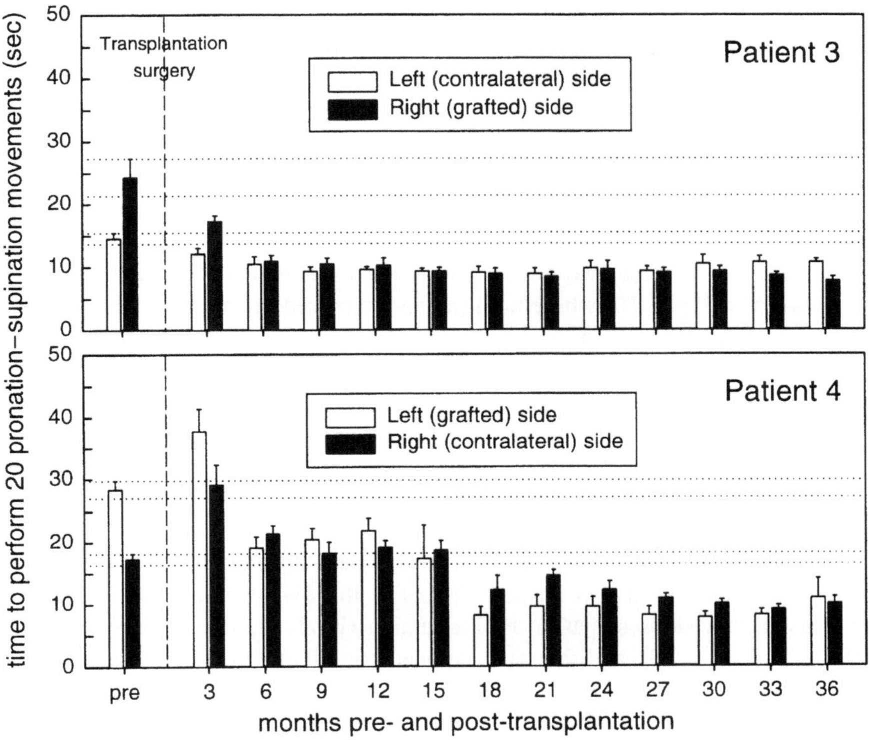

FIG. 5.9. Neurological testing in two patients receiving nigral grafts. The time taken to complete 20 pronation–supination movements is shown over 6 months before and up to 3 years after transplantation. (Redrawn from Lindvall et al., 1994, 1997, with permission © Lippincott, Williams & Wilkins.)

patients, and more axial motor functions such as balance and posture benefit less well than do more distal functions. In the Swedish series, improvement in the gait is only seen in those patients receiving grafts in the caudate nucleus, whereas no improvement was seen on this measure in patients receiving grafts in the putamen alone (Lindvall, 1997). Thus, as illustrated in the experimental studies, graft placement is likely to be critical not only in the extent but also in the profile of graft function.

Fluorodopa PET scans

The third widely used assessment that lies at the heart of most assessment batteries such as CAPIT is the use of *in vivo* scanning to detect graft placement, survival, and function. MRI (magnetic resonance imaging), which can provide the highest resolution of structural detail, is now a standard component in the stereotaxic implantation protocols in most centres (Palfi et al., 1998), and is useful not only for detecting graft placement and the tracks of graft injection but the survival of a graft as a circumscribed mass of tissue. However, MRI alone cannot provide information on the cellular composition or functionality of a graft, and for this purpose PET scans take precedence. Although they yield much lower spatial resolution, PET is at present the only method that can provide information on the neuronal composition and in particular the survival of dopaminergic neurones within the grafts *in vivo*. This information is critical if we are to be able to interpret rationally the functional changes in the patient's clinical picture.

Examples from the two patients we have discussed in the Swedish series are shown in Fig. 5.10, where both patients received unilateral implants in the putamen only. Whereas the fluorodopa uptake signal continues to decrease with the progression of the disease in the untransplanted caudate nuclei and the contralateral putamen, there is a dramatic and highly significant restitution of signal in the grafted putamen. In the case of patient 4, who was the only member of the series to have completely ceased L-dopa therapy at 32 months after implantation, the signal had by the same time point returned to be fully within the normal range for age-matched non-parkinsonian control subjects (Fig. 5.11). Although the degree and extent of this improvement has been different for each individual, after the first two patients all participants in the Swedish series have showed increased fluorodopa signal on PET scanning (Lindvall, 1997; Wenning et al., 1997; Widner, 1998), and this has also been seen in other centres (Hauser et al., 1998; Rémy et al., 1995).

The demonstration of surviving grafts in patients, where the time course, laterality, and magnitude of changes in the PET signal mirror changes in the neurological picture seen in the patient, gives credence to our interpretation that clinical efficacy is directly related to the survival and integration of nigral grafts and not just to non-specific consequences of surgery, placebo effects, and heightened expectation and optimism. This is further supported by the limited post-mortem studies in patients receiving foetal nigral grafts.

Post-mortem studies on human foetal dopamine grafts

One of the strongest pieces of evidence that the foetal tissue is working by providing a specific dopamine replacement in the host striatum comes from the correlation of clinical improvement with fluorodopa PET scanning results. This contention of graft survival and effect with dopaminergic re-innervation of the parkinsonian striatum has been further supported by the post-mortem studies of a limited number of patients who have died after receiving foetal nigral grafts. This is in marked contrast to the situation with AM grafts, where the post-mortem findings greatly undermined the rationale and validity of the approach.

The first reported post-mortem cases of patients dying with foetal nigral grafts were unhelpful, as the patients were not followed with fluorodopa PET

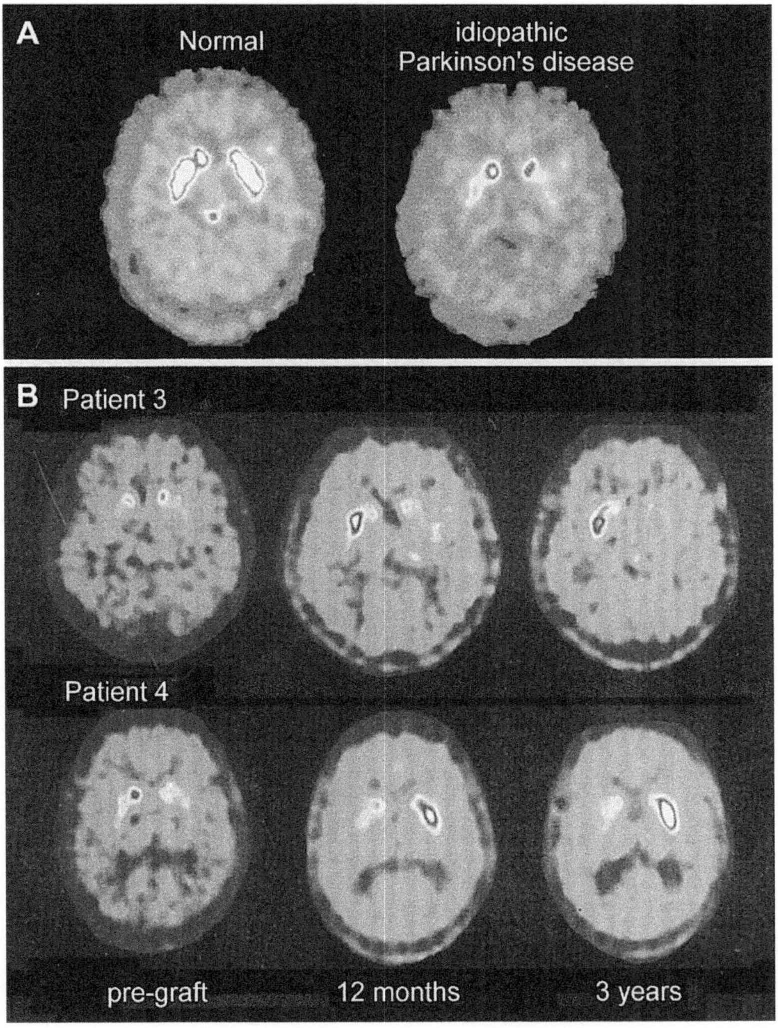

FIG. 5.10. PET scans of normal, Parkinson's disease, and transplanted brains, using [^{18}F]fluorodopa as the ligand to visualise the dopamine innervation of the striatum *in vivo*. (A) Reduced signal in the parkinsonian striatum in comparison to a normal control. (B) Surviving grafts seen in the left and right striata of patients 3 and 4 from the Swedish series, respectively. (Reproduced from Brooks et al., 1990, and Lindvall et al., 1994, with permission © Lippincott, Williams & Wilkins.)

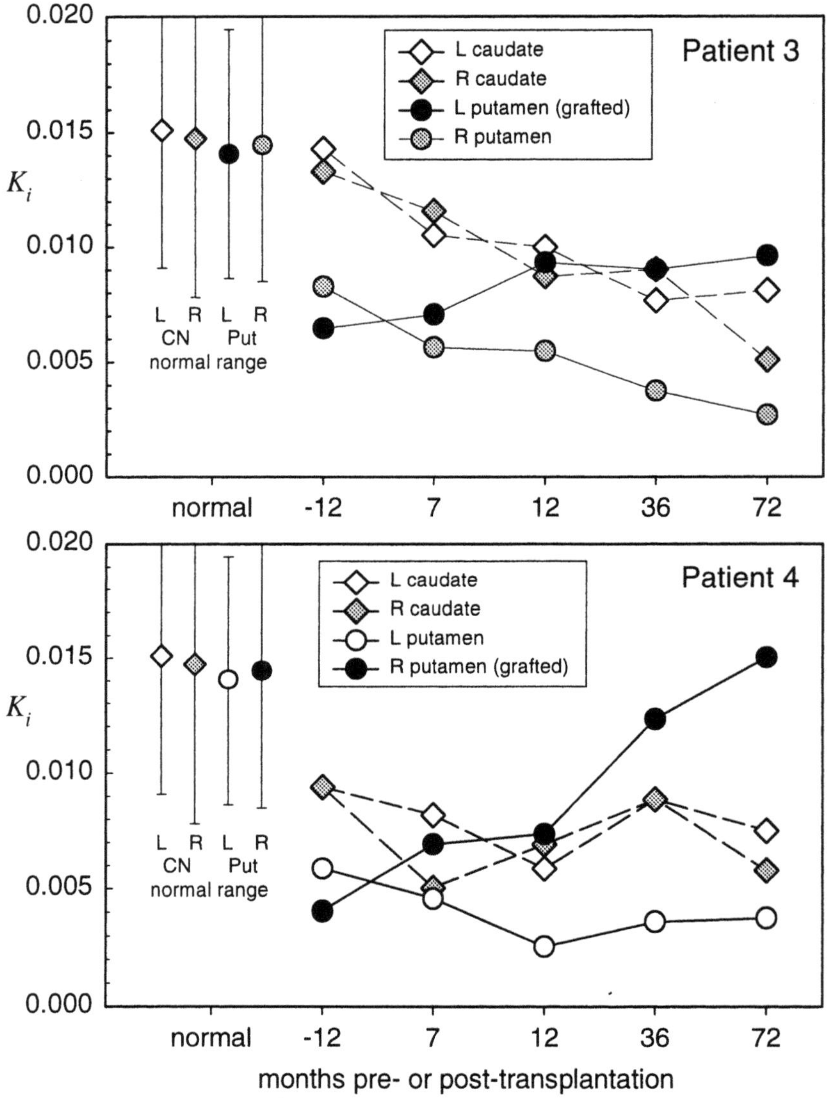

FIG. 5.11. Quantitative analysis of the fluorodopa binding in the sequential PET scans of two patients receiving nigral grafts. Note reversal of the binding constant into the normal range only in the grafted putamen, but a continuing decline with progression of the disease in other non-transplanted sites. (Data from Lindvall et al., 1994, with permission © Lippincott, Williams & Wilkins.)

scans and showed only minimal benefit from the procedure. The first of these post-mortem cases was in 1990 and failed to show any surviving dopaminergic cells within the graft, although neurones containing neuromelanin were identified along with synapse formation and some reactive glia and macrophages. No immune reaction was seen, which is of interest, as the patient's immunosuppression regime had had to be discontinued because of side effects. This patient was however unusual in that he had received cryopreserved tissue and turned out not to have PD but multi-system atrophy (MSA) (Redmond et al., 1990).

The second series of post-mortem cases were based on the patients operated on in the UK by Hitchcock's group and were again unhelpful, as no surviving grafted cells were found. However, the donor tissue was much older than that used in other centres, and this can readily explain the poor graft survival and the lack of any sustained clinical benefit in the patients (Hitchcock et al., 1990).

However, the most recent post-mortem studies from the American team based on a collaboration between South Florida and Chicago show healthy grafts with abundant cells and fibre outgrowth into the host striatum (see Fig. 5.12). Both patients, unlike those who had previously come to post mortem, had derived significant benefit from the grafts, and this correlated with an increase in fluorodopa uptake in the putamen on PET scanning (Kordower, 1998; Kordower et al., 1995). Their deaths were unrelated to the transplantation procedure, and occurred 18–19 months after they had received their grafts.

These latter cases therefore clearly demonstrate that embryonic ventral mesencephalon grafts can survive in the human parkinsonian brain, extend processes, and provide extensive dopaminergic innervation of the striatum. This is in agreement with the experimental findings for rat and monkey allografts, and supports the hypothesis that these grafts work by a comparable mechanisms in animals and man. As outlined in Chapter Four, the experimental evidence suggests that specific dopaminergic innervation in the striatum is central to graft function.

Factors critical for graft function

In spite of good recovery on many measures, all of the patients remain parkinsonian, even years after receiving a successful transplant (Lindvall, 1997). In the third group of patients from the Lund series, several cases merit particular mention, either because of the special nature of the PD disease (due to MPTP in patients 5, 6, and 11, see Table 5.5) or because they have shown a rather poor response to transplantation (patients 8 and 9).

The three cases of transplantation in MPTP-induced PD are particularly interesting (Widner, 1998; Widner et al., 1992), not only in their own right, but also because they allow us to address the issue of whether the progressive nature of idiopathic Parkinson's disease may be detrimental to the long-term survival of the grafts. The disease in these young addicts was induced acutely by ingestion

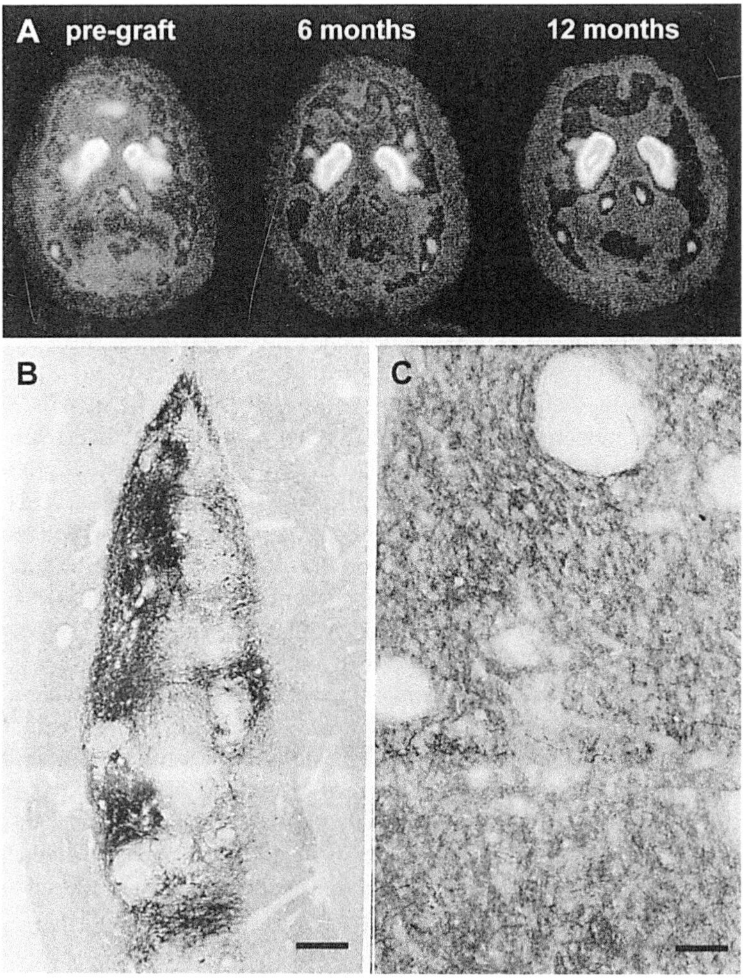

FIG. 5.12. Histology from the post-mortem of a patient receiving a nigral graft who died 18 months after transplantation. (A) Pre- and post-operative PET scans showing bilateral surviving grafts while the patient was alive. (B,C) Tyrosine hydroxylase staining of a surviving graft (B) and its innervation of the host striatum (C) in the post-mortem brain. (Reproduced from Kordower et al., 1995, with permission © Lippincott, Williams & Wilkins.)

of the toxin MPTP, which, whilst remaining only transiently in the body, nevertheless causes massive cell death that is permanent, non-progressive and relatively specific to the dopaminergic system. These patients should therefore represent the closest correlate to the animal models in which the transplantation methodology was developed, and by so doing should derive the greatest benefit from the transplant procedure. Indeed, all three patients have shown good graft survival in PET and sustained recovery of symptomatic performance on a wide range of tests, including improved speed of movement, reduced rigidity, and improved "off" performance (Widner, 1998), as in the idiopathic patients described above. So far, the recovery in the successful idiopathic patients, which is now approaching 10 years after the initial transplantations, appears rather comparable in time course and efficacy to that seen in the three MPTP patients. In particular, there is no sign of a selective downturn in the benefit provided after long-term survival in the former group, suggesting that the fears about grafts being able to survive and function in an environment of progressive neurodegenerative disease in idiopathic PD were unfounded.

In the remaining patients with parkinsonism, the first two patients had grafts that survived poorly as a consequence of a sub-optimal implantation technique (see previously). There have been two other cases in which the functional recovery was also less good than in other patients in the series. Patient number 8, whilst reporting some initial benefit, deteriorated 3 months after grafting. Moreover, the rate of progression of the disease coupled to the development of new symptoms in this patient raised the question as to whether he may represent a case of MSA rather than idiopathic Parkinson's disease. MSA is a disorder in which there is degeneration in a number of CNS sites, including the substantia nigra and striatum. It runs a more aggressive clinical course than PD, and because the pathological process involves the striatum, the patients show a non-sustained response to L-dopa therapy (Wenning et al., 1994). MSA can be very difficult to distinguish from PD, especially in the early stages of the disease when the L-dopa response is most apparent, and indeed one patient from the USA who died having received an ineffectual nigral graft was also found to have this condition (Redmond et al., 1990—see above). Moreover, although patient 8 has failed to show any sustained clinical improvement following grafting, his PET scans show clear evidence of good graft survival. Therefore his failure to improve is not simply a consequence of a graft that has failed to survive.

The second case deserving specific mention is patient number 9. In this case the patient developed a dementing illness that made assessment impossible. The patient eventually died from an intracerebral haemorrhage but, unfortunately, the brain was not retrieved for histological analysis. In this case the question as to whether the patient had Parkinson's disease with dementia or some other parkinsonian syndrome is therefore unresolved. However his PET scans did reveal a functioning graft.

Both these cases highlight some of the difficulties in clinical trials of this nature, namely the difficulty in being certain of the diagnosis (in contrast for example to Huntington's disease, where the diagnosis can be made with certainty) and the problems of long-term follow-up and assessment.

The major limitation on the progress in these studies is the relatively poor yield of dopamine cells in nigral grafts, requiring multiple foetal donors per recipient in all effective transplantation series (Olanow et al., 1996). In the fourth group of patients in the Swedish series, therefore, following successful demonstration of the efficacy of antioxidant treatment of experimental graft tissues in rats (see Chapter Four), lazaroid pre-treatment of the graft tissues has been introduced into the clinical series also. At this stage it is too early to say whether the use of lazaroids will make a substantial difference to the success of foetal transplants in either their clinical expression or ability to increase the yield of dopamine cells per foetus. Indeed, this reliance on large amounts of foetal tissue is still a major problem in the future adoption of this technique as a routine procedure.

A second fundamental technical issue that remains unresolved relates to the role of immunosuppression. Several of the patients treated in Sweden have developed complications as a result of this therapy. Freed and colleagues in Colorado, USA, have attempted to address this question empirically by giving alternate patients immunosuppression to compare the functional efficacy between those receiving it and those not (C.R. Freed et al., 1990, 1992). They report that all patients show improvement following transplantation, irrespective of whether or not they are immunosuppressed. However, it is difficult to draw any strong conclusion from this study of any clinical effect of the graft, since they are only implanting foetal tissue from a single 7–8-week-old ventral mesencephalon into each patient, and most of the patients have not received sequential PET scans. In the one patient who did receive scans before and after transplantation there was a significant increase in fluorodopa uptake bilaterally in the putamen at 3 but not 9 months after grafting, suggesting a lower yield of dopaminergic tissues in the grafts than is achieved in centres using multiple donors.

The successful use of foetal transplants in PD has now been shown by a number of other groups, most notably those based at Florida, USA, and Paris, France. The group in Florida have recently published their 12–24 month follow-up results on six patients with PD who received grafts of embryonic nigral neurones from donors aged 6.5–9 weeks post-conception implanted specifically into the post-commissural putamen as the area directly involved in mediating corticostriatal motor functions (Freeman et al., 1995a; Hauser et al., 1998). All patients improved following transplantation on a series of neurological tests, and the clinical improvement was matched by increased striatal fluorodopa uptake. Several patients experienced minor peri-operative complications, and two have subsequently died for reasons unrelated to transplantation surgery (see post-mortem results, already discussed). Similar results have been published by the French group (Peschanski et al., 1994; Rémy et al., 1995).

A dozen or more other groups around the world have now undertaken transplants in PD with foetal tissue (see Table 5.5), although the documentation of the procedure is often inadequate and consequently any conclusions of benefit uncertain. As emphasised in the introduction to this section, standardised test and assessment batteries are now available and well described (e.g. CAPIT-PD—see Chapter One), and there is no good reason why all patients entering into a clinical transplant programme should not be properly assessed. Only by providing such data will it be possible to evaluate the efficacy of any particular procedure or centre, and provide a standard for comparison of alternative treatments between centres. Sadly, many centres still fail to sign up to this approach, which not only makes their own data extremely hard to interpret, but also compromises the development of the field.

Conclusions from clinical trials on embryonic nigral transplants in humans

It is clear that patients with PD can improve with grafts of foetal nigral tissue and that this improvement can be correlated with increased dopaminergic activity in the striatum as evidenced by fluorodopa uptake on PET scanning. Therefore, in contrast to AM grafts, foetal nigral grafts almost certainly work by restoration of dopaminergic activity within the striatum as a consequence of graft-derived dopaminergic re-innervation. Although the target site for implantation is important, especially as in PD the dopamine deficiency is greatest in the putamen (Kish et al., 1988), the preparation of the tissue and the age of the donor are also critical in the success of the graft. In this respect Freeman et al. have demonstrated that the optimal ages for human nigral suspension and solid grafts range from post-ovulatory day 37 to 56, and 65 days, respectively (Freeman et al., 1991, 1995b). Therefore, groups that use embryos of gestational age greater than 9 weeks are already working with sub-optimal tissue. This tissue may then be further compromised by either a delay from the time of abortion to implantation and/or the preparation of the tissue prior to grafting, for example by cryopreservation.

The role of immunosuppression in patients receiving grafts of embryonic nigral tissue is currently unresolved (Widner & Brundin, 1988). Those groups who have generally not used such treatment have had disappointing results, which may however be more a reflection of the age of donor tissue and the site of implantation than of any rejection process.

SUMMARY

Under appropriate conditions, human foetal nigral grafts can produce substantial improvements in patients with PD, especially if young embryos (6–8 weeks gestation) are bilaterally grafted into both the caudate nucleus and putamen. The results world-wide, though, are very variable, which reflects a non-uniformity of transplantation technique and assessment despite the recommendation that all centres use the CAPIT-PD protocol. Furthermore, the technique of bilateral grafts to the caudate and putamen requires the use of at least 6–12 foetuses (Widner et al., 1992), which clearly is a major practical limitation on the widespread adoption of this technique irrespective of the major immunological and ethical problems with it (Calne & McGeer, 1988; Garry et al., 1992; Hoffer &

Olson, 1991). These issues highlight the pressing need for the identification of techniques either to expand the limited tissue that is currently available or to provide alternative more widely available tissue. These are issues that will be explored further in Chapter Nine.

CHAPTER SIX

Striatal grafts: Circuit reconstruction and Huntington's disease

INTRODUCTION

The detailed discussion of grafting neural tissues in parkinsonian animals and patients has yielded two main conclusions:

(1) Dopamine-rich grafts in the striatum can restore many, but not all, of the symptoms arising from forebrain dopamine depletion in animals and man.
(2) Neural grafts can work by a number of different mechanisms of action.

It has therefore been hypothesised that one of the main reasons for this inability of grafts to restore all functional deficits is that when placed in an ectopic site, they are not in a position to reconstruct the damaged circuitry of the striatum. This interpretation has gained weight through the study of a related model system: implantation of embryonic striatal tissue into the striatum. It has turned out that these striatal grafts have a greater capacity to reconstruct damaged striatal circuits than do nigral grafts, which is accompanied by a correspondingly broader spectrum of functional recovery. Moreover, in addition to their theoretical interest, striatal grafts have recently attracted considerable clinical attention because degeneration of intrinsic cells of the striatum is the primary pathology in Huntington's disease. This inherited neurodegenerative disorder is the second main neurological disease to be addressed in transplantation trials, although these are still in their early stages at the time of writing.

HUNTINGTON'S DISEASE (HD)

Huntington's disease (HD) is the commonest neurological disease with a simple (autosomal dominant) pattern of inheritance, affecting approximately 1:10,000 individuals in the UK. An excellent account of the disease can be found in Peter Harper's major review (1996). The disease typically first becomes apparent in middle age, often after the affected gene has been passed on to the patient's children, and progresses over a number of years to a profoundly debilitating form of "subcortical" dementia and movement disorder.

Until recently, neurologists and neuropsychologists paid closest attention to the motor symptoms of the disease, as indeed did George Huntington in his initial description of this chorea. However, whereas these overt dyskinetic symptoms may be characteristic, they are by no means always present throughout the disease or in all patients. In fact, the symptoms typically fall into three main classes, of which the motor may be the least debilitating for the patients and their families.

Motor. Uncontrollable abnormal movements ("dyskinesia", including chorea) may predominate early in the disease, but a poverty and inability to initiate movement (similar to hypokinesia or parkinsonism) is more apparent in advanced disease.

Cognitive. Patients can manifest profound intellectual impairments, in particular in tests of the "frontal" type involving the ability to plan and select appropriate patterns of goal-directed action. For example, HD patients have pronounced deficits on the classical test of prefrontal cortical function, the Wisconsin card sorting test, and more modern automated equivalents. The cognitive deficits in HD have been characterised as a form of "subcortical dementia" similar to that seen in a variety of diseases of subcortical origin such as Parkinson's disease and supranuclear palsy, and distinct from the more mnemonic deficits of supposed cortical origin characteristic of Alzheimer's disease and multi-infarct dementia (Filoteo et al., 1995; Lange et al., 1995).

Psychiatric. Although not so obvious, perhaps the most debilitating symptoms for many patients and their families are the personality and emotional changes associated with the disease, with depression, mania, and suicide all being common early features of the disease that persist throughout the illness.

Post-mortem analyses of the HD brain reveal widespread neuronal loss, the extent of which is dependent on the severity and chronicity of the condition. Although observable pathology in early and middle stages of the disease is restricted to the caudate nucleus and putamen, in advanced stages of the disease neuronal loss and atrophy spreads throughout the brain, to produce widespread degeneration in the neocortex and in other nuclei of the basal ganglia and brainstem. It remains unclear to what extent all the primary symptoms can be explained by the striatal pathology and the contribution of dysfunction in extrastriatal systems. Moreover, the extent to which the cortical pathology is a secondary retrograde consequence of degeneration in subcortical striatal targets rather than an independent process of cell death in the disease is also unclear. Both of these issues will influence the extent to which any strategy of therapy based on targeting the striatum for repair can be effective.

At the macroscopic level, the lateral ventricles become enlarged as the striatum degenerates, and this can be easily detected in brain scans such as magnetic resonance imaging (MRI) (see Fig. 6.1A,B). The two main nuclei of the neostriatum—the caudate and the putamen—both show progressive shrinkage and atrophy as the disease progresses, although of the two the caudate nucleus is affected earlier and to a greater extent than the putamen. The progression of shrinkage has been categorised into a series of stages, graded from 0 to 4, by Vonsattel et al. (1985), which provides a system that is very widely used for descriptive and neuropathological staging of the disease (see Fig. 6.1C).

At the microscopic level, the greatest cell loss is of the "medium spiny" population of neurones, which constitute the major input and output neurones of the striatum, and which use the inhibitory amino acid γ-amino butyric acid (GABA) as their primary neurotransmitter. By contrast, the interneurones of the striatum, characterised by larger spiny and aspiny morphology, and using somatostatin, neuropeptide Y, and other peptide neurotransmitters are less affected by the disease.

Our potential for understanding the cellular and molecular basis of HD changed dramatically in 1993, with the identification of the gene for the disease. The huntingtin gene includes a region at its tail end in which the triplet of DNA nucleotides (CAG) that codes for the amino acid glutamine is repeated approximately 20 times in normal individuals. By contrast in HD patients this repeat undergoes a 2–3-fold expansion to 40–60 copies on one gene (Huntington's Disease Collaborative Research Group, 1993). Little is yet known of the normal function of the huntingtin gene, nor of the mechanism whereby the faulty huntingtin gene (which carries an expanded CAG trinucleotide repeat) leads to selective degeneration of neurones in the basal ganglia even though it is expressed ubiquitously both within and outside the brain.

However, what the gene does provide is a reliable basis for diagnosis of HD in affected individuals, which allows for the inclusion of definitely affected individuals within experimental and clinical trials even at a presymptomatic stage of the disease. Moreover, the recent identification of aggregations of the cleaved peptide as distinctive intranuclear inclusions, in both the human disease and transgenic mice expressing the expanded CAG repeat fragment of the huntingtin gene (S.W. Davies et al., 1997; DiFiglia et al., 1997), provides new clues to the pathogenic mechanism underlying this disorder.

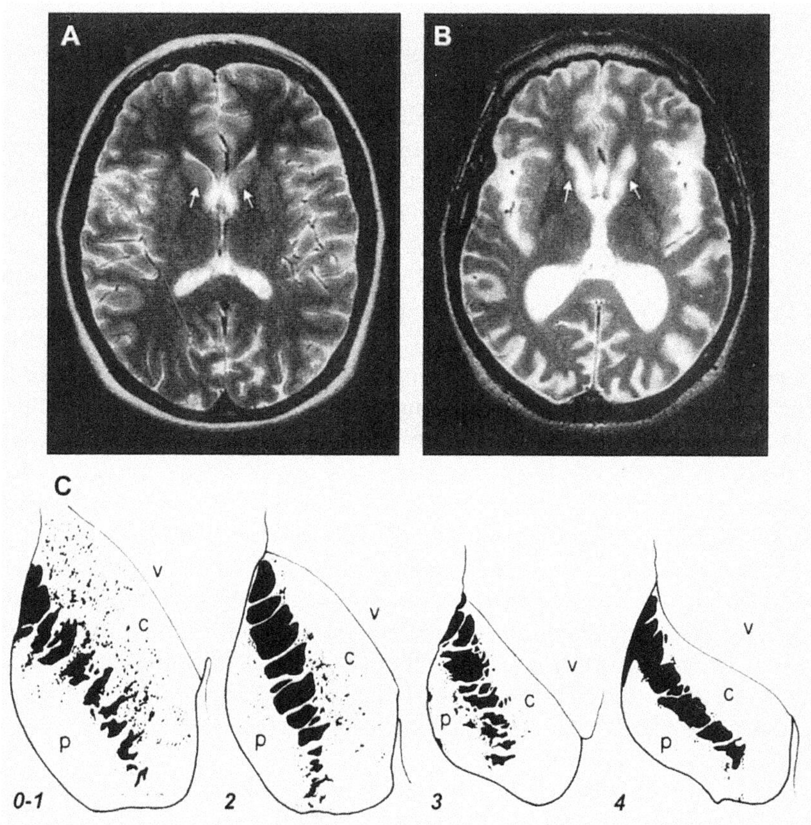

FIG. 6.1. Post-mortem neuropathology in Huntington's disease. (A) MRI of normal brain. (B) MRI scan of a patient with Huntington's disease. Note enlargement of the lateral ventricles and massive atrophy of the basal ganglia, in particular the caudate nucleus (arrows). (C) The neuropathological grading of striatal atrophy in Huntington's disease as defined by Vonsattel et al., 1985, from absent (stage 0) to maximum (stage 4). c, caudate nucleus, p, putamen, v, lateral ventricle. (Reproduced from Harper, 1996, with permission © WB Saunders.)

ANIMAL MODELS OF HD

Striatal lesions

Experimental lesions of the striatum in animals produce both cognitive and motor deficits akin to those seen in humans. However, until the past 20 years, research on the functions of this area of the brain progressed only slowly, owing to inadequate experimental techniques. In particular, when the only tools available were ablation or lesions via electrolytic, radiofrequency, or cryogenic probes, it was never possible to separate the effects of damage of the striatum itself from the effects of damage to fibres traversing these structures. For example, afferent and efferent pathways between the cortex and thalamus pass between and through the caudate and putamen nuclei of the neostriatum. Since cortical and thalamic damage produce well-characterised impairments in both the cognitive and motor realms, the attribution of any effects of such lesions to the neostriatum was always suspect (Laursen, 1963).

The turning point for psychobiological studies of the neostriatum came with the introduction of the excitotoxins as a technique for making specific striatal lesions while sparing axons of passage. The "excitotoxins" are a class of naturally occurring toxins that are glutamate receptor agonists, and include the compounds N-methyl-D-aspartic acid (NMDA), kainic acid, ibotenic acid and quinolinic acid. When administered into the brain above a certain concentration, excitotoxins bind to the glutamate receptors on neurones and induce a massive and prolonged excitation of those cells, leading to depolarisation, membrane collapse, and cell death.

Excitotoxins have several useful features.

(1) Glutamate is the predominant excitatory transmitter of the brain. Most neurones carry glutamate receptors, and so excitotoxins are effective toxins for most neurones. Glia do not carry many glutamate receptors, and are relatively unaffected by most excitotoxins.
(2) Glutamate receptors are predominantly located on cell bodies and dendrites. They are not found on the main shafts of axons, so that excitotoxic lesions in the brain destroy neurones at the site of injection but spare axons of passage.
(3) There are several different subclasses of glutamate receptors, each with differential sensitivity to the different excitotoxins. Since populations of neurones differ in the subclasses of glutamate receptors they carry, judicious selection of an excitotoxin can often provide lesions that are relatively selective to a subset of the neurones in an area.

In 1976, Coyle and Schwarcz first used kainic acid to make neurone-selective lesions of the neostriatum. They found that the injections resulted in a marked atrophy of the striatum viewed in histological sections, and a greater than 90% loss of the enzymes glutamic acid decarboxylase (GAD) and choline acetyl transferase (ChAT) which are convenient biochemical markers for GABA and cholinergic neurones in the striatum. At the same time, they confirmed that the myelinated axons of the corticothalamic pathways were spared by these lesions. In this first study, the authors noted the similarity of the changes in the lesioned striatum in rats to the histological and biochemical changes seen in HD, and explicitly proposed intrastriatal injections of kainic acid as an animal model of HD. In a follow-up study, Mason and Fibiger (1979) went on to show that bilateral kainic acid lesions produced locomotor hyperactivity in rats, which was considered to be equivalent to chorea in humans.

In subsequent years, these initial observations have been confirmed and developed in a number of important ways.

First, kainic acid has some marked side effects: It induces seizures that result in secondary degeneration in remote areas of the brain. Thus, after its injection into the striatum, remote damage has been reported in the piriform cortex, hippocampus, and amygdala. Although one way to overcome this problem is to suppress seizure activity with benzodiazepines (e.g. diazepam, Valium), an alternative and easier solution is to use other excitotoxins that are less epileptogenic. Therefore since the early 1980s ibotenic acid has been the excitotoxin of preference in the striatum for just this reason.

Second, both kainic acid and ibotenic acid are relatively non-selective, destroying all neuronal types in the striatum with equal facility. Recently, it has been proposed that quinolinic acid, which works at a different class of glutamate receptor, can produce a more selective lesion in the striatum, killing the GABA medium spiny neurones but sparing the neuropeptide Y (NPY) and somatostatin interneurones, reproducing the selective pattern of degeneration in HD itself. Quinolinic acid is less toxic than ibotenic acid, but also diffuses less well, so typically a focal quinolinic acid lesion involves several concentric zones of differing degrees of damage. At the site of the injection there is often non-specific damage and necrosis surrounded by a zone of total neuronal cell loss, around which lies a zone of relatively selective cell loss, and intact striatal tissue beyond that. If the purpose of an experiment is to study cellular degeneration at a microscopic level, then quinolinic acid can indeed reproduce circumscribed zones of damage in the striatum that mimic relatively well those seen in HD. However, if more extensive lesions throughout the striatum are required (either unilaterally or bilaterally), such as are needed to study the functional consequences of the lesions (and functional effects or anatomical connectivity of striatal grafts), then ibotenic acid remains the more reliable experimental option.

Third, the excitotoxins reproduce many aspects of the anatomical and biochemical pathology but do not mimic the pathogenic process of cell death in the human disease. There is accumulating evidence that the striatal degeneration in HD is associated with major impairments in mitochondrial function and cellular energy metabolism. There are now a number of "metabolic" toxins, including malonic acid and 3-nitroproprionic acid (3-NP), that reproduce the mitochondrial dysfunction and induce patterns of selective striatal degeneration akin to that seen in HD (Beal et al., 1993b). Daily dosing with 3-NP results in a major reduction in neuronal metabolism throughout the brain (as measured by a decline in succinate dehydrogenase activity) but a selective profile of neuronal degeneration that is restricted to the striatum (Beal et al., 1993a; Palfi et al., 1996). The reasons for this selective targeting of striatal neurones by these mitochondrial toxins are still poorly understood, but may be expected to yield new insights about the targeting of striatal pathology in HD. In the meantime, however, although 3-NP and related compounds may provide a better model of the pathogenesis of the human disease, the dosing regimes are more variable and unreliable than the conventional excitotoxins, making them less suitable as models for functional studies of strategies for repair.

Finally, the functional effects of the lesions have been analysed in considerably more detail since the early studies by Mason and colleagues, although our knowledge of this system still falls far short of that for damage to the nigrostriatal dopamine system (see Chapters Four and Five). Since our interpretation of the functional effects of striatal grafts is critically dependent upon our understanding of the functional organisation of the neostriatum itself, an overview of these more recent functional studies and the principles that have emerged requires a separate section in its own right.

Functional organisation of the neostriatum

Using excitotoxins to make selective lesions within the brain reveals that damage of intrinsic striatal neurones can produce motor, cognitive, and motivational impairments akin to all main classes of symptoms manifested by HD patients.

Cognitive. Bilateral excitotoxic lesions of the neostriatum in rats produce deficits in a range of cognitive tasks, including tests of maze learning, spatial navigation, delayed response, and temporal sequencing of behaviours in operant paradigms.

Motor. The deficits induced by striatal lesions include locomotor hyperactivity, disruption of performance of skilled motor tasks, impaired reaction times, and aspects of sensorimotor inattention and neglect. More detailed analyses have suggested that the impairment is one of selection and initiation of voluntary or goal-directed behaviours rather than an inability to execute particular movements *per se*.

Motivation. Although psychiatric deficits are more difficult to evaluate in animals, rats with striatal lesions exhibit impairments in the motivational control of behaviour. For example, striatal lesions disrupt the rats' ability to detect and adapt their response to changes in the value of reward, and change their reactivity to aversive stimuli.

From the specific studies of the effects of striatal lesions in rats and monkeys, some general principles arise.

Many of the deficits observed after striatal lesions are similar to those that have been described after damage in the cortex. Thus lesions in the head of the caudate in rats and monkeys produce deficits in a range of cognitive tasks (such as delayed response and spatial alternation) that were first described in the context of damage in the prefrontal cortex. Rosvold first recognised that since the caudate nucleus is a major output projection of the prefrontal cortex, the similarity of deficits following lesions in each of these areas suggests that they form part of a distinct "prefrontal system" (Rosvold, 1972; Rosvold & Delgado, 1956; Rosvold & Szwarcbart, 1964; Divac et al., 1967). Lesions within the caudate nucleus disrupt the major neo-cortical outflows, and are typical of what Geschwind (1965a,b) has termed a "disconnection" syndrome, in which cortical plans of action are separated from the downstream motor systems necessary for their execution.

In fact, it turns out that a substantial degree of topography is maintained in each projection within Rosvold's system. In the same way that the neocortical mantle is heterogeneous, with distinctive architectonic areas having different functions, so also for the related subcortical structures of the thalamus and neostriatum, which are inter-linked to the cortex in the form of corticostriatal loops, each of which has a distinctive function (Fig. 6.2; Alexander et al., 1986, 1990). The main development since Rosvold's original conception of this topographical organisation is one of extent. Corticostriatal loops apply throughout the whole neocortical mantle (all association and motor areas rather than prefrontal cortex alone) as well as the complete striatum (putamen and ventral striatum as well as caudate nucleus), and to all aspects of neocortical/striatal function (including motor and sensorimotor as well as purely cognitive).

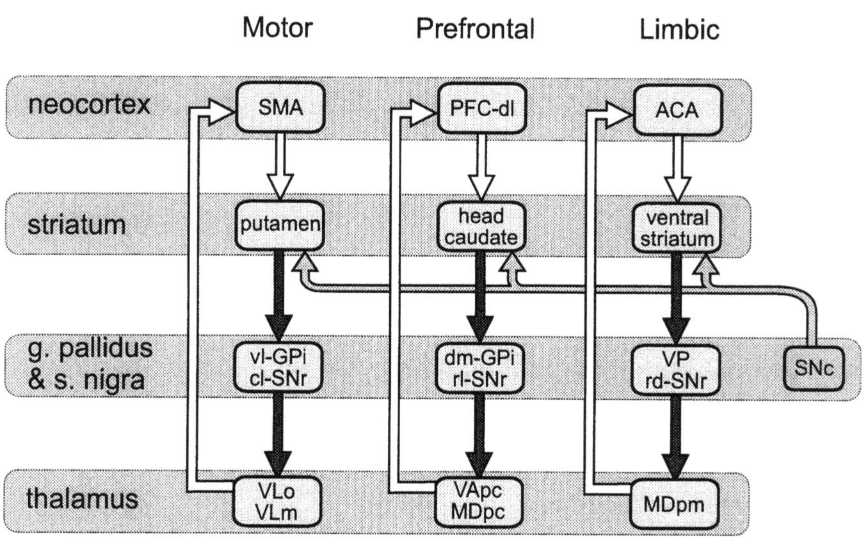

FIG. 6.2. Parallel cortical–subcortical loops through the basal ganglia. Abbreviations indicate anatomical subdivisions of each nucleus: ACA, anterior cingulate area of cortex; GP, globus pallidus, PFC, prefrontal cortex; SMA, sensory motor area of cortex, SNr, substantia nigra pars reticulata; VP, ventral pallidum. (Based on Alexander et al., 1986, 1990; for further details, see Dunnett & Everitt, 1998.)

STRIATAL GRAFTS IN EXPERIMENTAL RATS

The techniques of transplanting striatal cells into the excitotoxically lesioned neostriatum are essentially identical to those already described for grafting embryonic dopamine cells, and the same principles apply. Because of its deep site, most studies have used stereotaxic injection of dissociated cell suspensions rather than any of the various solid graft techniques. To be effective, the grafted tissue needs to be taken from the developing embryo at a gestational age of E14–E16 days in rats, at which stage the developing cells of the neostriatum are differentiating and migrating from the overlying germinal cell layer of the "ganglionic eminence" in the floor of the lateral ventricles. In contrast to the relatively poor survival that has characterised studies of nigral grafts, striatal grafts survive well, and typically only a single deposit from one striatal primordium is required per grafted animal. On subsequent histological analysis, the grafts are seen to undergo extensive growth to form a "mini-striatum" containing all major cell types and biochemical markers of the normal striatum in a patchy, rather than homogeneous, arrangement (Fig. 6.3).

The anatomy and biochemistry of these grafts will be described in more detail later. However, first let us consider the consequences of such grafts on the

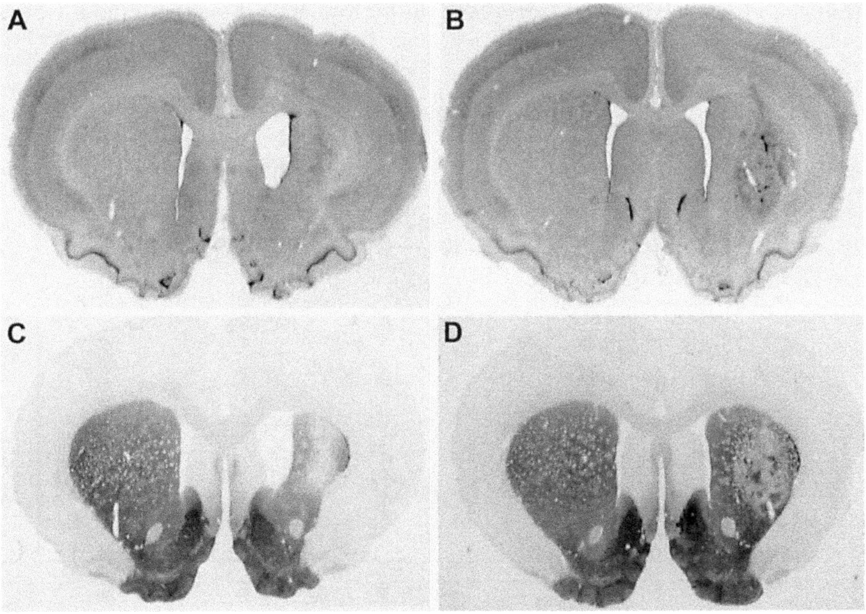

FIG. 6.3. Photomicrographs of the histological appearance of a striatal graft in the ibotenic acid lesioned rat striatum. Sections indicate brain sections of a rat with unilateral lesion of the right striatum (A,C) and a rat with an additional striatal graft (B,D), visualised with a general cresyl violet stain of cell bodies (A,B) and an acetylcholinesterase stain to highlight the striatal neuropil (C,D). (Original sections courtesy of Rose Fricker.)

behavioural deficits induced by experimental striatal lesions, because those data provide a functional framework for the levels of repair that have to be explained.

Functional studies of striatal grafts

Locomotor hyperactivity. The first functional studies of striatal grafts revealed that they are capable of reversing the hyperactivity seen with striatal lesions back down to control levels (Deckel et al., 1983; Isacson et al., 1984). In a subsequent study this effect of the grafts was found to be most marked during the night-time period when normal activity and lesion-induced hyperactivity both reach their heights (Isacson et al., 1986). Moreover, this latter study showed that the grafts were only effective if placed homotopically into the striatum and not when placed ectopically into the globus pallidus, suggesting that afferent connectivity of the grafts rather than simply re-innervation of their target may be important in their functional effects.

Delayed alternation. In that same study, Isacson et al. (1986) not only looked at locomotor activity, but also at the animals' ability to learn a delayed spatial alternation task in a raised T-maze. As shown in Fig. 6.4, striatal lesions totally abolished the ability to learn the alternation task and all animals of the lesioned group stayed at a chance level of performance throughout the 8 weeks

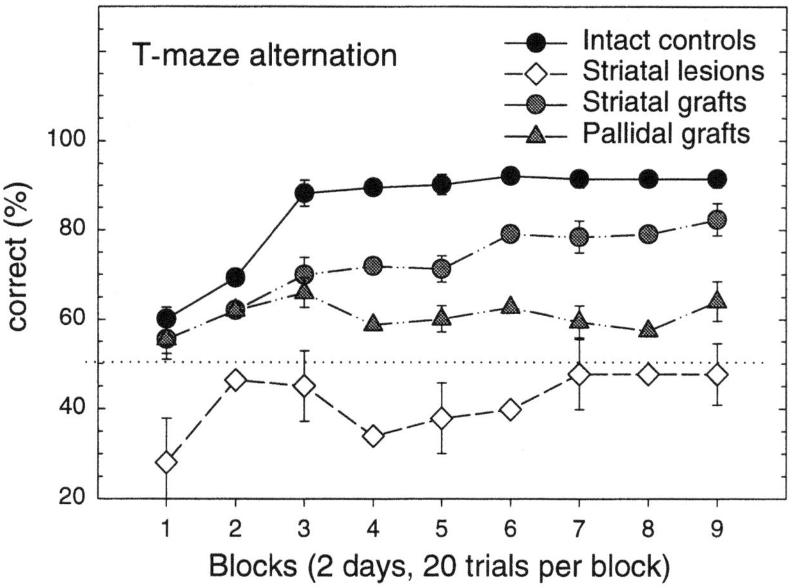

FIG. 6.4. Striatal grafts alleviate the deficits of rats with bilateral striatal lesions in a T-maze delayed alternation task. To be maximally effective the grafts of striatal tissue must be placed homotopically in the striatum ("striatal grafts"), rather than ectopically into the target areas of the globus pallidus ("pallidal grafts"). (Data from Isacson et al., 1986.)

of training. The animals with striatal grafts showed a substantial improvement, and although they were slower to learn than the intact controls, all but two of them reached an asymptotic level of performance above the 90% criterion by the end of testing. Again, although the group with striatal grafts implanted in the globus pallidus showed a small improvement they did not differ as a group from the lesion-alone control group, and no animals in the group with ectopic grafts reached criterion.

Rotation. Bilateral lesions in the neostriatum induce a hyperactivity syndrome, whilst the motor asymmetry induced by unilateral lesions can lead to rotation when the animal is activated, as by pharmacological challenges with apomorphine and amphetamine (see Chapter Four). Striatal grafts can reverse both amphetamine- and apomorphine-induced rotation in striatally lesioned rats (Dunnett et al., 1988c), although the pattern of reversal is different to that seen in rats with nigrostriatal lesions.

Since excitotoxic lesions of the striatum remove postsynaptic neurones of the nigrostriatal dopamine projection on the lesioned side, there can be no postsynaptic receptor supersensitivity. Thus in striatal-lesioned rats, rotation can be induced by apomorphine only at doses (0.5–1.0mg/kg) that act on normal receptors. Moreover, in contrast to the contralateral rotation seen in dopamine-depleted rats, apomorphine-rotation in rats with striatal lesions is in the ipsilateral direction, in agreement with preferential drug-induced activation of striatal outputs on the intact but not the lesioned side. The demonstration that striatal grafts can reverse apomorphine rotation, along with the demonstration from receptor binding studies (see later) that neurones in striatal grafts carry functional dopamine receptors, suggests that the grafts are able to restore balance between the output pathways on the two sides of the brain.

The loss of intrinsic neurones with striatal lesions and the corresponding asymmetry of functional outputs means that rats with striatal lesions will rotate in the same direction with the same dose of amphetamine challenge as is seen in the nigrostriatal-lesioned rat. Amphetamine does not act directly on striatal neurones but indirectly, by stimulating dopamine release from dopamine nerve terminals in the striatum, which then produces its effect through postsynaptic (i.e. striatal) dopamine receptor activation. Moreover, host dopamine fibres do grow into striatal grafts to make contact with the striatal output neurones (see later) and by so doing promote recovery of amphetamine-induced rotation. This suggests that the host dopaminergic inputs to the striatal grafts are functional and can interact with the graft regulation of striatal outputs so as to restore balance between the two sides.

Although rotation is a rather artificial behavioural test, these observations provided the first clear suggestion that information could be relayed from host via the graft back to the host; i.e. there was a functional incorporation of the grafted neurones into the neural circuitry of the host brain.

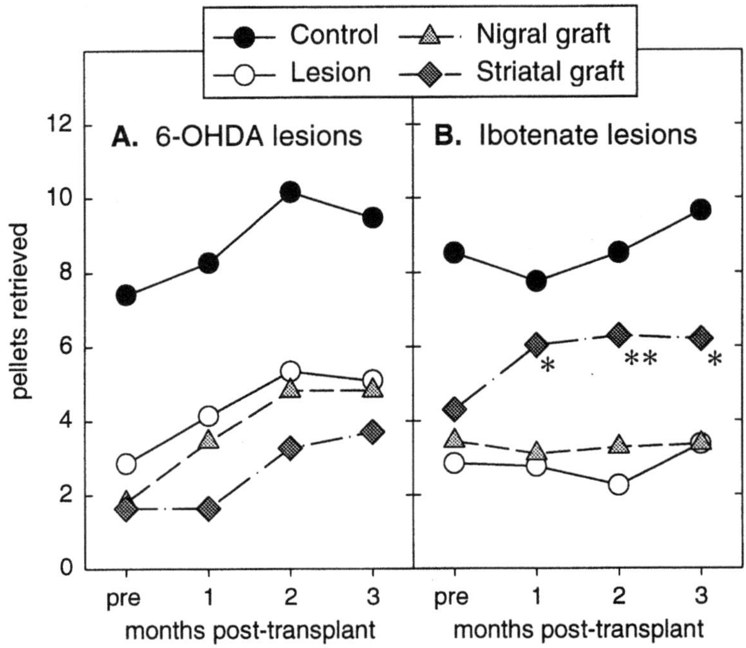

FIG. 6.5. Selective recovery of skilled paw use by grafts in the staircase reaching task. Rats received either (A) nigrostriatal lesions or (B) neostriatal lesions. The nigral graft is relevant and the striatal graft a control procedure for the nigrostriatal lesions, and vice versa for the striatal lesions. Paw reaching deficits were only alleviated by the relevant (homotopic) striatal grafts in the striatal lesion model, and not by the relevant (ectopic) nigral grafts in the nigrostriatal lesion model nor by either control graft. *,** indicate significant improvements with respect to the corresponding lesion group. (Data from Montoya et al., 1990.)

Skilled paw reaching. A more interesting set of tests to compare the skilled motor capacity of rats with nigral and striatal grafts is provided by tests of skilled paw reaching. As described in an earlier chapter, unilateral nigrostriatal lesions produce marked deficits in the co-ordination and accuracy with which a rat can use the contralateral paw to reach for and retrieve food pellets. This has always been one of the deficits which is resistant to alleviation by grafts of embryonic nigral tissue or other dopamine-secreting tissues. By contrast, several studies have shown a significant alleviation of the paw reaching deficit induced by excitotoxic lesions of the neostriatum in rats with striatal grafts (Dunnett et al., 1988c; Fricker et al., 1997; Montoya et al., 1990).

The clearest demonstration of this efficacy of striatal grafts is provided by the fully counterbalanced study of Montoya et al. (1990), in which he compared the effects of nigral and striatal grafts in rats with either 6-OHDA (6-hydroxydopamine) lesions of the nigrostriatal pathway or ibotenic acid lesions of intrinsic striatal neurones. As shown in Fig. 6.5, neither nigral nor striatal tissue grafts alleviated the nigrostriatal deficit when implanted into the dopamine-depleted striatum. By contrast, although *a priori* the striatal lesion may be considered to produce more extensive damage of multiple pathways than lesions of nigrostriatal inputs alone, this deficit was alleviated by striatal grafts implanted into the same striatal site. In this case the graft was homotopic, in contrast to the situation with nigrostriatal lesions, where both types of graft are ectopic to the loss induced by this lesion. The specificity of the striatal graft action is confirmed by the fact that nigral grafts were without effect.

Interpretations of striatal reconstruction

It appears that placement of striatal grafts into a homotopic rather than ectopic site is important for their functional efficacy. It was proposed in Chapter Four that the failure of recovery in rats with nigrostriatal lesions and nigral grafts on some tasks may be due to the fact that although nigral grafts restore a diffuse dopaminergic activation of the striatum, they do not reconstruct the damaged nigrostriatal pathway. Consequently, although performance on tests that reflect dopaminergic activation and net striatal output may be restored (such as locomotor activity, rotation, somatosensory neglect, posture, and side biases), performance remained impaired on other tests involving complex co-ordinated action (such as skilled paw reaching, disengagement behaviour, food hoarding, or the aphagia/adipsia syndrome) because of a failure to reconstruct the damaged nigrostriatal circuitries and thus restore the input and output of patterned information.

Recovery in tests such as T-maze alternation, skilled paw reaching, and aspects of rotation in rats with intrinsic striatal lesions and homotopic striatal grafts suggests on functional grounds alone that a degree of circuit reconstruction must be taking place in this model system. A number of other observations converge to support that hypothesis.

First, although the recovery in locomotor activity could be attributable to a down-regulation of striatal overactivity at the level of striatal terminals in the globus pallidus, the T-maze alternation task provides a long-established test sensitive to disturbance of corticostriatal integrity. Therefore a deficit in this test and its recovery with homotopic striatal grafts means there is a reversal of the lesion-induced disconnection syndrome isolating the neocortex from its motor targets in the globus pallidus and beyond.

Second, no pharmacological treatments have been found to overcome the cognitive impairments of the prefrontal type after intrinsic striatal damage, whether due to neurodegenerative disease as in HD, or after experimental lesions in animals. Striatal grafts can therefore be seen to work not in a purely pharmacological way, but in terms of circuit reconstruction.

Third, in a number of tests, striatal grafts were ineffective when implanted into the main output target of the neostriatum, namely the globus pallidus. This is important, firstly because it indicates that the striatal grafts reconstruct the

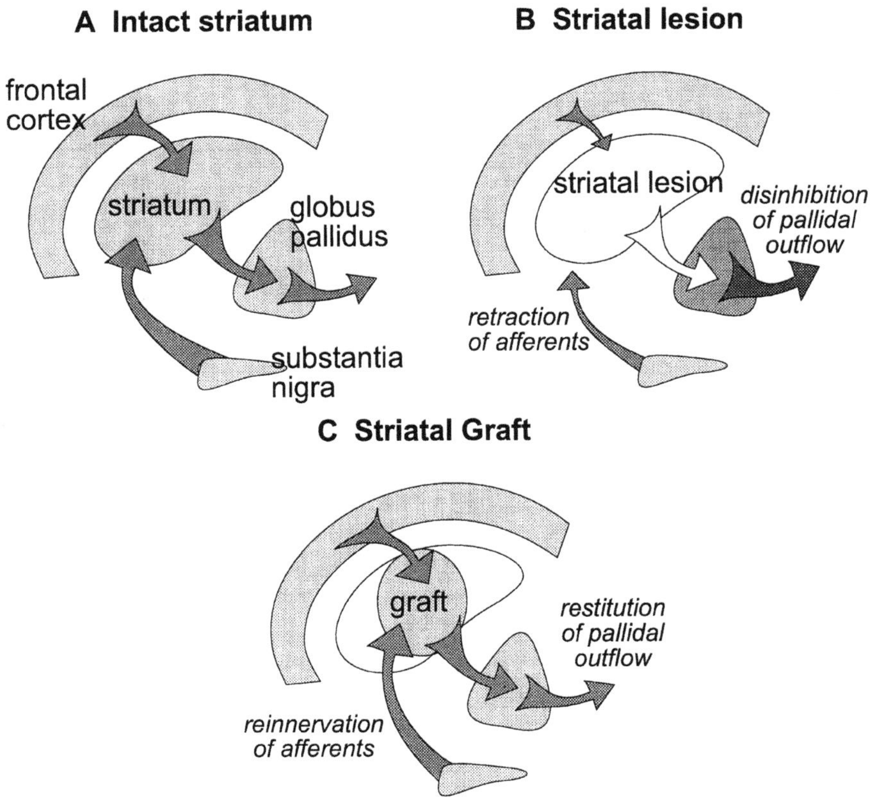

FIG. 6.6. Hypothesis of cortico-striatal circuit reconstruction with striatal grafts. (A) Normal cortical–basal ganglia circuitry. (B) Striatal lesions induce a disconnection syndrome within the cortical–striatal–pallidal loop. (C) Ectopic striatal grafts restore connectivity of the cortical–basal ganglia circuit. See Fig. 4.2. for further details of the simplified striatal circuitry shown here.

circuitry appropriate to this structure; and secondly because attempts to use striatal grafts to mimic the circumstances in which nigral grafts are effective, namely ectopic placement in the primary target area, are unsuccessful.

The contrast between nigral grafts, which have their limited effect primarily when placed into the ectopic site, and striatal grafts, which have a more extensive effect when implanted into the homotopic site, suggests that quite different mechanisms of action must apply in the two models—diffuse re-innervation of denervated targets, tonic release of deficient neurochemicals, and trophic actions on the host brain in the case of nigral grafts, vs. a hypothesised reconstruction of damaged neuronal circuitry in the case of striatal grafts (Fig. 6.6).

This is a strong hypothesis that turns out to be difficult to demonstrate directly. However, the past 5 years have seen a newly invigorated research effort oriented towards identifying principles of circuit reconstruction, and the results

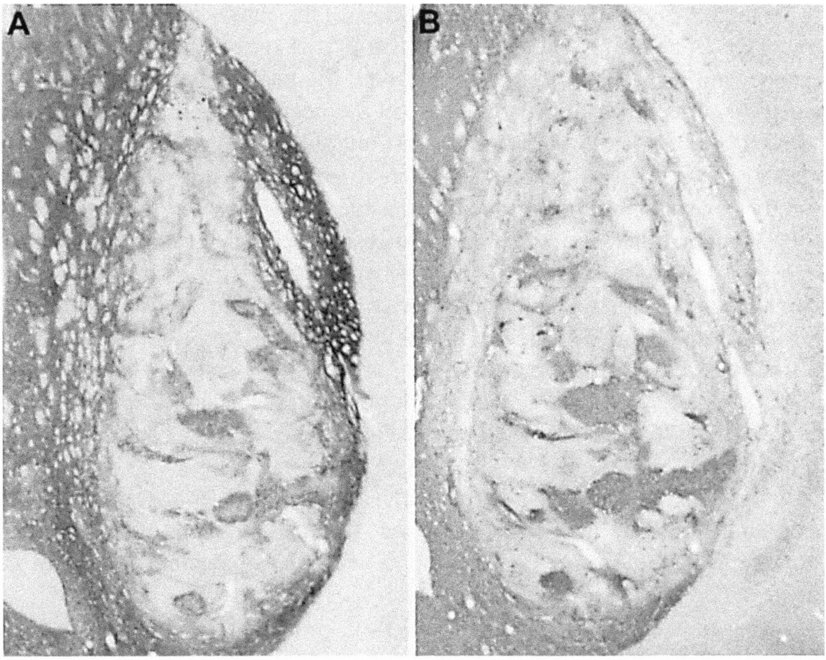

FIG. 6.7. Internal organisation of striatal grafts. (A) Acetylcholinesterase staining of striatal neuropil. (B) DARPP-32 labelling of intrinsic striatal neurones in adjacent section. Note the co-alignment of the "P zones" staining for different striatal markers. (Original sections with kind permission of Stefanie Thian.)

continue to support the hypothesis. Although the present volume adopts a primarily functional focus, the anatomical, biochemical, and physiological studies that give the hypothesis credence will be briefly considered.

Internal organisation of striatal grafts

The first grafts of striatal tissue into the kainic acid- or ibotenic acid-lesioned striatum were seen to survive well (see previously). In post-mortem histology, the grafts were primarily composed of neurones when stained with simple cell body stains as well as a number of simple markers of striatal tissue, e.g. the enzyme acetylcholinesterase. However, from the earliest studies it became clear that although there were neurones throughout the grafts, stains that are characteristic of the normal neostriatum show a distinctly patchy pattern (see Fig. 6.7). Moreover, when stains for different markers of striatal tissue are used on adjacent sections, the patchy zones are aligned. Thus, it turns out that "striatal" grafts contain patches—the so called "P (patch) zones" (Graybiel et al., 1989)—containing all the cell types, neurotransmitters, enzymes, and receptors of the normal striatum (Björklund et al., 1994).

This then invites the question: So what are all the cells seen in the intervening areas of the grafts—the so called "NP (non-patch) zones"? It turns out that the NP zones are also rich in neurones, but with the characteristics of non-striatal populations of cells such as those found in the neocortex and globus pallidus.

Striatal grafts therefore contain both striatal-like and non-striatal-like populations of cells. It is not possible to separate these populations at the time of graft dissection because they all originate from the same germinal cell layer in the embryonic ganglionic eminence. The non-striatal cells then migrate through the deeper striatal layers to reach their ultimate targets. Nor is it possible with present techniques to separate the different populations of cells in suspension prior to implantation. The problem is that although the fate of the cells is largely determined at the time of dissection, they are all small, round, relatively undifferentiated cells at this stage and are not yet expressing the differences in cell size or distinctive molecular markers on the cell surface that could be used for cell sorting.

Although the grafts contain a mixture of striatal and non-striatal cells, the important feature for their function is that the cells organise themselves into distinct striatal-like P zones as the grafts develop. It remains unknown how this is achieved:

(1) Do the striatal and non-striatal cells migrate and self-aggregate into clusters of cells of similar types?
(2) Is there a selective cell death of neurones whose neighbours are of a dissimilar type, resulting in a selective survival of similar cells together?
(3) Is the phenotype of each cell itself modified or regulated by its neighbours?
(4) Whichever is the process, by what mechanisms do the different cells recognise their neighbours?

Although we have no answers to these theoretical issues, the practical fact is that the cells in striatal grafts contain the developmental programmes to organise and reorganise themselves into structures akin to the normal neostriatum, which is almost certainly necessary if they are to be engaged in any meaningful functional processing of their inputs and to relay sensible output information to their targets.

Anatomical connections of the grafts

As well as reorganising itself as a new "mini-striatum", a striatal graft would need to develop appropriate input and output connections with the host brain if it is to be functionally effective. The extent and specificity of the reciprocal connections that are seen to form between graft and host is perhaps the most remarkable feature of this model system (see Wictorin, 1992 for review).

The outputs of a graft have been visualised anatomically in a number of different ways. Retrograde tracers can be injected in the host brain, anterograde tracers can be injected into the grafts, and xenografts of human or mouse striatal tissues have been implanted in the rat striatum and their connections demonstrated using species-specific antibodies. All have shown extensive axon outgrowth from striatal grafts coursing in a caudal direction towards the globus pallidus, which is re-innervated in most cases. Furthermore, in many cases the axon outgrowth is seen to extend even further caudally to reach the other major output nucleus of the basal ganglia, the substantia nigra pars reticulata (see Fig. 6.8). Retrograde tracing from the putamen and nigra shows that these outputs all originate from the striatal-like P zones of the grafts. Similarly, the inputs to the grafts can be visualised using anterograde and retrograde tracers as well as markers for the afferent dopaminergic input from the SN (substantia nigra) (Fig. 6.5B).

Excitotoxic lesions of the striatum destroy intrinsic neurones but leave the terminals of the input axons intact. These input axons will eventually atrophy, but for a period of several months are able to sprout into any appropriate new target tissue. Striatal grafts provide a very effective stimulus for inducing this sprouting and by so doing allow ingrowth of all the normal major inputs to the striatum, including cortical, thalamic, serotonergic, and dopaminergic projections. As one might expect from the nature of the grafted tissue, some inputs (such as those from the neocortex) grow into both the P zones and the NP zones of the grafts, whereas other inputs (such as the dopamine inputs) preferentially innervate the P zones in a manner that one would expect developmentally.

Perhaps the most dramatic demonstration of reconstruction of striatal circuits in striatal grafts is provided by the electron microscope studies of Debby Clarke (Clarke & Dunnett, 1993; Clarke et al., 1994). In the electron microscope, the actual form of the synaptic contacts can be observed. In the first place Golgi staining and GAD immunohistochemistry were used to identify cells in the grafts that were GABAergic and of the medium spiny neurone type. Then a combination of other techniques was used to show the connections of these cells (Fig. 6.9). First, the retrograde tracer horseradish peroxidase (HRP) was injected into the globus pallidus: The presence of HRP crystals in the cells of the graft showed that it was the medium spiny neurones that gave rise to the pallidal outputs. Second, lesions were made in the neocortex: Degenerating terminals of corticostriatal axons were seen making contact with the same medium spiny neurones in the grafts. Third, the sections were further stained with a TH (tyrosine hydroxylase) antibody: This showed that dopamine inputs to the grafts made synaptic terminals onto the dendritic spines of GABA medium spiny neurones. Indeed in some cases, the corticostriatal and dopaminergic nigrostriatal inputs were seen to converge onto the same output neurones.

From these various anatomical studies, we now have convincing evidence that striatal grafts do have the capacity to reconstruct striatal input and output

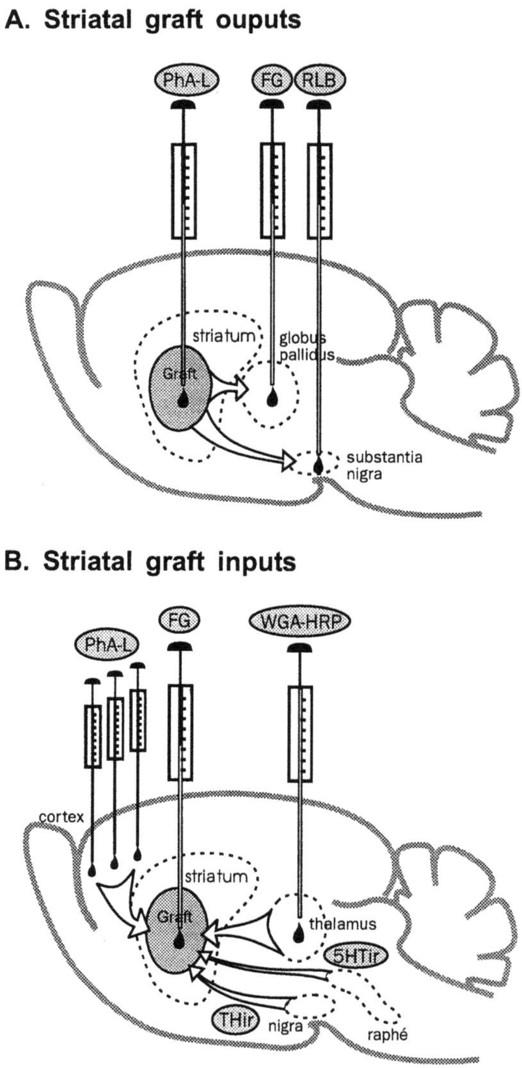

FIG. 6.8. Anatomical connectivity of striatal grafts. (A) Strategies for labelling fibre outgrowth from striatal grafts to the host brain. (B) Strategies for labelling fibre connections from the host brain into striatal grafts. All methods have revealed extensive reciprocal afferent and efferent graft–host connectivity. FG, fluorogold; HRP, horseradish peroxidase; ir, immunoreactivity; PhA-L, *phaseolus* leucoagglutinin; RLB, rhodamine-labelled microbeads; TH, tyrosine hydroxylase; WGA, wheat germ agglutinin; 5HT, serotonin. (Redrawn from Wictorin, 1992.)

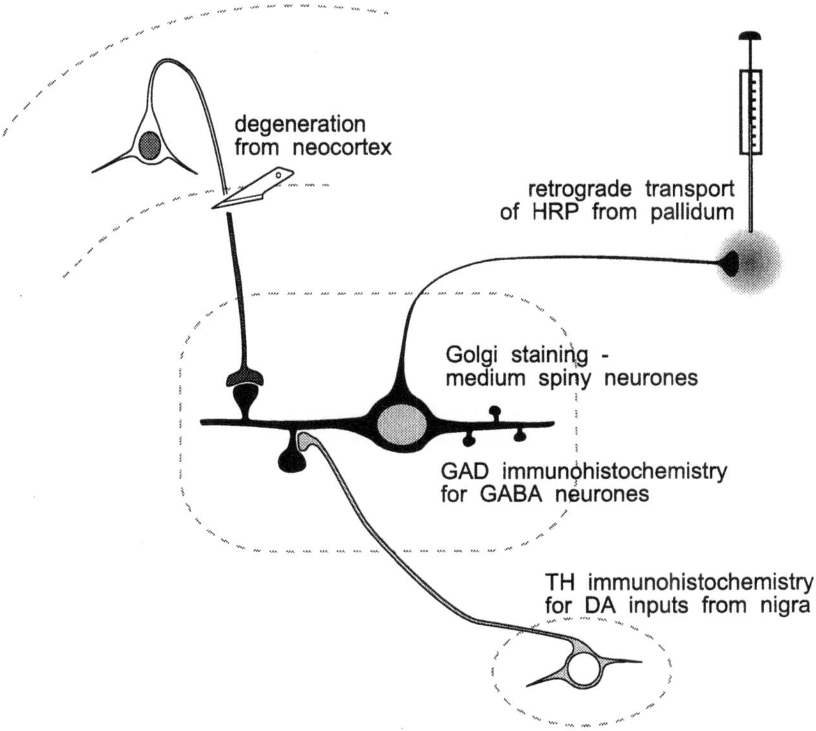

FIG. 6.9. Synaptic connectivity of striatal grafts visualised in the electron microscope. Individual neurones and their connections were identified by a combination of degeneration, tracing, Golgi, and immunohistochemical labelling. (Based on Clarke & Dunnett, 1993.)

circuits through the grafts. Indeed the evidence of circuit reconstruction is perhaps now stronger for this model system than any other. The more difficult issue is to determine the association between the structural and functional levels of analysis—just because grafts do reconstruct a damaged circuit does not mean that this is the basis for their functional effect.

Physiological and biochemical indices of circuit reconstruction

How are we to determine if the observed anatomical connections are in any way functional? One approach has been electrophysiological. This has so far been little investigated, but two studies have shown that stimulation in the host cortex or thalamus can be detected by recording electrodes placed within striatal grafts (Rutherford et al., 1987; Xu et al., 1991). Moreover, the recorded cellular firing patterns exhibit the characteristics of monosynaptic inputs, suggesting that the projections from the host brain to the grafts have the capacity to relay basic patterned electrical information.

A second approach is to monitor changes in gene expression in cells in responses to changes in their inputs. In the normal striatum, the level of expression of two peptides co-localised in the medium spiny output neurones, enkephalin and substance P, is regulated by the dopamine input to the striatum. If the nigrostriatal inputs are lesioned, expression of enkephalin increases whereas expression of substance P decreases. Similarly in striatal grafts, normal levels of enkephalin and substance P expression are seen within the P zones, whereas following lesion or blockade of the dopaminergic inputs enkephalin expression again increases and substance P expression decreases (Campbell et al., 1992). Thus the levels of expression of genes related to peptide neurotransmitters in the grafts is regulated by the host dopaminergic input in exactly the same manner as in the normal striatum.

A third approach is to use *in vivo* measurements of neurotransmitter turnover to monitor the activity of inputs and outputs of the grafts. For example, the graft projection to the globus pallidus is GABAergic. Sirinathsinghji and colleagues (1988) used a push–pull perfusion cannula to monitor GABA release in the globus pallidus of control, striatal lesion only, and grafted striatal lesion rats. The lesions produced a 97% loss of GABA release in the ipsilateral globus pallidus, which was restored to approximately 30% of normal levels in the graft-re-innervated pallidum. Of particular interest in this study was the observation that activation of dopamine inputs to the normal striatum induces a large brief surge of GABA release in the pallidum. This response was completely abolished in the pallidum ipsilateral to a striatal lesion, but restored following re-innervation by a striatal graft.

These various approaches all suggest that the reformed host cortical, thalamic, and dopamine inputs making direct synaptic connections with GABA output neurones are indeed capable of relaying functional information from the host brain to neurones of the graft. Furthermore, the grafts can transduce that information so as to exert a reciprocal influence back onto the appropriate neuronal circuits within the host brain.

CLINICAL APPLICATIONS OF STRIATAL GRAFTS IN HD

Is HD a suitable candidate disease?

HD is under consideration as a suitable candidate disease for the development of the next phase of neural transplantation as a therapy, primarily because of the similarities between the neuropathology in humans and the available animal models, and the remarkable functional reconstruction provided by striatal grafts in these models. In addition, the relentless course of the disease in man, alongside the absence of any useful alternative therapies, emphasises the importance of any approach that attempts to halt or reverse the disease process.

The recent discovery of the gene defect in HD does not by itself render neural transplantation redundant. Although there is naturally a renewed effort in seeking to identify new gene therapies, no obvious strategy for treatment is even on the horizon. It is anticipated that there will continue to be similar numbers of patients developing the disease for the foreseeable future. Indeed, one main advance achieved by identification of the gene is that reliable and accurate diagnosis is now possible, in contrast to PD (see Chapter Five). This not only allows for the more efficient study of early and predisposing factors to the development of the disease, but means that it would be possible to include patients early in the disease or even at a presymptomatic stage in any novel treatment programme such as neural transplantation, without concern about inaccuracies in early diagnosis.

In deciding whether to pursue a neural transplantation strategy in HD, one major concern at present must be the relevance of the animal models to the human disease. The aetiology of the deficit in the human disease is clearly quite different from experimental excitotoxic lesions in animals. It remains completely unknown by what cellular and/or molecular mechanism the expanded CAG repeat in the huntingtin gene results in neuronal pathology, although there is continuing speculation that an excitotoxic or metabolic deficit may be a final common pathway of cell death (Beal, 1994). Even more perplexing is how a gene that is expressed ubiquitously results in selective death of just the striatal medium spiny neurones. One aspect of this issue is whether the gene defect leads to activation of non-neuronal events that target striatal neurones selectively or whether there is a change in gene expression selectively in striatal neurones that makes them vulnerable to cell death—i.e. are they killed or do they commit suicide? It is possible that transgenic mice that overexpress the HD gene may yield answers to these questions, as well as providing a more suitable model in which to evaluate striatal grafts (Duyao et al., 1995; Goldberg et al., 1996; Mangiarini et al., 1996; White et al., 1997), but that stage has not yet been achieved.

A second concern must be the paucity of primate studies to date on striatal lesions and grafts. Where should the grafts be placed? Should this be in the form of many small deposits or a few large ones? Can striatal grafts regenerate and connect over the much greater distances that apply in the human brain in contrast to the rat brain? Only in the larger primate brain will it be possible to evaluate experimentally such issues of critical clinical importance, and such studies are only now commencing (Dunnett et al., 1997; Hantraye et al., 1992; Isacson et al., 1989; Kendall et al., 1998; Palfi et al., 1998).

However, on the basis of the experimental background, clinical trials of striatal tissue transplantation in HD have now commenced in several centres world-wide (Peschanski et al., 1995; Kopyov et al., 1998). The first reports, whilst being very rapid to establish priority, provide no useful information to determine whether the grafts have survived or achieved any meaningful benefit to the patient (Madrazo et al., 1995; Sramka et al., 1992). Thus, Sramka and colleagues report: "Four patients with Huntington's chorea were transplanted with embryonal brain tissue. Intensive choreoathetosis with serious damage of the postural musculature and dystonia developed in these patients, mainly on voluntary movement, as well as in the lying position. They were in groups IV–V of the Hoehn–Yahr scale, and were not able to stand and walk. As yet it is not possible to make a final postoperative evaluation, but a reduction in amplitude and frequency of hyperkinesia has been observed."

In the second study, Madrazo and colleagues (1995) report on two patients using several pre- and post-surgical neurological rating scales. They reported first that the surgery was safe and without complication in both patients, and second that the grafts appeared to slow the rate of progression of the disease in the 16 to 33-month postoperative follow-up period. However, in neither of these cases is there objective quantitation of neurological performance or evaluation of graft survival, factors that we have seen were critical in establishing the viability of nigral grafts in Parkinson's disease (Chapter Five).

Methods of monitoring patient progress

Unlike for Parkinson's disease, there are no standardised test batteries for HD, in part at least because research in this area has not been driven by major trials of novel drug treatments. Nevertheless, it is clear from the experience of the first clinical trials of neural transplantation in Parkinson's disease that a major factor in the success of certain centres was the use of standardised assessment protocols to monitor the progress of patients in an unbiased manner. The particular problem confronted in a transplant study is that the numbers of patients are invariably small, and it is difficult to undertake proper blind control procedures. Consequently, tests are required which are reliable and which can be used to monitor the progress of the disease on an individual-by-individual basis. With this in mind, both US and European groups have been collaborating to develop standardised assessment protocols. As outlined in Chapter One, a new core assessment protocol for intracerebral transplantation (CAPIT-HD) is under development, based on the experience of the PD trials but emphasising aspects of particular relevance to HD (Quinn et al., 1996).

In the first round, experiments are now under way to provide normative data on the rate and stability of progress of HD in untreated cohorts of patients over time, to provide an index of the variability of the course of the disease and a baseline for assessment of patients included into new clinical programmes. Without such well-established and validated baseline data, it is extremely difficult to distinguish changes associated with the implantation surgery against a slow and variable progression of the disease.

Methods of monitoring graft survival *in vivo*

A second important factor in the success of clinical trials of neural transplantation in Parkinson's disease was the availability of good *in vivo* imaging facilities to monitor the extent of the disease, and the placement and survival of the grafts. A major component in the confidence that the nigral transplants themselves were the basis of the functional recovery in the later patients in the Swedish transplant

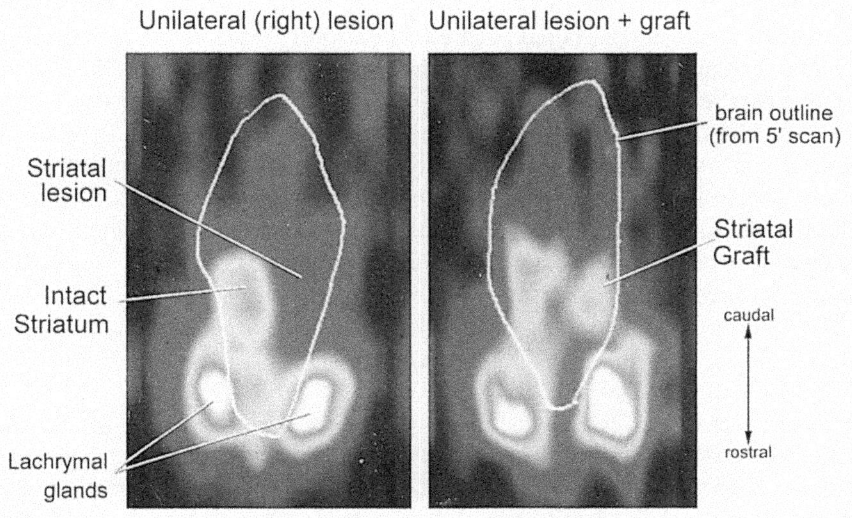

FIG. 6.10. PET scanning of D2 receptors in a striatal graft using ^{11}C-raclopride ligand in a small animal scanner. (Based on Torres et al., 1995.)

series was the demonstration of a close correspondence between the time course of functional recovery and the development of the fluorodopa signal from the grafts in the sequential PET (positron emission tomography) scans.

There have been a few studies using MRI (magnetic resonance imaging) and PET to image the striatal degeneration in HD, although as yet there are still no longitudinal studies to indicate whether these techniques can provide accurate assessment of the progress of the disease. The predominant ligand in the PET studies has been use of 2-fluorodeoxyglucose—a marker of general cellular metabolism. However, when it comes to monitoring the fate of striatal grafts, it would appear preferable to identify a ligand that can distinguish striatal from non-striatal cells, in particular because the viability of the striatal compartment rather than total neuronal survival within the grafts is likely to be fundamental to function.

In a preliminary series of studies, we have compared three ligands for detecting the viability of striatal grafts in rats in a small animal scanner (Fricker et al., 1997; Torres et al., 1995). In the smaller brain of the rat the [^{11}C] 2-deoxyglucose signal from the grafts was completely masked by the strong signal from the surrounding neocortex. Of more interest, were ^{11}C-SCH 23390 and ^{11}C-raclopride, which bind to D1 and D2 receptors respectively. The lesions produced a partial loss of the SCH 23390 signal and a complete loss of the raclopride signal in the lesioned striatum. However, since binding of these markers is relatively restricted to the striatum, the signal from the grafts was clearly demarcated without interference from surrounding areas of the forebrain (see Fig. 6.10). Not only was there a clear restitution of the binding potential to approximately 40% of normal levels in the grafted striatum, but also the recovery in the raclopride binding potential correlated closely with functional recovery in parallel tests of skilled paw reaching.

These results indicate that effective ligands are available for detection of striatal grafts and monitoring the viability of the striatal compartment within the grafts. In the light of these results, raclopride is now adopted as a core part of the CAPIT assessment in European trials, and we consider that no clinical trial should be undertaken without incorporating pre- and post-surgical *in vivo* scans as a core feature of the assessment protocol.

SUMMARY

Striatal grafts can reverse a wide range of complex cognitive and motor deficits induced by striatal lesions. This they do by establishing reciprocal input and output connections with the host brain, connections that are functional at both the electrophysiological and neurochemical levels. This recreation of the host circuitry allows homotopic striatal grafts to restore deficits following extensive striatal lesions that have proved resistant to alleviation by ectopic nigral grafts after the apparently more restricted nigrostriatal lesions. Indeed the observation that pharmacological or trophic strategies of treatment are ineffective in animals with striatal lesions or in patients with HD further supports this mode of action for striatal grafts, namely, that they reform reciprocal functional connections between graft and host and actually reconstruct damaged corticostriatal circuits in the host brain.

The remarkable level of reorganisation seen in experimental models in animals raises the issue of whether a similar pattern of functional recovery may be obtained in equivalent human syndromes, of which Huntington's disease provides the most obvious. This potential application is currently undergoing intensive research effort world-wide.

CHAPTER SEVEN

Alzheimer's disease: A difficult target for transplantation

One of the fundamental conditions for the development of a rational transplantation therapy is the identification of a target population or populations of cells central to the disease process, which one consequently seeks to replace. This provides the biggest problem for developing an effective transplantation strategy for human dementia, namely the failure to identify the primary basis and critical neuropathology of the disease process. Indeed, this problem restricts at present even our ability to determine whether such a strategy might ever be feasible.

THE PROBLEM OF DEMENTIA

Ageing is accompanied by a wide variety of structural and neurochemical changes that underlie the deterioration of virtually all physical and mental functions to a greater or lesser extent in later life. Within that general deterioration, dementia represents a more pronounced impairment in cognitive function, characterised by disorientation and impairments in intellect, memory, and new learning. The extent to which dementia represents a normal end-stage of the ageing process as opposed to a superimposed distinct disease is not clear, although a number distinct neurodegenerative disorders are associated with its development at a presenile age (e.g. Alzheimer's, Pick's, Huntington's, or Parkinson's diseases).

The extent of the changes within the CNS seen with both age-, as well as disease-related, dementia makes it impractical to attempt a complete repair process. Rather, the predominant research approach has been to seek to identify individual neuroanatomical or neurochemical systems that are either primary to the disease process or central to the functional deterioration. Such an identification allows for attempts at selective repair or replacement, which may then either inhibit the progression of the disease by blocking a critical initial pathogenic stage (e.g. by supplying a deficient trophic factor or by inhibiting amyloid deposition) or restore particular aspects of impaired function that are of particular importance to the patient (e.g. memory).

Experimental neural transplantation programmes for the functional amelioration of intellectual deficits associated with ageing and dementia have been guided by this strategy. However, the extent to which the animal models used in these studies are clinically relevant is controversial. So, for example, it is now well established than grafts of cholinergic neurones can ameliorate some learning impairments associated with lesions of cholinergic systems in the rat forebrain (see later). However, the relevance of this to Alzheimer's disease (dementia of the Alzheimer type, DAT) is unknown, given the uncertainty of the validity of the cholinergic hypothesis of DAT.

In this chapter the discussion concentrates in the first instance on a selection of the transplantation approaches that have been adopted to ameliorate cognitive deficits in experimental animal models. However, these animal models are often limited inasmuch as the induced deficits reflect only some distinct aspects of the dementia process. It is the applicability of such model systems to the human disorder of dementia that raises questions as to whether, through this approach, there is any hope for developing a viable therapeutic strategy for Alzheimer's disease or other forms of dementia. It is this issue that concludes this chapter.

CHOLINERGIC MODELS OF AGEING AND DEMENTIA

The cholinergic hypothesis of geriatric memory dysfunction

Of the wide variety of neurochemical systems that degenerate in the aged brain, one of the most marked and consistent is the reduction in forebrain cholinergic function. This was first noted as a decline in cortical and hippocampal choline acetyltransferase (ChAT) activity in the aged brain, and was followed by the observation that the basal forebrain neurones, from which the cortical innervation arises, also undergo ageing- and dementia-related atrophy (Bartus et al., 1982; Coyle et al., 1983). Of particular interest in the present context was the clinical observation of Elaine Perry and colleagues (1978) that there was correlation between the decline in cortical cholinergic activity and mental test performance in patients with dementia. These various observations, along with the deficits in learning and memory that have long been known to follow treatment with anticholinergic drugs in both animals and man, led to the formulation of the "cholinergic hypothesis" of geriatric memory dysfunction. This proposes that a deterioration in forebrain (and in particular cortical) cholinergic systems underlies the cognitive (and in particular learning and memory) deficits associated with ageing (Bartus et al., 1982). The cholinergic decline and the associated

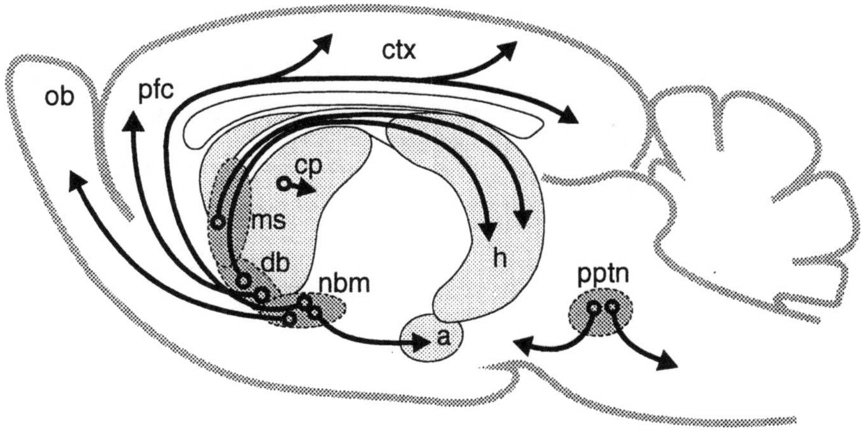

FIG. 7.1. Cholinergic systems of the basal forebrain, striatum and brainstem of the rat. a, amygdala; cp, caudate-putamen; ctx, neocortex; db, diagonal band of Broca; h, hippocampus; ms, medial septum; nbm, nucleus basalis magnocellularis; ob, olfactory bulb; pfc, prefrontal cortex; pptn, pedunculopontine tegmental nucleus.

mnemonic deficits reach their most severe in dementia, and so the cholinergic hypothesis may also account for the profound intellectual impairments of Alzheimer's disease (Coyle et al., 1983).

The explicit formulation of the cholinergic hypothesis has stimulated a decade of active research into the functional sequelae of lesions and pharmacological manipulations of forebrain cholinergic systems (see Fig. 7.1) in experimental animals. For example, excitotoxic lesions of the basal forebrain (made with kainic, ibotenic, or quisqualic acids) produce a variety of deficits in a number of relatively simple tests of learning and/or memory, such as passive avoidance and spatial navigation tasks. However, careful histological and functional analyses suggest that the consequence of cortical cholinergic lesions may be explicable more in terms of disrupted selective attention than an impairment in learning or memory *per se* (Dunnett et al., 1991). Nevertheless, the cholinergic hypothesis has provided the basis for an extensive search for cholinomimetic drugs that may provide a cholinergic replacement therapy for the cognitive deficits of ageing and dementia. The efficacy of these agents has largely been screened and tested for in animal models involving lesion or pharmacological blockade of the intrinsic forebrain cholinergic systems.

Cholinergic grafts in rats and monkeys with basal forebrain lesions

Cholinergic-rich ventral forebrain grafts can ameliorate some of the learning deficits associated with lesions of forebrain cholinergic systems. One of the first demonstrations of this phenomenon provides a good example of the general

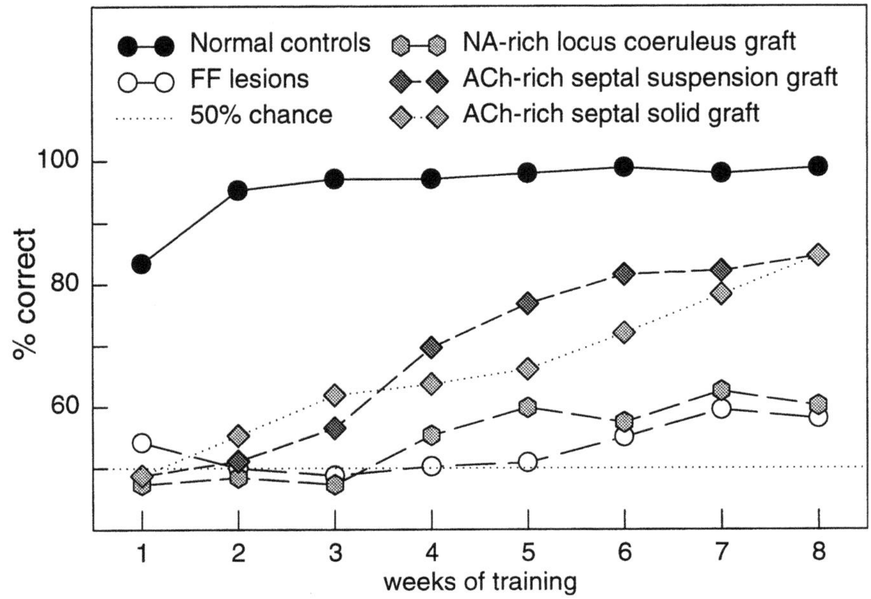

FIG. 7.2. T-maze alternation performance in normal rats, rats with fimbria-fornix (FF) lesions, and following transplantation of alternative tissues into the hippocampus. The controls rapidly learned the task to a high level of performance, whereas the lesioned rats were unable to learn the task. Noradrenergic (NA) grafts of locus coeruleus tissue did not alleviate the deficit. By contrast, cholinergic (ACh)-rich grafts of septal cells (both as solid grafts and as cell suspensions) enabled the animals to learn the task. Some but not all rats with cholinergic grafts eventually achieved the same high level of efficiency as intact control animals, but took considerably longer training to reach that level of performance. (Data from Dunnett et al., 1982.)

principles involved. In this study rats received lesions of the fimbria–fornix to deafferent the hippocampus of its main cholinergic (as well as noradrenergic and serotonergic) inputs, followed by grafts of either embryonic ventral forebrain (rich in cholinergic neurones) or of embryonic locus coeruleus (rich in noradrenergic neurones) implanted ectopically into the deafferented hippocampus (Dunnett et al., 1982). The lesions produced a profound deficit both in spontaneous exploratory behaviour (measured in terms of spontaneous alternation in a T-maze) and in the animals' abilities to learn a spatial alternation task in the T-maze. Whereas the noradrenergic grafts had no effect whatsoever on the animals' maze-learning deficit, the cholinergic-rich grafts provided a substantial and significant improvement in their ability to learn the alternation task (see Fig. 7.2).

Several features of this experiment are of note:

(1) The cholinergic-rich grafts were effective whether made by the solid or the cell suspension methods (see Chapter Three). This suggests that a

cholinergic re-innervation of the denervated hippocampus is sufficient to restore a limited degree of function, even though the full septo-hippocampal circuitry is not reconstructed.

(2) Cholinergic re-innervation of the host hippocampus appeared to be a necessary but not a sufficient condition for functional repair. In other words, overall the degree of recovery correlated with the extent of cholinergic fibre ingrowth into the host hippocampus, and all cases showing recovery did have good fibre ingrowth. However, there were individual cases in which good fibre ingrowth was not accompanied by functional recovery.

(3) Although the effective grafts improved performance significantly, even the best grafted animals still learned the task at a substantially slower rate than that achieved by control animals. Thus, function was not fully restored even though the septal grafts restored a normal density of cholinergic fibre inputs, and the ingrowing axons made normal synaptic contacts with the appropriate targets in the host hippocampus. This may reflect the fact that, although the grafted rats did eventually relearn the task, they showed only very limited spontaneous alternation in the initial phase of habituation to the T-maze environment, so learning of the reinforced contingency commenced from a very different baseline to that of the control rats (Dunnett et al., 1982).

These observations suggest that reconstruction of the cholinergic inputs alone is insufficient to restore normal performance. Further reconstruction may also be necessary for full functional repair; this could be in the form of either a better integration of the grafted neurones or by restitution of some other neural systems disrupted by the lesions (e.g. noradrenergic or serotonergic afferents to the hippocampus, or efferent projections coursing via the fimbria–fornix to subcortical sites).

Subsequent experiments have thrown further light on these issues. First, the ability of cholinergic grafts in the hippocampus to ameliorate deficits associated with fimbria–fornix or septal lesions has been replicated in a wide variety of learning paradigms, including T-mazes, radial mazes, the spatial water maze, and an operant Differential reinforcement of low rates (DRL) task (for detailed review, see Dunnett, 1990a, 1991; Sinden et al., 1994). In addition, similar principles have been found to apply also in the neocortex, the other major projection target of the cholinergic forebrain system. Thus, cholinergic grafts implanted into the neocortex have been found to ameliorate deficits induced by lesions of the basal forebrain in passive avoidance, water maze, T-maze and attentional operant tasks (Dunnett, 1990a, 1991; Sinden et al., 1994).

Second, several of these studies have used additional pharmacological manipulations to show that the graft-derived recovery is attributable to a specific cholinergic mechanism. Thus, Ola Nilsson and colleagues demonstrated that recovery in the Morris water maze induced by septal grafts could be blocked by treatment with the muscarinic antagonist, atropine, whereas this drug had no effect whatsoever on the rats with lesions alone (Nilsson et al., 1987). In a further comprehensive series of studies, Helen Hodges and colleagues have used a complex radial maze task that enabled them to identify lesion and graft effects separately on both working and reference memory components of maze learning, based on the use of both spatial and non-spatial cues (Hodges et al., 1991a,b). Grafts implanted into the hippocampus produced substantial amelioration of both spatial and cue-based reference memory and complete recovery of both spatial and cue-based working memory. Both the muscarinic agonist arecoline and the nicotinic agonist nicotine enhanced performance of the lesioned rats, but had no effect (arecoline) or actually impaired (nicotine) the already efficient performance of controls and rats with lesions plus cortical or hippocampal grafts. By contrast, antagonists at the two major classes of cholinergic receptors, scopolamine and mecamylamine, were found to disrupt the performance of the control and grafted rats while having less effect on the lesioned rats.

Third, these observations have recently been extended from rodents to a small New World primate, the common marmoset, in an elegant series of studies by Ridley and colleagues (1991). They have used an extended series of tasks, involving learning and reversal of simple and complex visual and visuospatial discriminations, to characterise the deficits that result from disruption in the septohippocampal system. They have found not only that conditional visuospatial discriminations appear to be particularly sensitive to fornix transection, but also that foetal marmoset cholinergic grafts (but not control grafts of cholinergic-poor tissues) implanted into the hippocampus of lesioned monkeys can alleviate those deficits (see Fig. 7.3).

Fourth, several recent studies suggest that the age of the graft donor may be critical to obtaining a good functional effect. Thus in rats, whereas grafts derived from embryos at all ages from E13 to E17 appear to give rise to good cholinergic re-innervation of the hippocampus, only host animals bearing grafts from the younger E13 and E14 donors appear to show good functional recovery in both radial maze and operant tasks (Cassell et al., 1991; Dunnett et al., 1989a). This has been taken to support the hypothesis that some neuronal connections other that just the cholinergic re-innervation must underlie the functional recovery.

Finally, a first clue as to which additional systems may be involved comes from the demonstration that co-grafts of serotonergic raphé tissue can yield a substantial promotion of the limited benefit associated with cholinergic grafts, even though the raphé grafts on their own are generally without significant effect (Nilsson et al., 1990). This supports Vanderwolf's (1987) hypothesis that the serotonergic system modulates cholinergic function in the hippocampus, and is compatible with his observations that blockade of both systems together induces far greater deficits than disturbance of either system alone.

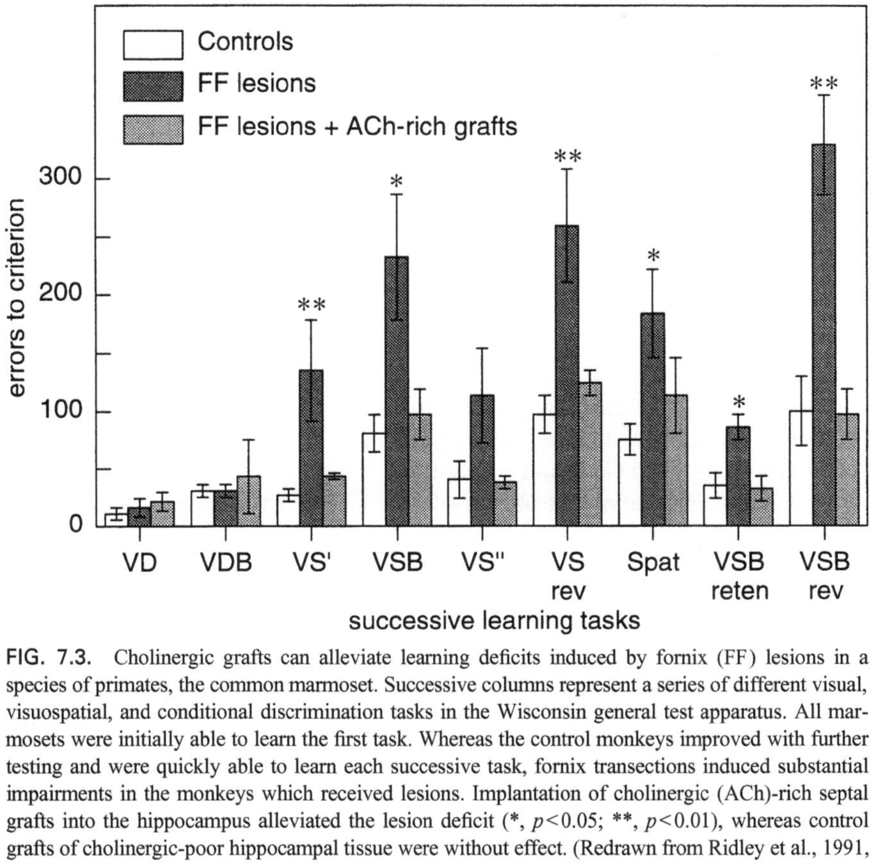

FIG. 7.3. Cholinergic grafts can alleviate learning deficits induced by fornix (FF) lesions in a species of primates, the common marmoset. Successive columns represent a series of different visual, visuospatial, and conditional discrimination tasks in the Wisconsin general test apparatus. All marmosets were initially able to learn the first task. Whereas the control monkeys improved with further testing and were quickly able to learn each successive task, fornix transections induced substantial impairments in the monkeys which received lesions. Implantation of cholinergic (ACh)-rich septal grafts into the hippocampus alleviated the lesion deficit (*, $p<0.05$; **, $p<0.01$), whereas control grafts of cholinergic-poor hippocampal tissue were without effect. (Redrawn from Ridley et al., 1991, with permission.)

Cholinergic grafts in aged animals

The observation that old rats and monkeys show similar deficits on many of the same tests of learning and memory as do animals receiving septo-hippocampal lesions or anticholinergic drugs has been taken as support for the cholinergic hypothesis of geriatric cognitive deficits and as such provides a rationale for testing potential cholinergic replacement strategies in old rats. Cholinomimetic drug therapies have provided significant effects in model systems, but generally the efficacy of both direct cholinergic receptor agonists and anticholinesterase inhibitors in aged animals has been disappointing. By contrast, a number of studies have revealed quite substantial benefits, albeit on selected tasks, of cholinergic-rich neural grafts in aged animals.

Graft studies in aged animals are more difficult to interpret than those conducted in younger individuals. In particular, whereas it is usually possible to achieve relatively consistent lesions with reproducible deficits in young animals, aged animals typically constitute a heterogeneous population with only some animals revealing deficits and others not differing from controls. Moreover, ageing is not a unitary process, with some animals showing more deficits "across the board" than other animals of the same age. Rather, different structural and neurochemical systems in both the brain and the rest of the body can undergo relatively independent deterioration, so that each animal will manifest an individual profile of normality and impairment across a range of functional tests. Thus, for many purposes, it is necessary to screen animals in advance and allocate only those with impairments to experimental and matched control groups. Although these principles are recognised as obvious to clinicians and scientists working with ageing human subjects, the heterogeneity of aged rat populations is frequently ignored completely in experimental animal studies.

In the first study of the functional effects of neural transplants on age-related learning deficits, Fred Gage and colleagues (1984) screened a large group of old rats in the Morris water maze task and selected 17 that manifested learning impairments greater than two standard deviations outside the range of performance of a group of young rats tested in parallel (Fig. 7.4). Some of these aged rats then received cholinergic septal suspension grafts implanted into the hippocampus, exactly as described for the lesioned rats above. Three months were allowed for the grafts to grow and integrate with the host brain before the rats were retested in the water maze task. The old rats with grafts showed a substantial improvement in their performance over their previous level of impairment, whereas the non-grafted rats showed no improvements whatsoever (Fig. 7.4). Indeed, even within the graft group, two of the 10 individual rats remained as impaired as the elderly non-grafted rats, which was accounted for in the subsequent histological analysis by a failure of the grafts to thrive in these two cases (Gage et al., 1984). By contrast, the other eight grafted rats all showed substantial recovery to a level where their performance was not significantly different from that of the young and unimpaired old animals.

Subsequent studies have extended these initial observations in similar ways to the developments in lesion models, described above.

First, the recovery in the water maze induced by cholinergic-rich septal grafts implanted into the hippocampus of aged rats is blocked by treatment with the anticholinergic drug atropine, even though atropine has no effect on the lesion-only animals (Gage & Björklund, 1986). This suggests that the recovery process is itself dependent upon a cholinergic mechanism.

Second, the benefits provided by cholinergic grafts in the hippocampus have been evaluated in tasks other than the water maze. One of the most interesting is an operant delayed matching to sample task that reveals a delay-dependent deficit in short-term memory of aged rats that is significantly alleviated by multiple septal graft deposits in the cortex and hippocampus (Dunnett et al., 1988a).

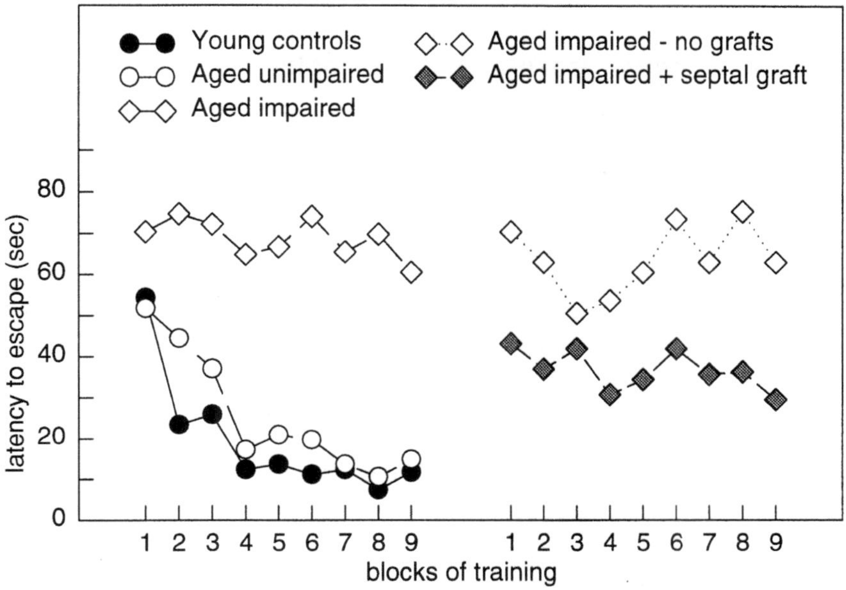

FIG. 7.4. Recovery of spatial navigation in the Morris water maze task in successive blocks of four trials prior to and following transplantation of septal tissues into the hippocampus of impaired old rats. Whereas young animals are efficient in learning to swim directly to the escape platform within 15–20 trials, 30–40% of 20-month-old rats are unable to learn the task (open diamonds, left panel). A subset of the old impaired animals then received septal grafts. The grafted rats manifested marked improvements in performance when retested 3 months later (filled diamonds), whereas the non-transplanted rats (open diamonds) showed no subsequent improvement even with further training (right panel). (Redrawn from Gage et al., 1984.)

Third, recovery on other types of task or classes of behavioural impairment can be obtained following implantation of other types of tissue into the hippocampus or other target areas in aged rats. Thus, for example, Collier and colleagues (1988) have shown that hippocampal implants of noradrenergic locus coeruleus grafts can ameliorate aged rats' deficits in acquisition and retention of a passive avoidance task. Conversely, intrastriatal implantation of dopaminergic nigral grafts can ameliorate age-related deficits in motor co-ordination and balance (Gage et al., 1983). Interestingly, this latter study was conducted in parallel with the above study of the effects of septal grafts on water maze performance by aged rats, and the patterns of recovery (in motor vs. spatial learning tasks) were quite specific to the transmitter type of the graft tissue and its site of implantation (Gage et al., 1983, 1984).

MODELS OF TROPHIC FACTOR DEFICIENCY

The role of nerve growth factor in trophic support

A tangential development of the cholinergic hypothesis has been the theory that the cholinergic deficit in DAT is due to a deficiency in specific trophic factors. This hypothesis has derived from the discovery that central cholinergic neurones are dependent upon target-derived nerve growth factor (NGF) for trophic support. Since these same populations of neurones decline in DAT, Hefti (1983) proposed the hypothesis that the loss of cholinergic neurones in the disease may reflect an insufficient availability of NGF to these cells. As one test of this idea, Fischer and colleagues (1987) gave chronic NGF treatment to aged rats and found that this would both reduce the atrophy of septal cholinergic neurones in the aged brain and ameliorate the impairments in retention of spatial navigation learning between blocks of test session. If this reasoning were correct, then NGF replacement might provide a potential therapeutic strategy for dementias such as Alzheimer's disease.

One problem with the trophic hypothesis, at least in it its strictest form, is that there have been difficulties in demonstrating any consistent reduction of levels of NGF, NGF receptors, or NGF expression in the cortex or hippocampus of the post-mortem Alzheimer brain. Moreover, there are considerable practical problems of delivery of a trophic factor treatment. NGF does not cross the blood–brain barrier, and so must be administered intracerebrally and chronically to be effective. Rather than attempting chronic intracerebral infusions, it is possible that the most effective way to deliver NGF or other trophic factors to the brain may be to transplant cells that secrete the target growth factor.

Transplants as NGF-delivery systems

A variety of sources of tissue that are naturally rich in NGF have been used as transplantable source of trophic factor. These studies have generally been conducted with one of two alternative purposes. The first is to promote the viability of other NGF-dependent cells following transplantation (such as the adrenal medulla) and has been considered in Chapter Five. The second purpose, relevant to models of dementia, has been to seek to inhibit degeneration of cholinergic neurones after axotomy.

The richest naturally occurring source of NGF is the mouse submaxillary gland. Implants of this tissue have been shown to increase the survival of septal and diagonal band neurones following fimbria–fornix transection (Fischer et al., 1988; Springer et al., 1988). However, even if these neurones survive, they are not able to regrow across the lesion cavity to re-innervate their hippocampal targets unless provided with a bridge of suitable tissue as a substrate for their regrowth. Messersmith and colleagues (1991) have recently attempted to combine these two graft functions using peripheral nerves (e.g. sciatic nerve), as they both provide a good substrate for axonal growth (see Chapter One) and also secrete relatively high levels of NGF. Sciatic nerve was therefore used to make bridge implants into the fimbria–fornix cavity, which resulted in an increased level of NGF accumulating in the host septum, and provided a substrate for substantial cholinergic fibre ingrowth.

An alternative source for achieving sustained delivery of physiological levels of NGF is directly to engineer cells for neural transplantation. Considerable preliminary success has been achieved in the transfection of fibroblasts and maintained cell lines with a variety of reporter and neuroactive genes, including the NGF gene. These engineered cells have been demonstrated to be capable of secreting NGF, and to have biological activity following transplantation. Thus, for example, intraventricular implants of NGF-secreting cells can rescue septal cholinergic neurones from the retrograde death induced by axotomy (Rosenberg et al., 1988), although the functional efficacy of such grafts is still largely unknown. This latter approach will be further discussed in Chapter Nine, since the major developments have all involved engineering cells to deliver growth factors into the brain.

THE CRITICAL NEUROPATHOLOGY OF ALZHEIMER'S DISEASE

The studies in the preceding sections have all been based on the view that degeneration in identified populations of subcortical neurones—predominantly cholinergic—underlies the relevant functional deficits of dementia. In summary:

(1) Experimental studies in animals certainly indicate that many deficits associated with selective lesions of basal forebrain cholinergic systems can be alleviated by grafts of cholinergic neurones implanted into the cortex and hippocampus.
(2) Similarly, certain aspects of cholinergic cell loss and atrophy induced by axotomy or related insults can be rescued by neurotrophic mechanisms, and grafts can be used as an alternative route for neurotrophic factor delivery.
(3) Some deficits in aged animals can be alleviated by embryonic grafts rich in different neurotransmitter-specific populations of cells (including cholinergic, noradrenergic, and dopaminergic neurones) placed in different forebrain sites, suggesting that at least some of the deficits in aged animals may be related to particular patterns of forebrain neurotransmitter loss.

Nevertheless, the applicability of this neurotransmitter-specific approach to Alzheimer's disease (and indeed to most other forms of dementia) has been subject to increasing challenge. The basic problem is that these changes are most probably secondary to the fundamental degenerative process in dementia. Consequently, it may indeed be possible to induce functional recovery with a pharmacologically specific (e.g. a cholinomimetic) treatment when experimental damage is restricted to disturbance of cholinergic regulation of the neocortex or hippocampus. However, it is quite unlikely that a similar treatment will have any beneficial effect when the cholinergic loss is accompanied by the widespread degeneration of cortical or hippocampal targets, as occurs in various dementing diseases, whichever component of the degeneration turns out to be primary.

Cortical and subcortical cell loss

Prior to the recent interest in identified neurochemical systems of the subcortical forebrain, dementia of whatever cause has classically been associated with neuropathology in the neocortex. This can include widespread cell loss, atrophy of the cortical mantle, and enlargement of the ventricles, as well as the classical senile plaques and neurofibrillary tangles of Alzheimer's disease and the multiple small foci of perivascular degeneration in multi-infarct dementia (Mann, 1985, 1997; Tomlinson et al., 1970). The symptomatology of dementia, involving a global impairment of intellect, reason, and personality, as well as pronounced deficits in memory and new learning, may best be considered as "the result of a more or less extensive destruction or disorganisation of the cerebral cortex" (Tomlinson & Corsellis, 1984). The bulk of evidence suggests that the subcortical cell loss in, for example, cholinergic systems is secondary to the cortical degeneration rather than its cause (Pearson & Powell, 1989).

Transplantation strategies have been used both to study this retrograde response and to attempt structural repair of the damaged neocortex. Thus, Sofroniew and Pearson (1985) used kainic acid and NMDA (N-methyl-D-aspartic acid) to lesion cortical neurones without inducing direct destruction of the afferent cholinergic terminals. Such lesions nevertheless result in retrograde atrophy of cholinergic neurones in the basal forebrain. However, the survival and healthy morphology of these cholinergic cells can be rescued by target replacement, achieved by implanting embryonic neocortical tissues back into the denervated neocortex (Sofroniew et al., 1986). Nevertheless, although these cortical grafts did attract sprouting and re-innervation by host cholinergic axons, as well as supporting survival of the host cholinergic neurones, the grafted cortical cells did not establish long-distance efferent connections with the host brain and they were consequently without effect on the functional deficits induced by the cortical lesions in the host animals (Sofroniew et al., 1990a).

Amyloid, plaques, and tangles in dementia

Over the past decade there has been a substantial switch in Alzheimer's disease research away from analysis of the cortical and subcortical degeneration in identified neurotransmitter systems towards the cellular and molecular analysis of the critical neurodegenerative elements of the disease. The senile plaque and the neurofibrillary tangle have been diagnostic hallmarks of Alzheimer's disease since the turn of the century. However, it has only been in the past 10 years that the amino acid structure of the βA4 amyloid protein (which constitutes the core of the senile plaque) has been identified, and the gene for the amyloid precursor protein (APP) from which it is cleaved has been located on chromosome 21, cloned and sequenced (Kang et al., 1987). In parallel, the contribution of tau and other neurofilament proteins to neurofibrillary tangles and their paired helical filament ultrastructure is now well described (Goedert, 1993; Goedert et al., 1988; Wischik et al., 1985). Furthermore, other genes, including the presenilins and isoforms of apolipoprotein E, provide genetic influences on the likelihood of developing Alzheimer's disease (Hardy, 1997; Strittmatter & Roses, 1996). These developments are leading to fundamental new insights into the ways in which abnormal expression, processing, and cleavage of normal proteins can lead to the cascade of events that end in the characteristic neuronal degeneration of Alzheimer's disease.

GRAFT MODELS OF THE CELLULAR PATHOLOGY

In the light of these developments in understanding the neuropathology of Alzheimer's disease and other dementias, several recent studies have employed neural transplants in the search for better models of the underlying neurodegenerative processes. To date, these models are restricted to the demonstration and analysis of the cellular pathology, and have not yet been developed into the realms of functional analysis or repair.

Cellular pathology in ageing grafts

One approach has been to employ neural transplantation strategies to investigate cellular ageing processes in isolated tissues, relatively separate from the global host environment. For example, Eriksdotter-Nilsson and colleagues (1989a,b) have followed the survival and anatomical development of cerebellar and hippocampal tissues over 22–23 months following transplantation into the anterior eye chamber. The aged grafts developed increased gliosis, and a marked accumulation of autofluorescent lipofuscin granules, both of which are characteristic features of the normal ageing process in the brain.

A second approach has been to focus on morphological changes in the neurones or glia of ageing grafts. One intriguing observation has been the demonstration of Hirano bodies and immunoreactivity with neurofilament antibodies (both of which are characteristic of tangle-bearing cortical and hippocampal neurones in Alzheimer's disease) in CNS (central nervous system) grafts isolated for greater than 6 months in a peripheral transplantation site (Doering & Aguayo, 1987). However, other markers of senile plaques or neurofibrillary tangles, such as staining with Congo red, thioflavin-S, or antibodies against paired helical filaments, were not observed in these grafts. Nevertheless, these observations provided a clear demonstration of the accumulation of individual features of the human neuropathology in isolated grafts, and offer model systems in which their development might be studied experimentally.

A third strategy has been to implant pathological tissues in an attempt to identify pathogenic processes in the grafts or host brain. For example, van den Bosch de Aguilar and colleagues (1984) transplanted fragments of temporal cortex from a post-mortem Alzheimer brain to the cortex of young adult rats. The grafts were seen to contain abundant neurofibrillary tangles and induced an extensive fibrous gliosis in the host brain. This included the occurrence of filament bundles in host brain astrocytes, which were considered to be structurally similar to Alzheimer's paired helical filaments, and were interpreted as suggesting either the incorporation of abnormal structural subunits into host cytoskeleton or the presence of some transmissible pathogenic agent within the diseased brain. However, no neurones were found to have survived within the xenografts, which is not surprising given the absence of any immunosuppression. Therefore, although this study employed neural transplantation, it is conceptually more similar to inoculation strategies using pathogens or pathogenic tissues such as have been used to identify neurodegenerative processes associated with toxins, prions, or slow viruses.

The trisomy 16 transplant model

A novel approach to the induction of Alzheimer-like pathology in grafts is based on the association between Down's syndrome and Alzheimer's disease. In addition to the physical features and mental subnormality that are the well-known consequences of the genetic defect in Down's syndrome, namely trisomy of chromosome 21, affected individuals also develop at 30–50 years of age the typical amyloid plaques and neurofibrillary tangles characteristic of Alzheimer's disease (Oliver & Holland, 1986). This suggests that overexpression of genes on chromosome 21 can lead to the neuropathology of Alzheimer's disease, and conversely that Alzheimer's disease may be due to abnormal expression of chromosome 21 gene(s). Since many genes and markers on human chromosome 21 map to chromosome 16 in mouse, trisomy 16 mice might provide an animal model not only of human Down's syndrome but also of the neuropathological features of Alzheimer's disease.

It has not been possible to test the trisomy 16 mouse model for long-term pathology, since trisomy 16 foetuses do not survive beyond term. However, using a neural transplantation strategy, pieces of embryonic trisomy 16 tissue can be implanted into the brains of normal host mice to study the long-term development of abnormal pathology in the tissue. Sarah-Jane Richards and colleagues (1991), transplanted neocortex and hippocampus from trisomy 16 embryos into the frontal and retrosplenial cortex, respectively, of normal young

TABLE 7.1
Patterns of neuropathological staining in Trisomy 16 grafts*

Antibody or stain	*Host*	*Control graft*	*Trisomy 16 graft*
Thioflavin-S	–	–	intracellular
Palmgren silver	fibres	fibres	fibres and intracellular
Amyloid precursor protein	–	–	intra- and extracellular
βA4 amyloid protein	–	–	intracellular
α1-antichymotrypsin	–	–	intra- and extracellular
Paired helical filaments (A128)	–	–	intracellular
Tau protein (monoclonal 6.423)	–	–	intracellular
Glial fibrillary acidic protein (GFAP)	astrocytes and processes	cell bodies	astrocyte processes
Ubiquitin	processes	processes	processes and occasional cell bodies

* Data from Richards et al. (1991)

adult host mice. Control grafts were derived from normal embryos from the same litters, and were subjected to the identical implantation and subsequent tissue processing as the grafts derived from the trisomy 16 donors. The development of any neuropathological changes in the grafts was then investigated after 4 months' survival. The trisomy 16 grafts were found to contain neuronal cells that were immunostained by a variety of antibodies that recognise pathological features in the Alzheimer's brain (see Table 7.1). In particular, abnormal staining with antibodies to both amyloid and tau was of a similar pattern to that observed in neurones in Alzheimer brain, and co-localised within the same cells. No similar immunoreactivity was seen either in control grafts taken from littermates or in the trisomic embryos.

Before the development of new transgenic lines, this graft paradigm provided the first viable animal model for monitoring the development of the cellular pathology involved in the human disease. However, because the neuronal pathology is seen developing within a self-contained graft tissue, there have as yet been no clear functional deficits associated with any pathology in the otherwise intact brain of the normal host mice.

Future prospects for better functional animal models

As noted above, transplantation models have so far been restricted to the development and analysis of the cellular neuropathology of Alzheimer's disease in experimental animals, and have not yet progressed to studies of the potential of grafts for functional repair in more valid models of that cellular pathology. In particular, there are several techniques for mimicking individual neuropathological features of dementia (Dunnett & Barth, 1991):

(1) *Scrapie.* Intracerebral inoculation of mice with certain strains of the scrapie virus can induce extensive spongiform encephalopathy and amyloid plaque formation, and deficits in passive avoidance can be detected even before the appearance of overt neuropathology.
(2) *Aluminium.* Intracerebral injection of high concentrations of aluminium salts has been seen to induce the formation of widespread neurofibrillary degeneration in rabbits, rats, and cats, and is associated with impairments in a variety of learning tasks as well as the pronounced ataxia and motor impairments that lead to rapid death in this model. However, neither the scrapie nor the aluminium model reproduces the actual pathological elements in the human disease, either in terms of the distribution of neuropathological changes or of the detailed molecular structure of the induced neurofibrillary deposits.
(3) *Transgenic mice.* A potentially better approach may be the recent development of strains of transgenic mice which overexpress particular isoforms of the amyloid precursor protein gene (Games et al., 1995; Quon et al., 1991), and at least one such strain of transgenic mice manifests mild but significant deficits in learning the Morris water maze spatial navigation task (Yamaguchi et al., 1991).

Although these various approaches may ultimately provide better functional models of particular aspects of the cellular neuropathology that underlies human dementia, unfortunately none is yet at the stage of producing convincing replication of the pathogenetic processes seen in human Alzheimer's disease, and none has yet been used to evaluate possibilities of repair by neural transplantation.

CLINICAL PROSPECTS IN DEMENTIA

To summarise the studies in experimental animals, neural transplants have been demonstrated to have at least a limited capacity to reconstruct identified neurotransmitter systems in the brain, and to provide functional recovery on relevant behavioural tests of cognitive function. This applies in particular to neuronal systems that are highly branched and diffuse in their distribution and which probably function to provide a regulation of their target structures (such as the cholinergic, adrenergic, serotonergic, or dopaminergic neurones of the isodendritic core), rather than to systems involved in the precise point-to-point relay of information between processing centres of the brain.

Such observations have been considered to be relevant to human dementia, in particular within the context of the cholinergic hypothesis of Alzheimer's disease. Indeed, clinical trials of central NGF administration to protect the cholinergic neurones have been attempted in Alzheimer's disease (Seiger et al., 1993). It may be argued that the limited success so far achieved with such a strategy relates to the problems of delivery of large molecules such as trophic factors across the blood–brain barrier into the central nervous system—problems which may in turn be addressed by new developments in transplantation (see Chapter Nine). Conversely, for reasons we have outlined, it may be the case that the generalised and widespread degeneration associated with the major dementias will never be susceptible to effective therapy by protection or replacement of a single neurotransmitter system.

It is the view of the present authors that the optimism for transplantation offering any major new opportunities in this area may be misplaced, other than (perhaps) in particular, circumscribed circumstances. Thus, the cholinergic deficit may indeed be central to some of the cognitive deficits in natural ageing, and it may also be relevant to certain dementias of subcortical origin. However, it is unlikely that transplantation surgery would be warranted in these conditions, either because the disorder is not sufficiently debilitating (as in the increased forgetfulness associated with normal ageing), or because the cognitive disorder is a secondary consideration to other more profound problems (as in the motor disorder of advanced parkinsonism).

By contrast, the available data suggest that the predominant dementing diseases of the Alzheimer's and multi-infarct types involve extensive degeneration and cell loss in the neo- and allocortex that cannot be attributed to a primary loss of circumscribed populations of subcortical regulatory systems. It may never be feasible to consider reconstruction of such widespread target degeneration by the replacement of individual regulatory inputs.

To date, the experimental repair of complex cortical circuits by neural transplantation in adult animals has proved to be of only limited success, and in those cases where benefit has been positively demonstrated it is almost certainly due to relatively non-specific trophic repair processes rather than the reconstruction of the damaged circuitry by the grafts (Kolb & Fantie, 1994). It should be noted that extensive reconstruction in complex neural circuits such as the neocortex is not ruled out in principle, as evidenced by the degree of recovery that can be achieved following transplantation in neostriatal systems (see Chapter Six). Rather, the conditions for similar patterns of repair have not yet been identified in the neocortex.

It is likely that our rapidly expanding understanding of the molecular and genetic events that give rise to the cellular degeneration and abnormal amyloid and neurofibrillary deposits in Alzheimer's disease will lead to the identification of novel strategies to inhibit and repair the neuropathology of dementia. Indeed, neural transplantation techniques are contributing to the development of new models of these processes, and it is plausible that they may also come to play a role in the treatment of dementing diseases. However, such advances must remain purely speculative until we can identify the principal neuronal elements and primary pathological events that constitute Alzheimer's disease and other dementias.

SUMMARY

In this chapter we have concluded that Alzheimer's dementia and related diseases involve a widespread cortical and subcortical pathology, involving cellular degeneration for reasons that are still not well understood. It is possible to mimic many of the features of this disease in animals, and indeed some of the neuropathological models themselves involve cellular transplantation. Similarly, it is possible to alleviate many particular aspects of cellular degeneration by cell transplantation, including selective degeneration of cholinergic and noradrenergic systems of the forebrain. However, to the extent that the human disease is widespread in both the classes of cells and the areas of brain affected, it is not plausible in the foreseeable future to achieve cellular repair other than of selected components of the disease, and there is at present little evidence that this will lead rapidly to substantial therapeutic benefit.

CHAPTER EIGHT

Spinal cord injury: The ultimate challenge

SPINAL CORD INJURY

For many, spinal cord injury represents "the big one"—the ultimate challenge for repair of damage in the CNS (central nervous system). Not only is the challenge tinged with magic—making the lame walk—but success also involves regeneration and precise reconnection of some of the longest axons of the nervous system—the corticospinal and ascending sensory tracts. If we can achieve regeneration over these distances of this order with functional benefit then perhaps anything is within our grasp.

Of course it turns out not to be that simple: different types of damage have been considered, with different graft strategies appropriate for each, and many different models have been pursued with a varying amount of success. As a starting point we should consider the consequences of spinal cord injury, to identify the nature of the problem to be addressed.

Severe spinal injuries resulting in paralysis affect approximately 750 people per year in the UK, numbers that are even more devastating when it is realised that the majority of those affected are teenagers and young adults, in particular following riding and motor cycle accidents.

The basic elements for repair of spinal injury are illustrated in Fig. 8.1.

First and foremost, spinal injury is a pure "disconnection" syndrome (Geschwind, 1965a,b)—disconnecting the descending fibre tracts of the corticospinal motor pathways to the spinal cord motor neurones and the ascending somatosensory inputs from the periphery and spinal cord to the brain. Intrinsic circuits of the spinal cord below the transection are left intact, including the primary motor neurone connections with the muscles, but they are now disconnected

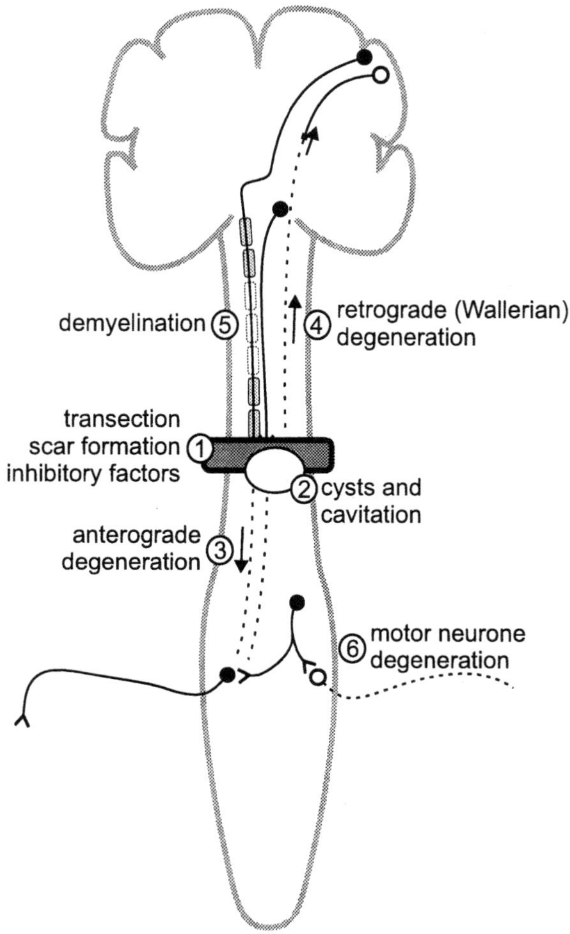

FIG. 8.1. Degenerative consequences of spinal cord injury and disease. (1) Transection injuries result in a disconnection of ascending and descending axons and scar formation at the site of injury. (2) Cysts form at the site of injury which can expand along the cord rostral and caudal to the site of injury. (3) The distal portions of cut axons degenerate by necrosis. (4) The proximal portion of cut axons may degenerate by loss of target support. Other more selective cell loss can result in specific diseases, including, (5) demyelination in multiple sclerosis, and (6) degeneration of motor neurones in amyotrophic lateral sclerosis.

from all descending control, resulting in paralysis: either solely in the legs (paraparesis) or all four limbs (quadriparesis) depending on the level of injury. Similarly, all afferent information concerning touch, pain, and joint position sense are lost to the supraspinal somatosensory areas of the brain, resulting in anaesthesia, although under some circumstances additional secondary sensory sequelae can develop, such as phantom limb pain. Since the primary spinal cord lesion is one of axotomy, the primary goal of any therapy is not so much to replace lost neurones as to stimulate axons to regenerate in both ascending and descending pathways to re-innervate their appropriate distal targets.

As a transected axon degenerates, there is necrotic degeneration of the distal axon following disconnection from the cell body. In addition to which axotomy can also result in retrograde degeneration of the axon (Wallerian degeneration), which in part is mediated through a loss of target-derived trophic support (see Chapters One and Two). Furthermore, the spinal insult precipitating axonal loss is typically associated with an inflammatory reaction and the formation of astrocytic scar tissue, which provides a physical barrier for regenerative regrowth. This, coupled to changes in the capacity of glial cells to secrete and remove toxic molecules from their environment, further impedes the regenerative process.

In addition to the axotomy and glial scar a further event takes place in the cord that needs to be considered. As cellular tissue dies, cysts filled with cerebrospinal fluid (a so-called "syrinx") form at the site of spinal injury; these can expand in a rostral as well as a caudal direction, resulting in further development of symptoms as progressively more levels of the cord are affected.

Thus all of these events need to be addressed when considering spinal cord repair after trauma. However, the spinal cord can be affected in other ways, most notably in multiple sclerosis (MS), in which there is focal demyelination of axons in the spinal cord (as well as other more rostral sites such as brain, brainstem, optic nerve, etc.), and amyotrophic lateral sclerosis (ALS) in which there is a selective degeneration of motor neurones resulting in a rapidly progressive motor decline leading to death within 2–3 years. In these neurological conditions the repair strategy will be different, as selective subpopulations of cells need replacing—namely, oligodendrocytes within MS and motor neurones within ALS.

SPINAL CORD GRAFTS

Potential mechanisms of spinal cord repair

The variety of degenerative processes contributing to the functional deficits associated with spinal cord injury means that a variety of approaches have been adopted to promote spontaneous regeneration as well as explicit repair. Many of these strategies involve transplantation of tissue either to replace lost neurones and/or to act as a stimulus for host regeneration. Therefore to date the following main strategies have been adopted (Fig. 8.2):

(1) Grafts as a source of trophic or anti-inhibitory molecules: To stimulate host axons to regenerate back to distal targets and overcome the inhibitory influences of the host glial environment.
(2) Grafts to inhibit cyst development: To fill cysts and reduce the pressures leading to cyst development, thereby reducing the slow progression of the symptoms from syrinx expansion.

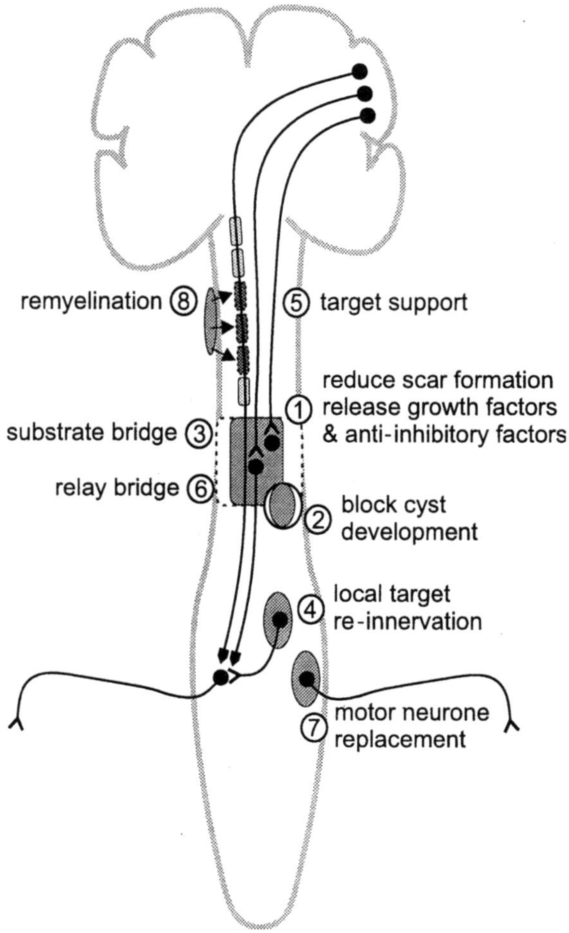

FIG. 8.2. Strategies for graft-derived repair in the injured (or diseased) spinal cord. (1) Grafts as a source of reparative molecules to reduce scar formation and to release growth and anti-inhibitory factors. (2) Grafts to inhibit cyst development. (3) Grafts to provide a growth substrate for regeneration of host axons. (4) Grafts to provide a local re-innervation of deafferented distal targets. (5) Grafts to provide target-derived trophic support against retrograde degeneration. (6) Grafts to provide a relay bridge to reconnect distal targets. (7) Grafts to replace lost motor neurones. (8) Grafted glial cells to remyelinate demyelinated axons.

(3) Grafts as substrate bridges: The graft provides a substrate for axon regeneration, enabling penetration through the astrocytic scar and across the site of transection.

(4) Grafts as a source of local afferents: Even if long-distance regeneration is not achieved, some aspects of reflex control may be provided by local re-innervation of regulatory afferent systems (e.g. of catecholamine or indoleamine neurones).

(5) Grafts provide target support: Grafts can provide alternative sources of target support for axotomised axons, preventing or reducing retrograde degenerative changes.
(6) Grafts as relay bridges: As an alternative to using bridges of tissue that provide a substrate for long-distance regeneration of host axons, distal targets may be reconnected using bridges of embryonic neural tissue which are not only capable of acting as substrate bridges but also as a source of local afferents. Furthermore, embryonic neurones in grafts may have a greater capacity for growth into the distal stump than have the transected axons of the adult brain. This will restore the circuitry so long as the grafted neurones are themselves innervated by local sprouting of host afferents.

Evidence for each of these processes will be explored in turn. Moreover, as individual strategies become refined, the argument turns out not to be whether one approach is better than another, but rather how the different approaches can be optimally combined. Finally, we will want to consider two special types of spinal cord lesion in which identified populations of cells are lost as a consequence of disease, namely:

(7) Grafts to replace lost motor neurones in various forms of motor neurone disease in which the grafted cells have a different requirement, i.e. to replace the lost motor neurones of the ventral horn that innervate skeletal muscles.
(8) Grafts to replace lost glia: The selective loss of oligodendrocytes results in demyelination and dysfunction of long-distance axon pathways in the CNS in MS. Recent evidence suggests that it may be possible to remyelinate central axons by implants of oligodendrocyte precursors resulting in restitution of axon transmission and thus function.

Grafts as a source of trophic or anti-inhibitory molecules

In Chapter One, we identified several of the factors that limit axon regeneration in the adult mammalian CNS, of which one of the most important is the inhibitory glial environment. As a result, Martin Schwab and colleagues raised antibodies ("IN-1") against an inhibitory fraction of CNS white matter and demonstrated that the antibody blocked the contact inhibition exerted by oligodendrocytes on growth cones in tissue culture (Bandtlow et al., 1990), and by so doing allowed axons to grow over their surface. Moreover, when applied *in vivo*, following partial transection of the spinal cord, animals treated with the IN-1 antibody showed much greater axon regrowth into the distal segment of the spinal cord than was seen in control animals (Fig. 8.3; Schnell & Schwab, 1990, 1993),

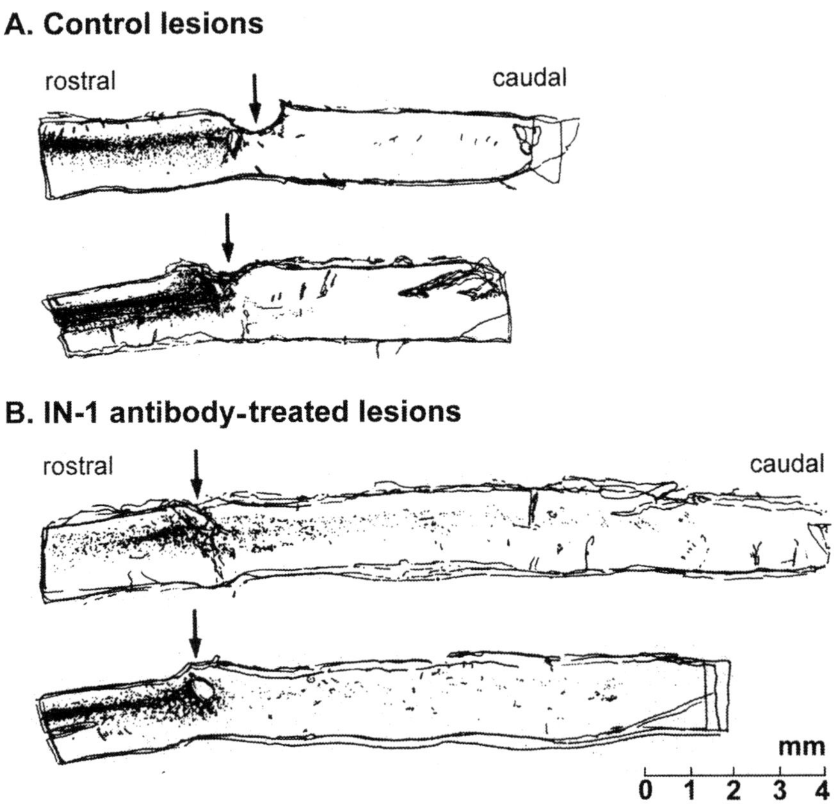

FIG. 8.3. Regeneration of host corticospinal axons in the distant segment of the hemitransected spinal cord is promoted by treatment with the anti-inhibitory IN-1 antibody. Chronic delivery of IN-1 is achieved by implantation of antibody-secreting hybridoma cells into the brain ventricle. (Reproduced from Schnell & Schwab, 1990, reprinted with permission *Nature* © Macmillan Magazines Limited.)

with some recovery of specific reflex and locomotor functions (Bregman et al., 1995).

In these studies, in order to deliver IN-1 into the spinal cord, antibody-producing hybridoma cells were implanted as a tissue graft into the third ventricle of the brain. Thus, although the mechanism of action is effectively the pharmacological delivery of a molecule, the function of which is to promote plasticity of damaged host axons, the pharmacokinetic problems of delivery of such large molecules lead to the use of tissue transplantation as the preferred method of targeted delivery into the CNS.

A similar strategy is likely to apply to the delivery of other trophic as well as anti-inhibitory molecules into the damaged spinal cord. For example, several neurotrophins, in particular NT-3, can also enhance regeneration of corticospinal axons following axotomy, and this trophic influence is additive to the effects of the IN-1 antibody treatment (Schnell et al., 1994). Thus combining both treatments to promote axon survival, growth, and sprouting, as well as blocking the inhibitory effects of the host environment, results in a more effective therapy than either treatment alone. Although in this study, the IN-1 antibody was delivered by grafting, the growth factor molecules were injected centrally. As will be seen in the context of amyotrophic lateral sclerosis (q.v.), cells engineered to deliver growth factors are under active development, and the combination of trophic and anti-inhibitory influences in co-grafts represents a technology primed for development.

Nevertheless, the degree of regeneration and recovery achieved by such pharmacological manipulations alone remains somewhat limited, both at the level of axon regrowth and functional recovery. Moreover, this strategy is more obviously effective in situations of partial injury where individual spinal pathways are cut but the continuity of the cord remains, as opposed to situations of total transection and complete disconnection of the proximal and distal stumps.

Grafts inhibit cyst development

In clinical terms, the problems associated with spinal cord injury can be exacerbated, over and above the deficits associated with the primary spinal trauma, by the formation of fluid-filled cysts at the site of injury which then expand progressively into the rostral and caudal segments of the cord. This is particularly harmful when the expansion is in the rostral direction, impinging upon higher levels of the cord that were previously unaffected, with the associated rise in the level of dysfunction.

Seiger and colleagues have tackled this by grafting embryonic spinal cord into the cystic cavities, which has the effect of reducing their spread. This has so far been demonstrated to be effective in rats (Åkesson et al., 1998), and is now under initial clinical evaluation, although it is too early to say whether it is of clinical benefit.

Grafts as substrate bridges

One of the problems of regeneration in the CNS, as discussed in Chapter One, is that spontaneous axon regeneration is rather limited in the adult mammalian brain and spinal cord. However, since we know that axons do regenerate well along peripheral nerves, a peripheral nerve transplanted to the spinal cord could be used as a bridge along which central axons can grow (Fig. 1.6). David and Aguayo (1981) used such an approach and found that axons from neurones in the brainstem grew through the peripheral nerve and back into the distal part of the spinal cord, whilst axons of spinal neurones grew through the bridge and back into the spinal cord. It is therefore possible to stimulate central axon

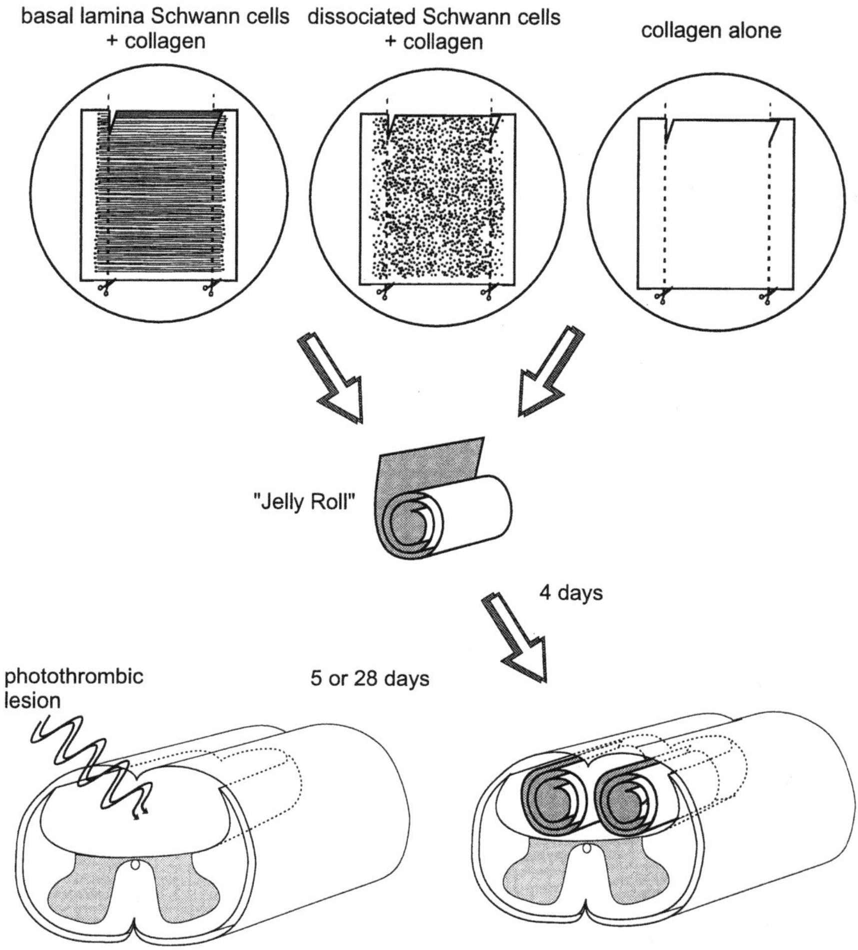

FIG. 8.4. Schwann cell matrix implanted into the photochemically lesioned spinal cord as a "jelly roll" bridge. (Redrawn from Paino et al., 1994, reprinted with permission.)

regeneration and bridge a spinal cord injury in both directions by providing a suitable growth substrate for regenerative axon growth.

As a consequence a search for more practical and suitable tissue substrates for CNS axon regeneration has been undertaken. The starting point as one might expect has been the Schwann cell, since this peripheral glial cell provides a powerful source of both growth factors and substrate molecules for axon growth.

Mary Bunge and colleagues have purified Schwann cells and packed them in a polymer tube that can be implanted directly into the site of transection (Fig. 8.4). The goal here is to reintegrate the cut ends of the injured cord, to inhibit the formation of a glial scar, to provide a suitable cellular substrate for regeneration of host axons between the cut surfaces, and to provide improved guidance of axons back to appropriate distal targets. So far it has been possible to stimulate axon growth into and through the peripheral nerve conduit, but as yet the outgrowth into the distal stump remains limited (Paino & Bunge, 1991; Xu et al., 1995, 1997). Again, combination strategies suggest themselves and so Guest and colleagues have combined the Schwann cell bridges with fibroblast growth factor (FGF) and IN-1 antibody treatments to enhance the extent of regeneration across the cavity (Guest et al., 1997).

It is clear that peripheral glia provide a substantial stimulus for axon regeneration in the injured spinal cord, but there are two main limitations of this technique:

(1) Only neurones very close to the point of insertion of the peripheral nerve grow in, and certainly not those located at a distance (such as the pyramidal neurones of the motor cortex).
(2) Once axons have traversed the peripheral bridge they do not continue to grow back to their appropriate targets in the host brain or spinal cord, but appear to stop in the less hospitable CNS environment.

Although it is now clear that Schwann cell bridges can stimulate sprouting and regeneration of remote cell bodies, including ingrowth from the descending pyramidal tract neurones, the extent of outgrowth remains considerably limited. Although the extent of plasticity that has been achieved should not be undervalued, the limited axon regeneration of mature nerve sprouts once they have penetrated back into the distal cord stump is at present the biggest problem with the primary peripheral glial graft approach.

Grafts as a source of local afferents

A potentially simpler strategy for spinal repair may be provided by a restricted replacement of neurochemical inputs which modulate local reflexes. The spinal cord, apart from containing highly organised descending motor and ascending sensory pathways that transmit complex information, has within it a large number of local neuronal circuits which are modulated by regulatory inputs from a number of diffusely innervating brainstem nuclei. These inputs may prove easier to replace than some of the more complex circuits found within the cord (Nógrádi & Vrbová, 1994). For example, control of the bladder or ejaculation are under descending regulation from noradrenergic and serotonergic systems of the brainstem and, although their restoration will not allow a paralysed patient to walk, the possibility of restitution of bladder control or reflex sexual capacities would nevertheless represent substantial benefits to such individuals. Moreover, although the intention and commands to initiate walking and other voluntary actions are of forebrain origin, the co-ordinated sequencing of locomotion is in part organised in local reflex circuits (central or locomotor pattern generators) at

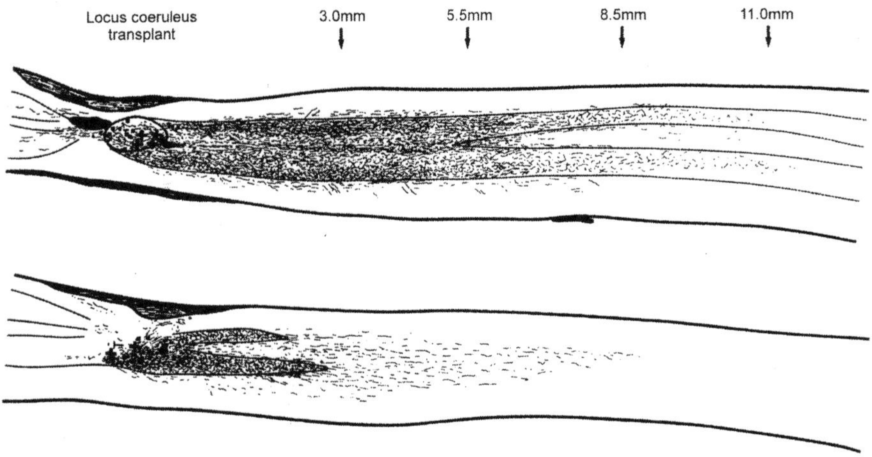

FIG. 8.5. Extensive noradrenergic re-innervation of the 6-OHDA denervated spinal cord by locus coeruleus grafts. (Reproduced from Nornes et al., 1983, with permission © Springer-Verlag.)

the level of the spinal cord itself. It is therefore plausible that local regulatory inputs can influence and modify pattern generators even if they do not restore voluntary actions.

Akin to nigral grafts in Parkinson's disease (discussed in Chapter Four), one primary strategy at this level of repair has been to implant embryonic monoaminergic neurones ectopically into the lower spinal cord, and investigate consequent changes in tonic control and reflex function. Spinal cord transection will completely remove the rich noradrenergic and serotonergic innervations of the spinal cord that normally originate in the brainstem, and grafts of brainstem neurones can provide an effective and extensive replacement of these local innervations (Foster et al., 1990; Nornes et al., 1983; Privat et al., 1989) (Fig. 8.5).

Moreover, the implants restore a degree of reflex function. Thus, for example raphé grafts in the distal cord below a transection can restore penile erection and ejaculation reflexes in rats (Privat et al., 1988). Perhaps even more impressive are the observations that implants of noradrenergic neurones can restore certain placing and withdrawal reflexes, and increased reflexive stepping not only after selective 6-hydroxydopamine (6-OHDA) lesions (Buchanan & Nornes, 1986; Moorman et al., 1990) but also after spinal transections at the level of the thoracic cord (Yakovleff et al., 1989, 1995).

Grafts provide target support

Grafts can provide alternative sources of target support for axotomised axons, and by so doing prevent or reduce retrograde degenerative changes. This is particularly true when the damage is sustained early in life at the time when developing neurones are particularly dependent upon trophic support from their targets to define and maintain appropriate patterns of connectivity (see Chapter Two).

A clear example of this graft-derived protection has been demonstrated in the red nucleus. Spinal cord damage in neonatal rats results in massive retrograde degeneration of the rubrospinal tract, and cell atrophy and loss within the red nucleus itself. Bregman and Reier (1986) therefore grafted embryonic spinal cord tissue into a midthoracic spinal cord lesion and found an almost complete rescue of the rubral neurones: Cell numbers decreased from a control level of 3500 in the intact red nucleus to 1500 in lesion animals, and returned back up to 3400 cells in the ipsilateral red nucleus of grafted animals. Back-labelling with horseradish peroxidase (HRP) indicated that at least some of the red nucleus axons grew through the grafts to reach distal spinal targets (the grafts serving as a substrate bridge), and whether these axons formed functional synapses was not addressed in this experiment. Subsequent studies have now shown that a similar pattern of rescue can be observed in the adult animal, although at this age only about half, rather than all, the neurones are saved (Mori et al., 1997). However, it should be realised that these embryonic neuronal grafts also receive synaptic inputs from other brainstem nuclei (Himes et al., 1994; Itoh et al., 1993).

Grafts as relay bridges

If embryonic spinal cord grafts can receive inputs from the host and if they can project out into the host cord, then it is possible that the grafts can act to restore ascending and descending spinal circuits by acting as an active relay rather than just a passive bridge for reformation of connections (see Fig. 8.6). If so then the goal will be to utilise the greater regenerative capacities of embryonic graft neurones to target outgrowth (Bregman, 1994; Bregman et al., 1993).

The reason for believing that spinal cord grafts act as neuronal relays rather than passive bridges arises from a comparison of the patterns of axon regrowth and functional recovery after spinal cord injury in the neonatal versus the adult spinal cord (Bregman et al., 1993). Bregman and colleagues implanted embryonic spinal cord into cavities that were made in one half of the spinal cord and reported clear evidence for functional recovery both in neonatal and in adult animals. By contrast, the anatomical regrowth differed considerably between the two different ages of the animals. Following neonatal damage, spinal cord grafts promote extensive re-innervation not only into the graft but also through the graft and back into the host brain (Bregman & Reier, 1986; Bregman, 1987; Bregman et al., 1993), whereas after adult damage there is modest ingrowth into the grafts but very little back into the adult host cord (Bregman et al., 1993—see previous section on substrate bridges). Thus Bregman reasons that whereas following neonatal injury the recovery may be by either type of bridging mechanism, recovery in the adult animal is most plausibly attributable to grafts providing a relay reconstruction of the damaged circuits (Bregman et al., 1993).

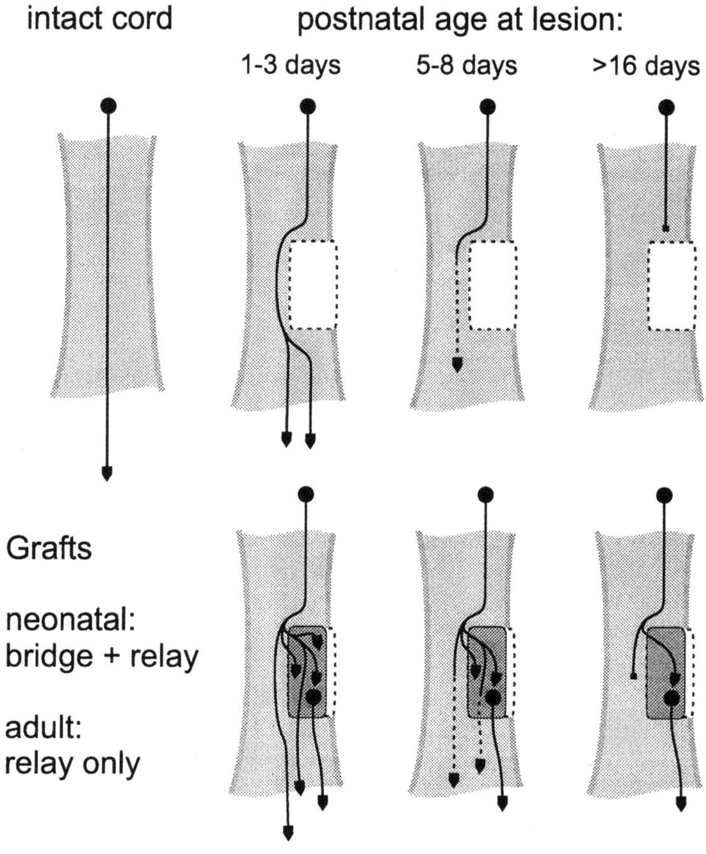

FIG. 8.6. Comparison of two possible mechanisms for circuit repair in the injured spinal cord. Following neonatal lesions, spinal cord grafts provide both a source of neurones to receive and *relay* inputs to distal targets, and a cellular *bridge* that allows regeneration of host axons back to their targets. By contrast, grafts in the adult CNS appear only capable of restoring a relay-type function. (Based on Bregman et al., 1993.)

In this context, then, it is appropriate to consider briefly the extent and limits of functional recovery that have been observed, and seek to identify the factors that determine success. For example, in developing animals, many aspects of accurate locomotion are seen to be restored in animals that received spinal cord grafts after spinal injury at birth, including measures of base support, stepping on a treadmill, hindlimb rotation, etc. (Bregman, 1994). Importantly, the recovery is dependent upon the anatomical contiguity between the grafts and the host spinal cord at the lesion site. In the adult animal, Kunkel-Bagden et al. (1993) have reported that the reduced stride length induced by hemitransection is restored to normal in rats with spinal cord implants, as is the accuracy of foot placement when crossing a grid or a raised runway. Indeed, the precise pattern of recovery after spinal cord grafting can differ considerably between adult and neonatal lesions, reinforcing the hypothesis that different mechanisms may apply (Bregman et al., 1993). Locomotion on treadmill stepping tests is of course susceptible to reactivation of local spinal circuits. Recovery on more complex and voluntary tests such as climbing over objects and reaching has been demonstrated in grafted rats that sustained neonatal spinal cord injuries (Diener & Bregman, 1998), but not as yet in animals that sustained their injury as adults.

However, these reports of recovery in mature animals were all obtained in the hemitransection model. It is plausible that control of spinal locomotor pattern generators was generated entirely via descending pathways on the intact side, and the grafts may have replaced some tonic balance between the two sides rather than restoring any descending control. Whereas there is good evidence that spinal cord grafts can restore aspects of muscle tone and stepping following complete spinal transection in neonatal animals, there is as yet no good evidence for restitution of voluntary motor control based on spinal grafts alone after complete lesions in the adult.

Combination strategies

Increasingly it is being realised that restitution of function after adult spinal cord lesion will only be achieved if a variety of approaches are combined, given the number of reactive events induced by such a lesion (see Fig. 8.1). Specifically, Fawcett and Geller (1998) argue that four different strategies will be required together:

(1) Trophic factor stimulation to promote regrowth of CNS axons and plasticity of connections.
(2) Blockers of myelin inhibition, for example using the IN-1 antibody, to reduce the inhibitory nature of the host CNS.
(3) Counteracting the glial scar, based on the recent recognition that reactive astrocytes can prove as inhibitory to growth and regeneration as the oligodendrocytes (S.J.A. Davies et al., 1997).
(4) Grafts of bridging cells, whether involving substrates for axon regrowth or embryonic neurones for relay of connections.

The first studies attempting to combine these strategies are showing considerable optimism. Thus Cheng et al. (1996) bridged complete spinal cord transections with the following combination of therapies (see Fig. 8.7):

(1) Peripheral glial bridge based on multiple segments of intercostal nerve (18 fine nerve implants per gap).
(2) Re-routing of the pathways by running the bridge from white to grey matter so as to avoid the inhibitory influence of central myelin.

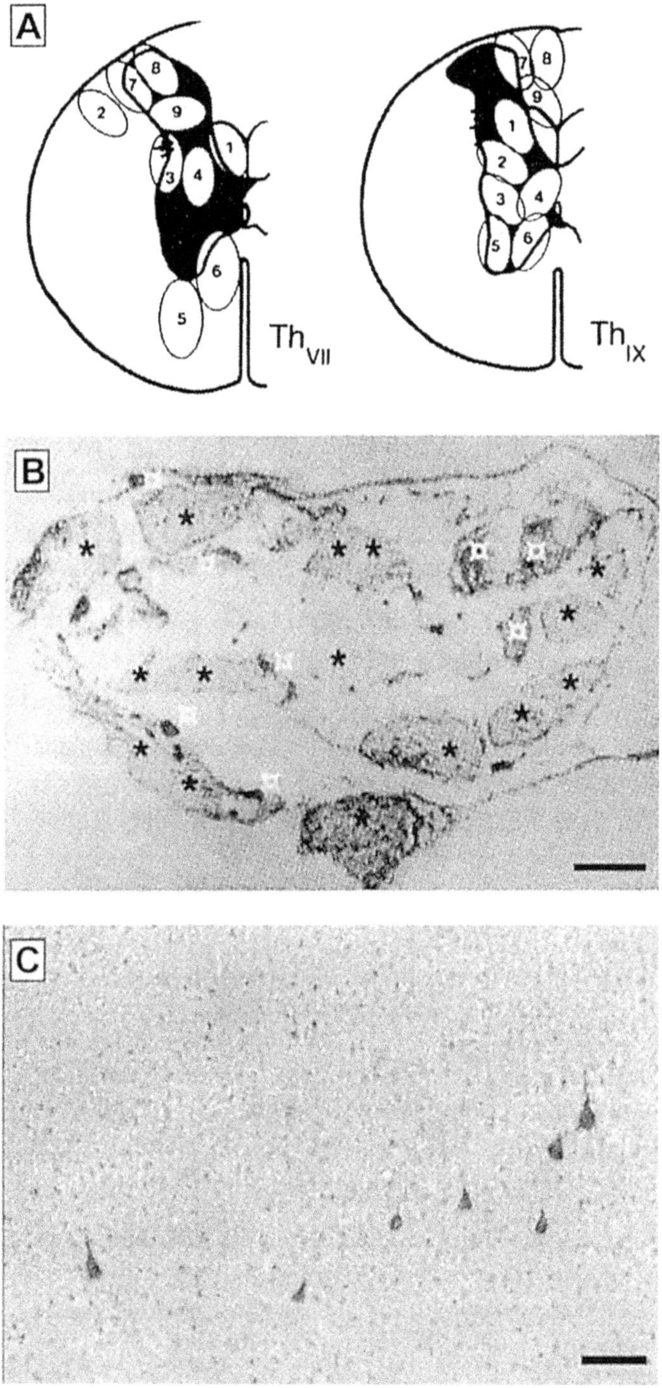

FIG. 8.7. Reconstruction of injury at thoracic (ThVII–ThIX) levels of the spinal cord by implantation of multiple segments of intercostal nerve combined with suturing, stabilisation in fibrin glue, and additional growth factor treatments. (A) Location of proximal and distal ends of nerve segments. (B) Histological visualisation of intercostal nerve segments (asterisks) in cross-section. (C) Retrograde labelling of cortical neurones projecting through the graft to innervate distal spinal cord. (Reproduced from Cheng et al., 1996, with permission © American Association for the Advancement of Science.)

(3) Stabilisation of the lesion and graft by fibrin glue, to which had been added the growth factor, acidic FGF.
(4) Fixation of the whole reconstruction to prevent flexion damage by the wiring of the spine into a rigid dorsiflexion position.

In this study the spinal transection resulted in total loss of hindlimb postural support in the control lesion rats, with the limbs extended and rotated outwards. Bilateral return of functional postural support was seen in 28% of the combination graft rats, with unilateral improvement seen in all others and occasional additional improvements (as evidenced by a partial return of locomotion involving stepping of all four limbs, the ability to support body weight). A variety of control procedures were without functional effect, and this included intercostal grafts alone or the full combination but with white-matter-to-white-matter bridging. Anatomical studies in three animals showing recovery employed the retrograde tracer HRP, which was injected into the lumbar spinal cord distal to the lesion. In two of these cases many pyramidal neurones were back-labelled in the motor cortex, providing a clear demonstration of restitution of the corticospinal tract.

Although partial functional recovery had been seen previously in a variety of spinal cord lesions (hemisection, crush, contusion, and other partial lesions), a degree of ambiguity remained about the nature and mechanism of recovery in such cases. By contrast the study by Cheng et al. (1996) offers the first clear evidence of significant functional alleviation in rats with complete transection. Indeed, the authors did not just cut the exposed cord but removed a whole 5mm segment, which was then subjected to histological verification to confirm completeness. This experiment therefore unambiguously made the point that these grafts can restore and facilitate anatomical and functional connections in the damaged spinal cord.

Inevitably, the procedures can be further improved. Thus alternative sources of more permissive cells for bridging may become available (Li et al., 1997), more specific and potent combinations of growth factors can certainly be achieved, and the technology of bridging matrices is clearly at an early stage. However, after more than two decades of active research, the apparently intractable problem of spinal injury does at last appear to be yielding to transplantation, and clinical trials of the new combination strategies cannot be far away (Fawcett & Geller, 1998).

MOTOR NEURONE DISEASE

Motor neurone degeneration and replacement

In addition to mechanical or traumatic injury, a second major class of neurological problem arises from neurodegenerative diseases of the spinal cord, such as amyotrophic lateral sclerosis (ALS—a form of motor neurone disease). Several features of this disease make it a more suitable candidate for transplantation. First, it is a circumscribed type of neurone that degenerates (the motor neurones), a situation that favours neural transplantation (see for example Chapters Four and Five). In addition, whereas the grafted motor neurones have to reconnect with distant target muscles to be functional, this re-innervation is via axonal growth along peripheral nerves, a situation that one would expect to be more conducive for regeneration.

Grafts of motor neurones have been investigated in two models of ALS. In the first, motor neurones are lesioned by injection of excitotoxic amino acids directly into the ventral horn in rats, whilst the second model employs a mutant mouse strain in which the motor neurones undergo early degeneration rather like that seen in ALS. Grafts of embryonic motor neurones have been employed in both models, with comparable results: The grafted neurones not only survive but also are seen to generate axons that grow out along appropriate peripheral routes and under certain circumstances can even re-innervate distant target muscles.

The clearest series of studies of motor neurone transplantation are provided by Vrbová and colleagues at University College London. In these studies, the authors crush the sciatic motor nerve in rat pups at birth, which results in total retrograde degeneration of the motor neurones in lumbar segments L4 and L5 that project via the sciatic nerve to the hindlimb musculature (Fig. 8.8A). Grafts of bromodeoxyuridine (BrDU)-labelled motor neurones taken from embryos at the age of their neurogenesis are then implanted into the spinal cord. Although the grafted neurones are unable to grow axons through the host CNS to enter the ventral nerve routes, if the nerve root is itself reimplanted into the host cord adjacent to the grafts, then the graft neurones are able to generate axons that grow through the peripheral nerve to innervate target muscle (Sieradzan & Vrbová, 1994). The motor neurone phenotype is confirmed by its staining for the cholinergic marker acetylcholinesterase (AChE) and for calcitonin gene-related peptide (CGRP), and its graft origin confirmed by the BrDU label. Muscle re-innervation was demonstrated by back-labelling the grafted neurones in the spinal cord with the fluorescent tracers diamino yellow and fast blue injected into the muscle. Back-labelled motor neurones were observed in the host ventral horn as well as within the graft deposit, but since many of these were double labelled with BrDU it appears that the grafted neurones migrate into appropriate areas in the adult host brain, rather than remaining exclusively within the graft tissue mass (Clowry & Vrbová, 1992).

The major problem of this approach remains the fact that neurones grafted into the spinal cord do not spontaneously regenerate axons into the ventral root, at least not in the adult CNS. This is thought to relate to the inhibitory nature of the glia that make up the central white matter. In the earlier studies this was overcome by transplanting a separate piece of muscle and its own peripheral nerve (Fig. 8.5B). However, recent studies by Nógrádi & Vrbová (1996) have modified the procedure simply to involve a detour of the relevant ventral root directly to

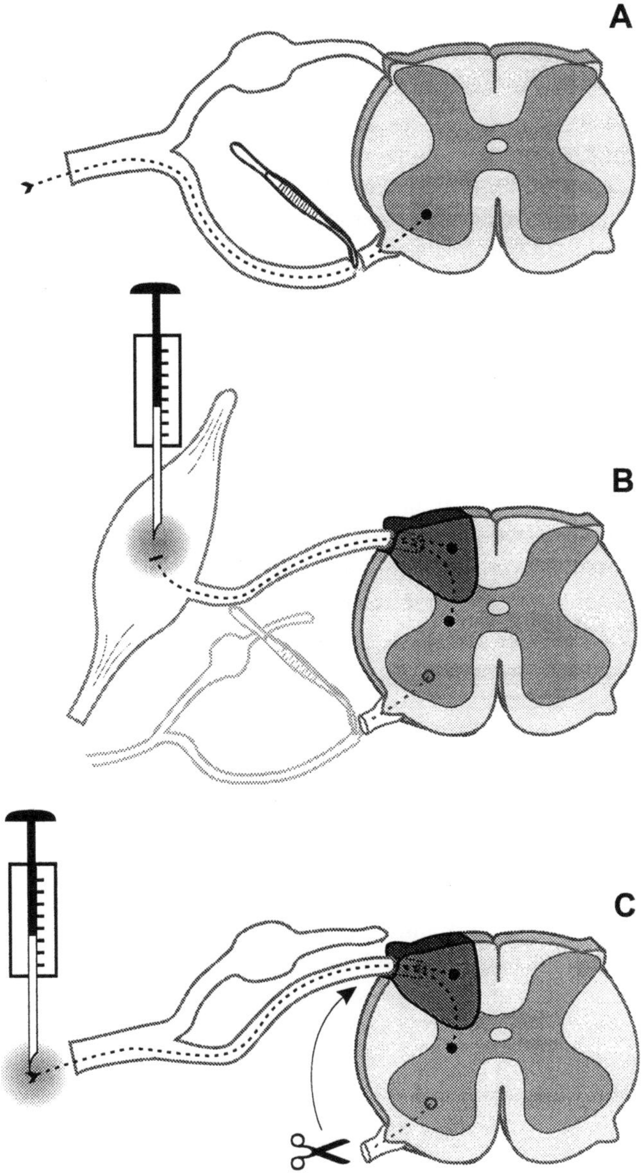

FIG. 8.8. Motor neurone implants in the spinal cord. (A) Motor neurone depletion by crush of ventral root of the sciatic nerve. (B) Embryonic motor neurones are implanted in the dorsal spinal cord and attached to a transplanted soleus muscle via its attached nerve root (after Clowry & Vrbová, 1992, with permission © Springer-Verlag). (C) After ventral root avulsion, embryonic motor neurones are implanted into the dorsal spinal cord and the ventral root re-attached (after Nógrádi & Vrbová, 1996, with permission © Blackwell Science.)

the graft, leaving the peripheral nerve and target muscle *in situ* (Fig. 8.5C). This model is effective in restoring a graft-derived motor neurone innervation of the target muscle with much higher numbers of back-labelled motor neurones as well as improved tetanic tension in the target muscles and motor function. Thus, whereas animals with ventral root avulsion and re-implantation alone had marked deficits both walking and standing the grafted rats walked almost without visible deficit 3–4 months after the implantation.

However, in ALS the motor neurone degeneration is not confined to a single site within the CNS but involves the majority of motor neurones throughout the spine, brainstem, and cerebral cortex. Therefore, the disease is not amenable to simple replacement therapy with neural transplants of motor neurone-rich tissue. Instead, alternative strategies have been pursued which aim to promote motor neurone survival through neurotrophic factors.

Motor neurones have been shown to be protected in tissue culture, and their selective degeneration in a mutant *pmn/pmn* mouse with progressive motor neuropathy can be reversed by growth factor treatments using ciliary neurotrophic factor (CNTF) or glial cell line-derived neurotrophic factor (GDNF) (Sagot et al., 1995; Sendtner et al., 1992) (see Fig. 8.9). However, in the clinical domain the situation is complicated by the fact that trophic molecule administration via a peripheral route is associated with a rapid inactivation of that factor (a few minutes with CNTF, for example), yet also by the development of pronounced side effects such as hepatotoxicity with CNTF. Recent trials have therefore sought to implant cells engineered to secrete CNTF into the thecal cavity at the base of the spinal column, using novel cell encapsulation technologies (described in detail in Chapter Nine). There is now clear evidence that such trophic implants can reduce motor neurone cell death in the murine models of human ALS (Sagot et al., 1995), which has led on to the first clinical trials of this technique in Switzerland. Six patients with ALS have received implants containing CNTF, which has been shown to be released in a sustained fashion over 14–17 weeks into the CSF, with no entry into the blood stream, so avoiding peripheral side effects (Aebischer et al., 1996). At the time of this first report there was no clear evidence for slowing of the progression of the disease on a clinical ALS rating scale. However, the authors emphasise that the small number of patients and short observation period preclude a proper assessment of efficacy in this initial safety trial, and data from a more extended efficacy trial have not yet been released.

PAIN

A further interesting area for consideration in spinal cord transplantation relates to a topic of considerable clinical importance: The discovery that transplantation of adrenal medullary chromaffin cells can provide a novel and effective route for analgesia in intractable pain, in particular that associated with terminal cancers.

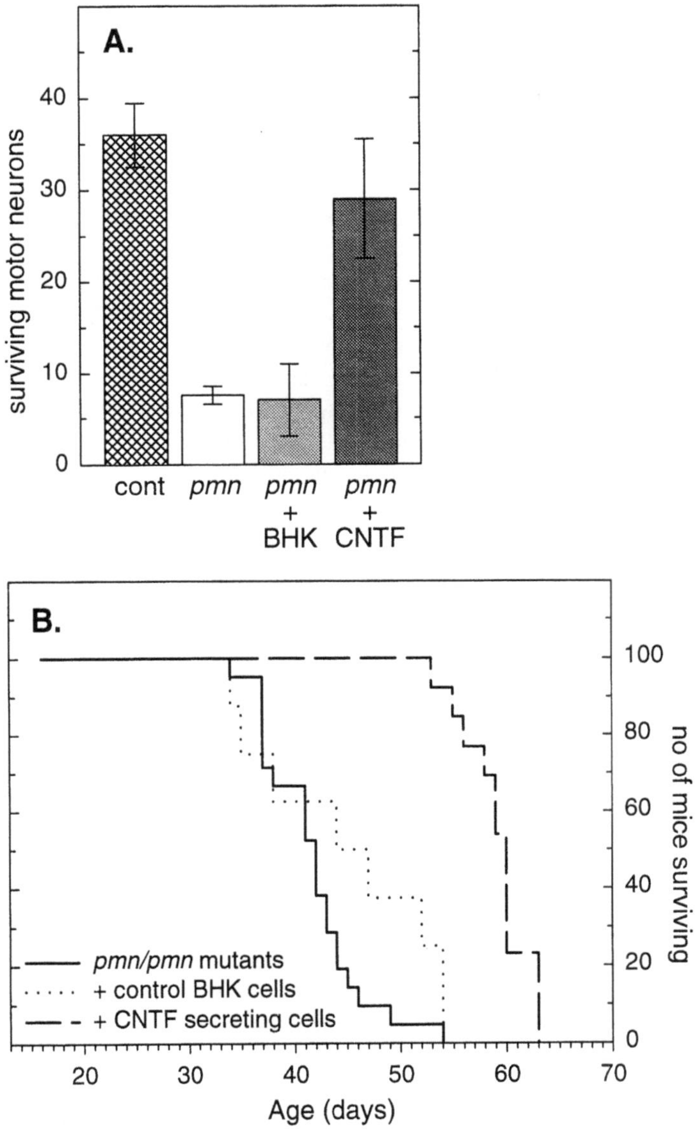

FIG. 8.9. Motor neurones rescued in mutant *pmn/pmn* mice by chronic administration of CNTF delivered by implantation of encapsulated baby hamster kidney (BHK) cells engineered to secrete the trophic molecule. (A) Survival of motor neurones in the facial nucleus. (B) Survival curves for mutant mice are significantly extended for the mice with CNTF-secreting implants, but not in mice with control implants. (Data from Sagot et al., 1995, with permission © Blackwell Science.)

This topic of research arose from the realisation that adrenal cells, as well as secreting catecholamines, also produce and release a wide variety of peptides, including opiate-like substances. Indeed, one of the stranger and completely unexpected outcomes in the initial clinical trials of adrenal medullary grafts in Parkinson's disease (see Chapter Five) was the observation that grafted patients required surprisingly low levels of postoperative analgesia in contrast to what would have been expected for a major abdominal operation to remove one adrenal gland (Drucker-Colín et al., 1990; Penn et al., 1990).

Sagen et al. (1986b) were the first to demonstrate that implantation of adrenal chromaffin cells into the subarachnoid space in the spinal cord of rats produced a highly significant reduction in pain sensitivity on a variety of simple nociceptive tests (e.g. hot plate, tail flick, and paw pinch) (see Fig. 8.10). This analgesic action of the graft is dependent on the release of both catecholamines and opiate-like substances (especially enkephalin)—an effect that can be enhanced by stimulating the chromaffin cell through its nicotinic cholinergic receptor.

Subsequently, the ability of adrenal grafts to induce analgesia has been extended to experimental models of chronic pain which may better reflect situations of clinical concern. For example, intradermal injections of *mycobacteria* into the base of rats' tails produces a chronic arthritis which is manifested by weight loss and increased vocalisations, both of which are substantially alleviated by adrenal grafts but not control grafts in the spinal cord (Sagen et al., 1990). Similar results are obtained with chronic neuropathic pain induced by denervation of sensory inputs from the hind paw. In this model the reduction in behavioural abnormalities associated with the pain is correlated with graft survival and catecholamine release (Ginzburg & Seltzer, 1990).

If these grafts are to find clinical application then a suitable source of adrenal cells needs to be identified, as patients with chronic pain syndromes or terminal cancer are not ideally suitable for autotransplantation of their own adrenal glands. Sagen and colleagues have therefore systematically explored the use of xenografts of bovine adrenal tissues, since this potential source of chromaffin cells is readily available in relatively large supply. Thus, bovine adrenal xenografts placed into the subarachnoid spaces of the rat spinal cord reduced acute pain sensitivity using the same three tests as had previously been used to assess the efficacy of rat cells (Sagen et al., 1986a). The xenografts appeared to survive up to 4 months in the spinal cord, their efficacy was similarly promoted by nicotine treatment, and their analgesic effects appeared to be mediated by release of both catecholamines and opiate-like substances from the grafts, since analgesia was blocked by both phentolamine and naloxone. However, the long-term survival of xenografts is not optimal, although this can be improved by the use of immunosuppressive agents such as cyclosporin A (Czech & Sagen, 1995).

The clinical trials of adrenal medulla grafts to the subarachnoid space of the spinal cord have so far been undertaken for terminal cancer pain, in patients for whom strong pharmacological analgesia has proved ineffective. Winnie et al.,

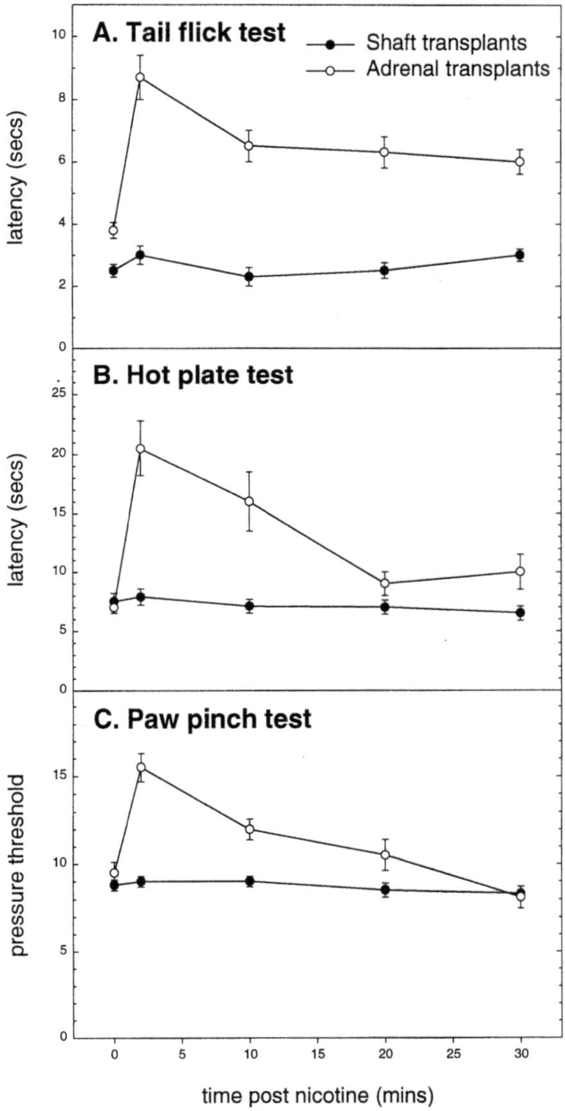

FIG. 8.10. Adrenal chromaffin cells reduce acute pain in rats, as indicated by an increased latency to respond in tests of tail flick (A), hot plate (B) and paw pinch (C). The effects are particularly strong when the cells are stimulated with 0.1 mg/kg nicotine, injected subcutaneously. (Reproduced from Sagen et al., 1986b, with permission © Elsevier Science.)

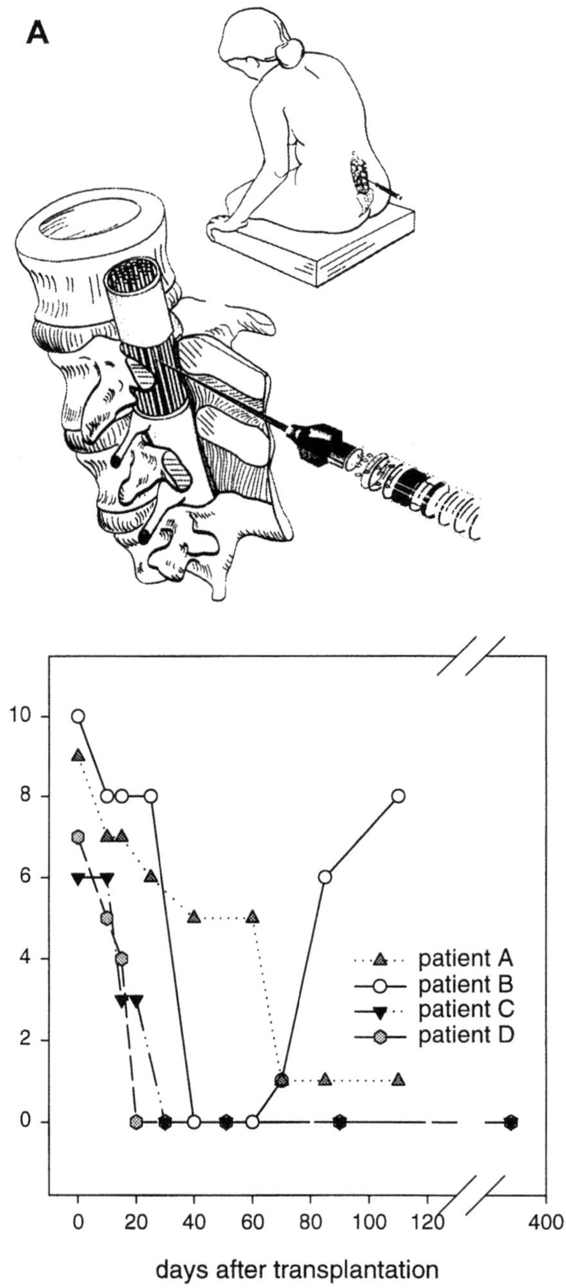

Fig. 8.11. (A) Surgical procedure for subarachnoid injections of human chromaffin cell allografts in the spinal cord. (B) Reduction in the ratings of subjective pain in four terminal cancer patients. (Reproduced from Czech & Sagen, 1995, with permission © Elsevier Science.)

(1993; see also Czech & Sagen, 1995) collected human adrenal cells from cadaver donors, dissected the chromaffin cells and maintained them in culture for at least 7 days before transplantation. Small pieces of allograft tissue were then implanted into five patients via a lumbar puncture needle into the subarachnoid space at level L4–L5 (see Fig. 8.11A). Of the four patients followed up, all showed a good alleviation of severe pain and substantial reductions in their subjective ratings as monitored by visual analogue scales (Fig. 8.11B). Similar results have been reported by a separate group using a similar procedure (Pappas et al., 1997; Tkaczuk et al., 1997), with histological evidence of graft survival at post mortem (Bès et al., 1998).

An alternative approach with xenogenic cells is to encapsulate them using a similar technology to that just described for CNTF delivery in ALS and described in more detail in Chapter Nine. This approach protects the cells from immunological rejection and again yields functionally effective and neurochemically specific grafts (Sagen et al., 1993) that have now also progressed to clinical trial, with some early promising results.

DEMYELINATION AND REMYELINATION

A second major disease that can affect the spinal cord and that involves predominately the loss of a single cell type, the oligodendrocyte, is multiple sclerosis (MS). Multiple sclerosis is the commonest neurological disease of young adults and is characterised by episodes of inflammation and demyelination at different sites of the CNS at different times (Scolding et al., 1998). The cause of this condition is unknown, but a critical event in genetically susceptible individuals is the immune targeting of oligodendrocytes, probably in response to an environmental trigger (McDonald et al., 1992; Scolding et al., 1998). Oligodendrocytes are the glial cells in the CNS that provide the myelin sheaths that insulate the axons of long-distance pathways of the brain and spinal cord (see Chapter One). The oligodendrocytes targeted by the autoimmune inflammatory event produce focal "plaques" of demyelination throughout the white matter, which are clearly visible as high-signal lesions on magnetic resonance imaging (MRI) as well as at post mortem (see Fig. 8.12). The loss of oligodendrocytes and the resultant demyelination, as well as the release of cytokines in the inflammatory process, causes an impairment in nerve impulse conduction along the axon (Moreau et al., 1996; Redford et al., 1997). Consequently, the symptoms of the disease, at least initially and at the time of acute relapses, reflect impaired conduction both in the brain and in the major ascending sensory and descending motor pathways of the brainstem and spinal cord. However, with time, the chronically demyelinated axon starts to degenerate, such that the long-term disability with this disease is more related to secondary axonal loss than demyelination (Davie et al., 1995; Ferguson et al., 1997).

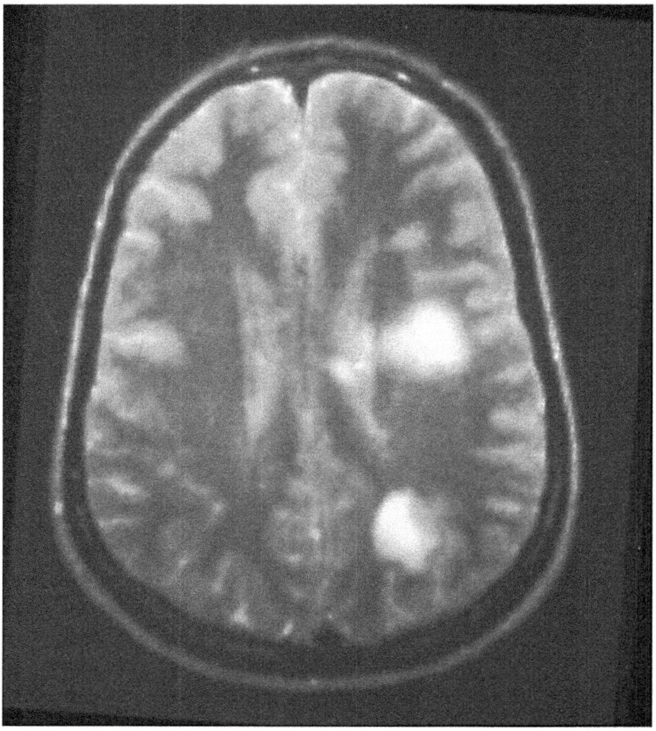

FIG. 8.12. MRI of a patient with MS showing the characteristic white matter lesions that represent areas of demyelination. (Original scan courtesy of Dr Neil Scolding.)

Early in the disease, the acute inflammatory demyelinating lesion can remyelinate by the recruitment of normal oligodendrocytes and their precursors in the CNS. In addition in the spinal cord, Schwann cells, which have considerably greater remyelination potential, can migrate into the CNS. However, as the disease progresses, the ability of plaques to repair themselves diminishes, and as new inflammatory episodes occur, the patients relapse and remit with secondary progression.

Since the numbers and migratory capacity of oligodendrocyte precursors in the mature CNS is limited, leading to the breakdown of mechanisms for spontaneous repair, there has been considerable interest in the extent to which it may be possible to employ a transplantation strategy for explicit replacement of lost oligodendrocytes or the relevant precursor cells. Success in this enterprise has arisen not least from the fact that the developmental lineage of oligodendrocytes and type II astrocytes from "O-2A" precursor cells is one of the best worked out in mammalian CNS. Successful transplantation and remyelination of demyelinated central axons has now been demonstrated using two fundamentally different model systems.

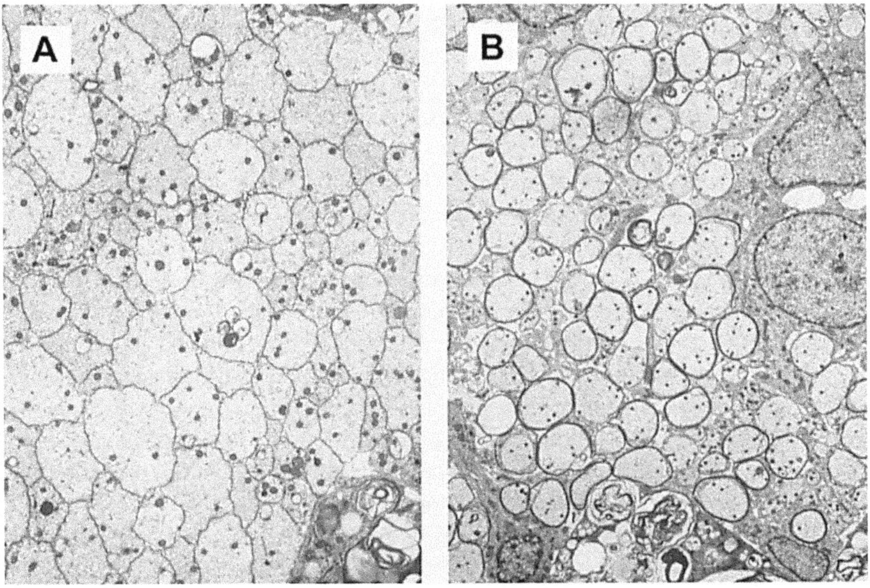

FIG. 8.13. Electron micrographs of the dorsal column of the spinal cord to visualise single axons in cross-section and their myelination, seen as a ring of electron-dense material. (A) Ethidium bromide injection and X-irradiation eliminate all myelination of the axons in the dorsal column. (B) Grafts of oligodendrocyte precursors produce remyelination of the axons. (From Groves et al., 1993, with permission *Nature* © Macmillan Magazines Limited.)

In the first model system, Blakemore and colleagues have made demyelinating lesions of the dorsal columns in the spinal cord of rats by injection of the glial cell toxin ethidium bromide, which results in extensive demyelination of axons over several segments of the cord (Blakemore & Franklin, 1991). If no further treatments are undertaken, the cord will spontaneously remyelinate, primarily as a result of the inward migration of Schwann cells, which can be prevented by local X-irradiation of the affected area. In this model a variety of different types of cell have been implanted and the most effective appears to be not oligodendrocytes themselves, but the O-2A precursor. The grafted precursor cells migrate and integrate through the area of demyelination and form new myelin sheaths wrapping round the central axons, with all the appropriate morphological features of normal central myelin when viewed in semi-thin and electron microscope sections (Groves et al., 1993, Fig. 8.13).

The second main model system has employed mutant strains of mice and rats with a genetic deficiency in myelin production. The first studies were done with the shiverer mouse, which is characterised by an absence of myelin basic protein. In this model implants of oligodendrocytes can migrate over long distances and myelinate axons not only in the brains of neonatal animals (Gumpel et al., 1993) but also in the spinal cord and brain of adults (Friedman et al., 1986; Gout et al., 1988), a result that has also been seen in other mutant strains of animals including the myelin-deficient rat (Tontsch et al., 1994).

However, several key issues need to be addressed before any clinical transplant programme of remyelination can be considered. First, the grafted cells have to be able to migrate to the sites where they are required, namely to recognise and be attracted to the site of the lesion before differentiation and remyelination can take place. To date though, both oligodendrocytes and their precursors retain only a limited capacity for migration (Vignais et al., 1993).

Second, since multiple sclerosis is an autoimmune inflammatory disorder it will be necessary not only to repair the damage but also to halt the disease process. In recent years there have been advances in identifying the immunological processes involved in the pathogenesis of MS, and new selective antibody therapies show considerable promise (Moreau et al., 1996). However, the recent realisation that much of the long-term disability in MS is due to secondary axonal loss raises many questions as to the timing and value of transplants designed solely to remyelinate CNS axons.

Third, it is clear that in rats and mice, O-2A progenitor cells provide the most effective cells for transplantation. However, the lineage of human oligodendrocytes and the relevant markers for their identification and selection have not until recently been known. However, with an explicit view towards prospective transplantation, the active characterisation of the human oligodendrocyte lineage is now under active investigation (Scolding et al., 1995).

Finally, remyelination has to be shown to be effective, and, remarkably, given the extensive literature on the anatomy of glial grafts in demyelinating lesion models in animals, functional studies are rather sparse. Nevertheless, the situation is slowly being rectified. At the neurophysiological level, Ian Duncan and colleagues have shown that conduction velocities are markedly slowed and action potentials exhibit abnormal frequency-response properties in the dorsal column of myelin-deficient rats, both features of which are almost completely alleviated following remyelination of the dorsal column (Utzschneider et al., 1994). Indeed, the authors were able to conclude that "transplantation of exogenous glial cells into amyelinated spinal cord results in restoration of normal conduction properties". At the behavioural level, Jefferey and Blakemore (1997) have shown so far that, if Schwann cell migration is not blocked, spontaneous remyelination is accompanied by a return of motor function in a series of beam balance tests. Furthermore, there are some preliminary reports that suggest a similar alleviation of the behavioural deficits can be observed after transplantation of O-2A precursors.

Thus, whilst glial cell transplantation has not yet reached the point of clinical application, there is some suggestion that the various components necessary for developing an effective clinical therapy are slowly being put in place.

SUMMARY

In this chapter we have described rapid advances in a variety of novel strategies for promoting regeneration and repair in the spinal cord, not only in situations of traumatic injury and spinal disconnection, but also in diseases involving particular cell types, such as the motor neurones in amyotrophic lateral sclerosis and the oligodendrocytes in multiple sclerosis. Grafts can be used to replace lost neurones and facilitate circuit repair as well as as an alternative source of trophic and other neuroactive molecules. The delivery of neurotrophic factors through a graft can both protect neurones against disease processes of cell death and promote intrinsic plasticity, and has the advantage of providing a more effective route for the CNS delivery of these agents whilst minimising their peripheral side effects.

As each of the model systems has been developed, so has the number of preliminary clinical trials employing a variety of new strategies. Each can certainly be improved both in terms of the technology and application, but functional reparation in the spinal cord is likely to provide radical new opportunities for treatment in the next decade.

CHAPTER NINE

Other sources of cells for transplantation

INTRODUCTION

In the preceding chapters we have considered the development of neural transplantation for application in a variety of human neurological diseases. The most obvious and advanced applications are to Parkinson's disease, but it is clear that important applications are already under consideration and development for a variety of other human neurodegenerative conditions. The strategy has been to identify the cells which are lost and to assess the efficacy of their replacement in animal models of the human disease. For the most part, the most effective techniques have been to seek replacement by primary neurones taken from embryos: i.e. replacement is with the same population of neurones that are lost, but harvested from a donor at an early stage in development when the cells are dividing and growing processes to their appropriate targets in the adult host brain. This strategy has proved remarkably successful when assessed experimentally in the laboratory and gives every appearance of also having the potential for efficacy in the clinic. However, there is an obvious problem with this approach. The use of primary human foetal donors required by this strategy for clinical application raises a range of both practical and ethical problems. As a consequence there is an extremely limited availability of cells, which has proved to be the main restriction on a more rapid and widespread development of neural transplantation technologies into the clinic.

The ethical issues have been discussed elsewhere in this volume (see Chapter Five). Although a matter for individual consideration and decision, in our view there is no fundamental ethical problem with the use of human foetal tissues for research or therapy, provided that work complies with the legal requirements of the society in which the work is to be undertaken and follows clearly specified guidelines to ensure separation of the decisions of whether, when, and how an abortion is undertaken from the subsequent use of the foetal tissues. Such guidelines have been developed in most Western countries, and clear ethical guidelines have been adopted in the UK and elsewhere (Boer, 1994; Polkinghorne, 1989). Nevertheless, the use of tissues derived from elective abortion, however carefully regulated, remains controversial for many people.

Of more fundamental biological concern, there remains a range of practical issues that will always apply to use of tissues derived from human embryonic or foetal donors.

Age of donors. It is known that for any given population of embryonic neurones there is an optimal age and critical time window for their transplantation which corresponds to their period of normal development. In the case of dopaminergic cells of the substantia nigra this turns out to be at around 6–8 weeks of gestational age, which corresponds reasonably to the time when some (although not all) terminations of pregnancy are actually conducted. However, for other tissues this need not be the case, and so it is plausible that other cells that differentiate earlier or later in development will simply never be available.

Accuracy of dissection. Tissues derived from routine suction abortions are typically fragmented, so that accurate dissection is far more difficult and potentially imprecise than that which can be achieved under controlled experimental laboratory conditions using, for example, pregnant animals killed for the specific purpose of tissue donation. As a result the potential risk of transplanting non-neural tissue is a real one (see, for example, Folkerth & Durso, 1996).

Sterility and infection. All tissues destined for clinical transplantation have to be fully assessed for infectivity. The present protocols predominantly involve testing the maternal blood for viral infections, although there is currently no way of detecting early stages of HIV infection or prion disease. In addition, extensive washing protocols are required to reduce the risk of bacteriological infections, but the conclusive proof of sterility of donor tissues will only ever be assessed by culturing the tissue for several days, which presently cannot be achieved within the time constraints of neural transplantation.

Timing of donation and implantation. Present techniques require implantation of tissues within hours of being harvested. As a consequence the recipient has to undergo full neurosurgical preparation, before the availability of suitable tissue in sufficient quantity, and meeting all safety criteria, is known.

Numbers of donors. The poor survival of dopaminergic neurones and possibly other cells used for transplantation has required the use of multiple foetal donors for each recipient in all successful clinical trials to date. The effective co-ordination for the simultaneous collection of not just one but multiple donors, all within the correct developmental age window, compounds the practical difficulty of developing a feasible clinical transplantation programme.

Supply and demand. Even if each of these problems can be alleviated by application of improved strategies for collection, preparation, hibernation, and neuroprotection of graft tissues, the demand for suitable tissues for transplantation is likely to rise, whereas social changes, changes in ethical and legal regulation, and new methods of contraception and termination (including the rise in use of the "morning after" pill) are all likely to reduce the supply.

For these practical, legal, and ethical reasons, the development and widespread application of cell transplantation procedures based on human foetal donor tissues is likely to continue in a severely restricted fashion for the foreseeable future. Consequently, there is now growing interest and commitment of research resources into the search for alternative sources of tissue that may be used for transplantation in the treatment of Parkinson's and other diseases of the nervous system. This approach is currently one of the major issues, in that the conceptual framework that grafts can survive, integrate and restore function is now generally accepted.

THE NATURE OF REPAIR

Throughout the present account, we have considered the mechanisms by which grafts exert their effects. As well as its theoretical interest, this issue becomes of fundamental importance when we consider alternative sources of tissues for transplantation. The demands that a graft must fulfil to restore function will determine the alternatives we can consider. We considered a range of mechanisms of function in detail in Chapter Two and will return to this topic again in the next chapter. For present purposes, two main levels of functional action are relevant, molecular vs. neuronal replacement. The main techniques associated with each level are summarised in Table 9.1, and the principles of each approach are outlined in the following sections.

Molecular replacement

Some grafts may act by augmenting or replacing a missing molecule. We may consider the utility of this approach in a number of different situations.

In Parkinson's disease substantial benefit may be achieved by delivering dopamine at physiological concentrations to defined sites within the basal ganglia. Indeed, this was the original notion behind using adrenal transplants, an approach which we have already considered in some detail (see Chapter Five). In this situation, the aim is to replace a deficient neurotransmitter molecule. Although the disease involves loss of neurones, we know that a pharmacological reactivation

TABLE 9.1
Alternatives to primary foetal neurones for transplantation

Molecular replacement	*Neuronal replacement*
Peripheral neurones and ganglia	Peripheral neurones and ganglia?
Slow-release polymers and matrices	Neuronal cell lines
Secretory cell lines	Neurospheres
Encapsulated cell lines	Immortalised neuronal cell lines
Genetically engineered cells and cell lines	Xenografts
In vivo gene transfer	

of the dopamine receptor is sufficient to restore a substantial degree of function, as evidenced by the utility of L-dopa therapy in many patients early in the course of Parkinson's disease.

In chronic pain (discussed in Chapter Eight), it may be sufficient to deliver an appropriate cocktail of opiates and catecholamines into relay centres in spinal pain pathways. In this situation molecules which are themselves not deficient are being added to alter the regulatory control of information relay in the nervous system. In this respect the implantation of GABAergic neurones to increase neuronal inhibition in the control of epilepsy may prove to be a useful intervention.

Third, the delivery of neurotrophic or growth factor molecules may protect intrinsic host neurones against a progressive disease process or promote plasticity and recovery within damaged host systems. As we have seen, such a strategy is being actively considered in a variety of contexts: using glial cell line-derived neurotrophic factor (GDNF) and ciliary neurotrophic factor (CNTF) for protection of motor neurones in amyotrophic lateral sclerosis (ALS), using CNTF to protect striatal neurones in Huntington's disease; and using GDNF and/or neurotrophins to protect dopamine neurones in Parkinson's disease.

Although the mechanisms of action differ, the transplantation strategy in each case involves delivery of neuroactive molecules at physiological concentrations across the blood–brain barrier to targeted sites within the brain. In this context then, transplantation is being considered, in comparison to other pharmacological strategies, because of its ability to place the missing agent directly into the central nervous system (CNS) with the potential self-regulating and self-sustaining properties of a biological delivery system.

If the major action of a graft is to provide pharmacological support then it is important to consider what are the optimal features of the transplanted cells which allow it to perform this function. In this respect other features will have to be considered such as its availability, stability, practicality, and safety profile. For example an ideal cell would have many or all of the following features:

(1) It would be readily available, including the capacity for growth or preservation in the laboratory.
(2) It would be ethically neutral.
(3) It would be easy to graft, involving minimal neurosurgical complications.
(4) It would have ready survival following implantation.
(5) It would not be tumorigenic.
(6) It would not be capable of inducing an immunological reaction.
(7) It would have efficient and stable delivery of the relevant molecules.
(8) It would have the ability possibly to regulate the level of the target molecule's production.
(9) It need not be neuronal. For some purposes, the cells might adopt a neuronal phenotype and establish connections rather than simply function as a "minipump" in the host brain; but for other purposes this may be an actual disadvantage.

Needless to say, no cell has yet been identified that meets all these considerations; but as we shall see a number of promising strategies have been applied.

Neuronal replacement

In other situations, delivery of a biologically active molecule will not be sufficient. When damage or disease kills neurones there is a disruption of an integrated neuronal circuitry and so repair requires not only replacement of neurones but also restitution of their connections. This might be at the following levels.

(1) Diffuse non-synaptic re-innervation (e.g. dopamine in Parkinson's disease).
(2) Restoration of a regulatory or activational input that requires transmitter action at a synaptic site which may even extend to the regulation graft–host projection at the presynaptic level (e.g. spinal cord monoaminergic transplants).
(3) Restitution of afferent and efferent connections of the grafted cells into the host neuronal circuitry (e.g striatal grafts in Huntington's disease). In these situations, the requirement will not be simply for an appropriately secretory cell, but for one with a series of key neuronal properties to differentiate, connect, transduce neuronal inputs, and relay that information via synaptic contacts to target neurones. Logically, this need not be a neurone if all these properties can be transferred to a non-neuronal cell; but for all practical purposes neurones are required to achieve this level of repair.

Many of the features required for an ideal neuronal replacement cell mirror those required of an ideal secretory cell.

(1) It must be readily available, including the capacity for growth or preservation in the laboratory.
(2) It must be ethically neutral.
(3) It must be easy to graft, involving minimal neurosurgical complications.
(4) It must have ready survival following implantation.
(5) It must not be tumorigenic.
(6) It must not be capable of inducing an immunological reaction.

However, in this case we do not require efficient, stable, regulated delivery of relevant molecules. Rather, the cell needs to exhibit specific neuronal features necessary for it to fulfil its function of replacing lost neurones within connected circuits of the host brain.

(1) It must be able to differentiate into a particular neuronal phenotype.
(2) It must be able to express a particular neurotransmitter, including the development of the cellular machinery for transmitter synthesis, packaging, release, reuptake, and metabolism.
(3) It must be able to develop appropriate patterns of neurite outgrowth, both axonal and dendritic.
(4) It must be able to make synaptic contacts with appropriate host targets.
(5) It must be able to express appropriate growth factor and neurotransmitter receptors on the cell surface.
(6) It must be able to attract host sprouting and form synaptic contacts between host axons and graft dendrites and cell somata.
(7) The activity and transmitter release of the grafted cells must be able to be regulated by neuronal and hormonal inputs from the host.

Demanding as they may seem, many of these features are indeed re-established when grafting primary embryonic neurones, as for example has been well established for striatal grafts (see Chapter Six). The capacity of alternative cells and tissues to reform any or all of these neuronal features, even when derived from a neuronal lineage, will probably determine their functional efficacy, and consequently will prove key criteria for assessing their relative potential. As emphasised above, it is difficult to envisage the technology required to transform non-neuronal cells into ones with these features, and it is likely that for the foreseeable future suitable alternatives for repair at the neuronal level will be based on more readily available sources of neurones or neuronal cell lines.

Within the context of neural transplantation, we have also considered situations where glial cells are lost, as in multiple sclerosis, and the need for their replacement by oligodendrocytes. The strategies required in the search for alternatives to human foetal oligodendrocyte precursors fall within this second category of specific cellular replacement—namely, the isolation of a specific glial cell with distinct properties for migration, axon ensheathment and myelination, rather than replacement of identified secretory molecules.

SECRETORY CELLS AND TISSUES

Peripheral neurones and ganglia

In the case of Parkinson's disease, we have already considered the use of the adrenal medulla as an alternative source of tissue for transplantation, based on the facts that peripheral neural tissues and ganglia will regenerate throughout life, will survive transplantation in adulthood, and if taken as an autograft (i.e. from the recipient patient him- or herself) will overcome most ethical and immunological problems. As we have seen, though, this strategy did not prove particularly successful in the case of adrenal medullary autografts in Parkinson's disease, for a variety of practical reasons related in particular to the limited survival of the grafts and the unacceptable side effects of the procedure (see Chapter Five). Nevertheless, that particular failure does not preclude the possibility of other peripheral tissues being suitable in this or other diseases. In the case of Parkinson's disease, there are a variety of other catecholamine-containing tissues, such as sympathetic ganglia, which have until recently received relatively little attention despite the fact that they were among the earliest tissues to be transplanted into the adult CNS (Stenevi et al., 1976). This is due in part to the difficulties in obtaining large quantities of the tissue when compared to the adrenal chromaffin cell and to its lack of phenotypic plasticity. However, studies with this tissue have shown that it can survive transplantation (Itakura et al., 1988; Nakai et al., 1990; Stenevi et al., 1976), grow extensive fibre networks, continue neuropeptide synthesis after intraocular grafting (Stieg et al., 1991) and reverse drug-induced rotation in human xenografts to rats (Kamo et al., 1986; but see Yong et al., 1989); and it has even been the basis for an initial clinical trial in Parkinson's disease (Itakura et al., 1994).

A related ganglion, the carotid, has recently attracted more interest, since this uses dopamine rather than noradrenaline as its primary transmitter. Carotid grafts were first shown to be as effective as adrenal medulla grafts in the rotating hemiparkinson rat model over a decade ago (Bing et al., 1988), although efficacy was not as good as for PC12 or adrenal grafts. However, this topic has recently been revisited (Espejo et al., 1998) with an improved experimental technique. In this study it was shown that the survival of the total number of catecholaminergic cells implanted was close to 60% over 3 months and the grafted animals were seen to recover not only on tests of drug-induced rotation but also on several sensorimotor tests such as response to whisker scanning and thigmotaxis in an open field. Although very recent (at the time of writing), this study has already attracted much interest and commentary (Rosenthal, 1998). This is not least because the grafted neurones developed extensive dopaminergic neurites which grew back into the denervated striatum—i.e. like nigral grafts they appear to re-innervate the host brain. This would help explain the behavioural recovery seen in these animals, which is better than that obtained with other dopamine-secreting grafts and includes more complex sensorimotor behaviours that have previously only been alleviated by nigral grafts in the rat Parkinson's disease model. The recency and lack of confirmatory studies at this time prevent any recommendations of this technique, but it is certain to provide a new angle on the search for future transplant therapy in Parkinson's disease.

Slow-release systems

An alternative pharmacological strategy to the treatment of Parkinson's disease has been to improve the delivery of dopamine to the striatum. Whilst in the clinical domain this has led to the development of slow-release oral preparations of L-dopa, experimentally attempts have been made to graft in polymers rich in dopamine that release their contents over long periods of time, up to 12 months (Sabel et al., 1990; Winn et al., 1989). This approach has the advantage that the clinically effective treatment can be placed at the site where it is required, namely the striatum. Furthermore, it avoids the erratic uptake of L-dopa through the gut and blood–brain barrier that is important in the development of motor dyskinesias seen in the later stages of oral L-dopa therapy. The disadvantage of the approach is that it requires invasive surgery, is associated with significant trauma, and makes no attempt to recreate synaptic circuitry. Therefore whilst smoothing out the motor fluctuations of patients with advanced Parkinson's disease, it will never be a cure for the underlying disease.

The efficacy of L-dopa therapy in Parkinson's disease demonstrates that a basic strategy of direct dopamine replacement can be effective. The "on–off" and dyskinetic side effects associated with long-term pharmacotherapy and disease progression may in part be due both to the phasic availability of dopamine at its receptor with standard routes of drug administration, and to the associated accumulation of receptor supersensitivity. These problems may be overcome by sustained tonic central delivery of L-dopa or dopamine into the neostriatum. One strategy for identifying effective alternative therapies, whether by cell transplantation or gene manipulation, is therefore to seek to achieve specific central delivery of dopamine to its striatal receptors on a sustained basis and with the possibility of selective targeting to distinct striatal regions.

Hargraves and Freed (1987) first demonstrated the essential feasibility of this approach. They infused dopamine over a period of 2 weeks into the CNS via a striatal cannula attached to an Alzet® minipump, and showed that this was associated with a reduction in apomorphine rotation, providing a functional index of the down-regulation of striatal receptor sensitivity (Fig. 9.1). Nevertheless, such minipumps require regular change, and chronic intraparenchymal infusions are frequently associated with progressive tissue damage and inflammation at the site of delivery. Consequently, subsequent studies have sought improved

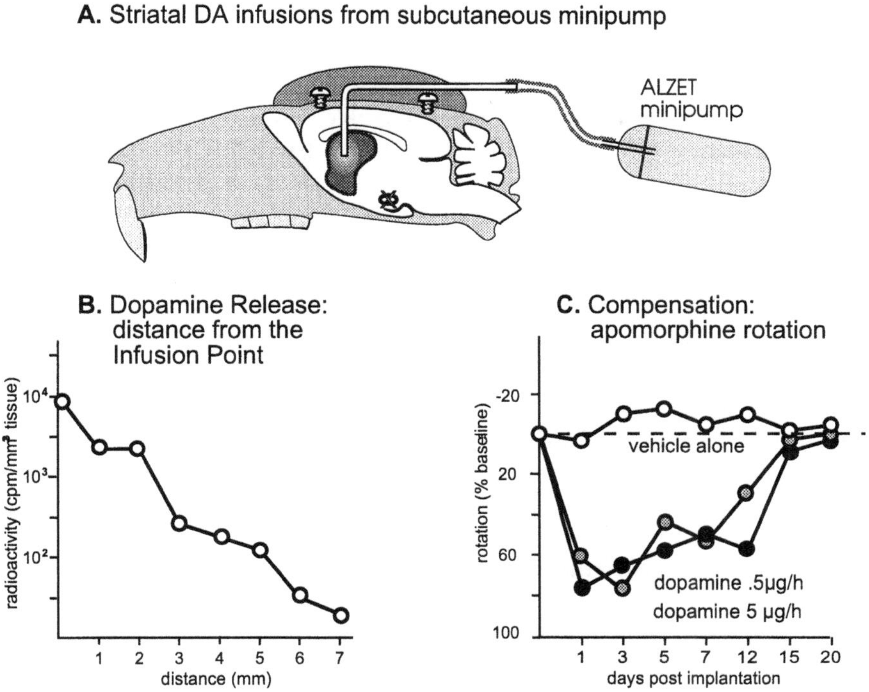

FIG. 9.1. Subcutaneous implants of minipump to deliver DA (dopamine) to the brain. (A) Schematic mode of delivery into the striatum via an intracerebral cannula. (B) Concentration gradient of dopamine diffusion at different distances from the point of delivery. (C) Compensation of apomorphine rotation lasting approximately 2 weeks, which relates to the capsule capacity and the duration over which dopamine is released. (Based on Hargraves & Freed, 1987, © Elsevier Science.)

implantation strategies for the chronic and sustainable delivery of dopamine into the CNS.

One strategy originating from polymer chemistry is the encapsulation of crystalline dopamine or L-dopa into a polymeric matrix that can then be implanted into the brain. The matrix will then slowly diffuse or dissolve, releasing the encapsulated dopamine into the host neuropil. This strategy has been attempted by a number of laboratories with some success in the standard rat parkinsonian model, including the demonstration of functional recovery on simple measures of apomorphine rotation (Becker et al., 1990; McRae et al., 1991, 1994). As well as technical problems of ensuring stable levels of delivery at a controlled level without unacceptable damage in the brain, implanted dopamine-secreting polymers suffer a similar problem to Alzet minipumps, i.e. the limited lifespan of the dissolving matrix before renewal is necessary. Clearly, the advantage of a grafting strategy is that cells that release dopamine have more possibility of being self-sustaining in the living brain and to delivering dopamine to the host receptors at stable physiological levels.

CELL LINES

Tumour-derived cell lines

It would certainly be appealing if it were possible to maintain cells permanently in the laboratory for transplantation rather than harvesting them afresh each time they were needed. Such cells could be characterised in detail, potentially manipulated to express just those features required of our transplant, tested for safety and the presence of pathogens, and collected for implantation as and when they were required at the convenience of the neurosurgeons and their patients.

In normal development, even a dividing cell will only undergo a limited number of divisions until it differentiates into its final cell type—the phenotype. There remains some debate whether there is an absolute limit to the number of times—say 30 or 40—any cell can divide, which may underlie fundamental principles of ageing. However, this issue is not in doubt in the CNS: Once committed to a given fate, neurones can neither change phenotype, or revert to a proliferative state and start dividing again. Indeed this lack of plasticity is one of the major reasons that we need to consider cell transplantation in the CNS when cell loss in many other organs and tissues has a much greater capacity for self-repair.

Under some conditions neurones can and do change into a proliferative state, although this is typically a sign of disease: Proliferating cells lead to unregulated growth and will form tumours, as well as often having the capacity to migrate away from their initial site of proliferation, yielding secondary spread of the cancer. Cells derived from brain tumours can typically be grown and maintained as cell lines in tissue culture, and express a variety of features of potential interest.

The most widely studied neuronal cell line is the PC12 cell, which was originally derived from a rat phaeochromocytoma (adrenal medulla) tumour. The cells of this tumour are similar to chromaffin cells, and so primarily secrete the catecholamines adrenaline and noradrenaline. They are easily maintained and expanded *in vitro* so that they can be readily available for transplantation at will (Fig. 9.2). However, without immunosuppression, PC12 cells do not survive well long-term following transplantation into the rat brain (Freed et al., 1986b; Hefti et al., 1985) although long-term survival can be achieved with a restoration of dopamine release and reversal of motor deficits in grafted animals given cyclosporin A (Bing et al., 1988; Okuda et al., 1991). However, as would be expected, PC12 grafts form tumours in the host brain, and so, despite their beneficial effects within the dopaminergic network, many animals die within a few weeks (Bing et al., 1988; Hori et al., 1993).

It is possible to reduce tumour formation by a variety of strategies, including treatment with antimitotic agents such as mitomycin C or X-irradiation, without adversely affecting their long-term survival and functional effects (Okuda et al., 1991). However, it is unlikely that simple cell lines of this type will ever be

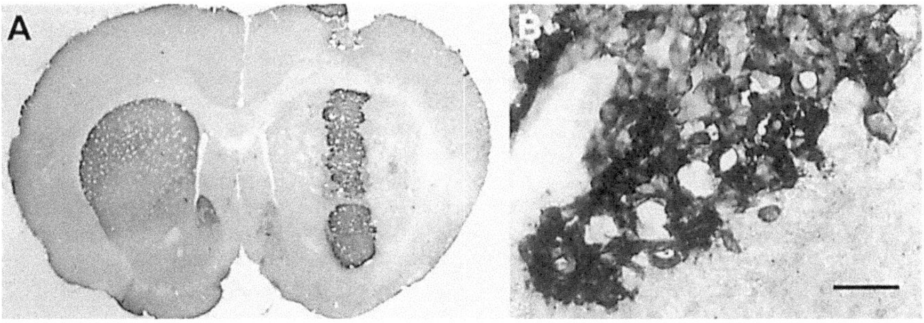

FIG. 9.2. PC12 cells grafted to the dopamine-depleted striatum of a hemiparkinsonian host rat. Catecholamine-secreting PC12 cells are visualised with tyrosine-hydroxylase immunohistochemistry at low (A) and high (B) magnifications. (Reproduced from Hori et al., 1993, with permission © Elsevier Science.)

accepted as an alternative source of cells for clinical transplantation because of the difficulty of ensuring absolute safety associated with such intrinsically proliferative cells.

Neurospheres

A second alternative is to increase the efficiency of harvesting human foetal cells for transplantation to the point that they can be more readily available and sustained in the laboratory until required. Interest in this possibility has come about through the development of strategies allowing for the large-scale expansion of multipotential stem cells from both embryonic and adult mouse brain (McKay, et al., 1990; Reynolds et al., 1992; Svendsen et al., 1995; Vescovi et al., 1993).

During development, there is a process of cell division and specialisation, with the early cells in the developmental lineage having a multipotential capacity. With time, however, the cells become committed to a certain phenotype. Some of these early cells are termed "stem cells" because: (1) they are *self-renewing*—i.e. they divide to form multiple copies of themselves, allowing expansion in cell numbers; and (2) they are *multipotential*—i.e. they have the capacity to differentiate into a variety of different cell types (see Fig. 9.3).

These cells, as they progress along a developmental lineage, pass through a number of progenitor cell stages which have a more limited multipotential capacity. At the final stages of differentiation, the precursors undergo a terminal cell division into cells not only with a committed neuronal fate, but also a particular phenotype.

Neuronal lineages are still poorly understood and the topic of active current investigation. Nevertheless, if embryonic brain tissue is harvested and grown in specific culture conditions in which newly born neurones die but stem and precursor cells survive, then the tissue is maintained in a dividing state, allowing

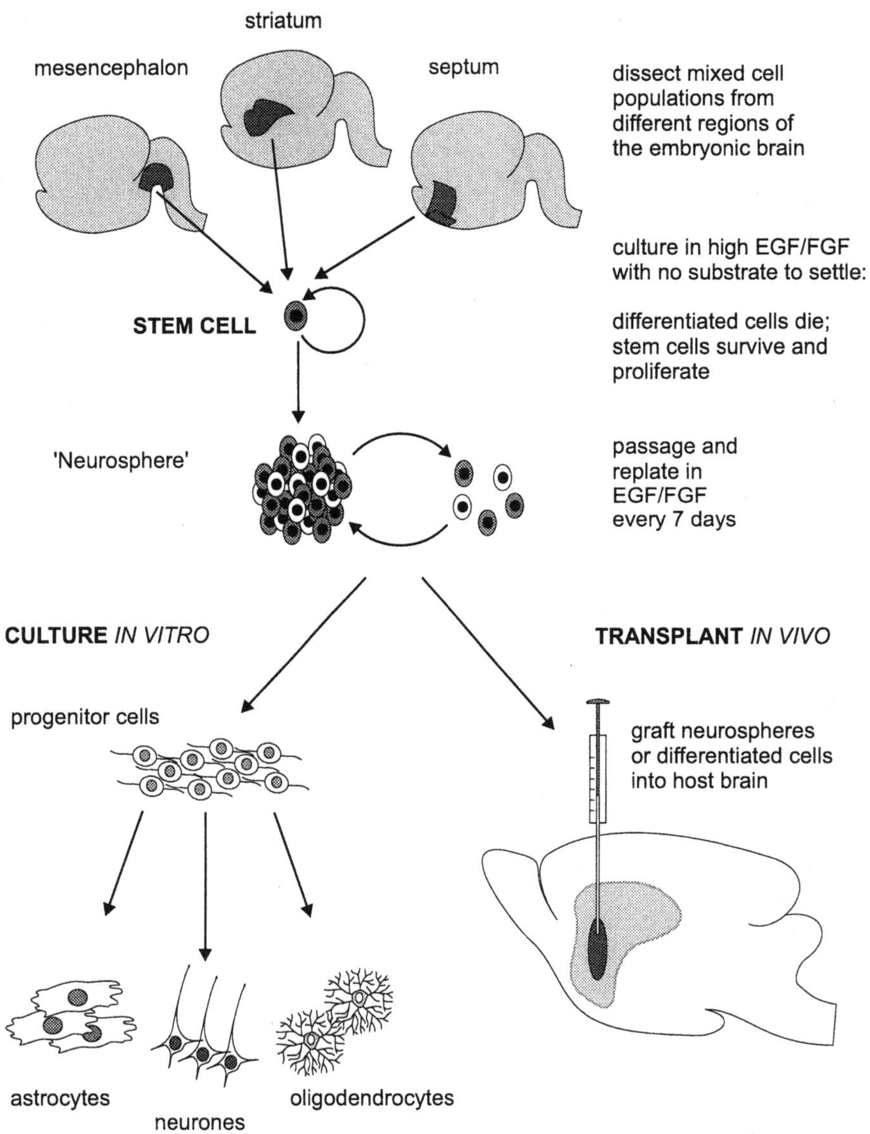

FIG. 9.3. Neurospheres and precursor cell lineages in culture and in grafts. EGF, epidermal growth factor; FGF, fibroblast growth factor. (Redrawn from Svendsen & Rosser, 1995, with permission © Elsevier Science.)

for the expansion of large numbers of neuronal precursors. These specific culture conditions are the absence of a substrate for the cells to settle on and the presence of specific neurotrophic factors. The cells are therefore kept free-floating in medium containing high doses of epidermal and/or fibroblast growth factors (EGF and FGF), and can be made to differentiate by the provision of a substrate to which the precursor cells can attach.

When grown under these conditions, the stem/precursor cells will proliferate exponentially to form growing spheres of dividing cells—"neurospheres". If the culture conditions are subsequently changed back to those favouring differentiation and development, the cells differentiate into neurones and glia but not other cell types. Although originally developed with mouse neural tissue, subsequent studies have shown that similar cells can be grown from rat, pig, monkey, and human embryonic tissues, and that altering the culture conditions can affect the proportion of neurones or glia that ultimately develop. However, many of the critical stages in the developmental process for these cells are not known, although there is a hope and expectation that it should be possible to differentiate neurospheres into distinct populations of specific cell types suitable for transplantation, for example dopamine, striatal, or hippocampal neurones or oligodendrocytes.

Cells expanded as neurospheres can certainly survive transplantation back into the lesioned rat central nervous system (Svendsen et al., 1996) and, as one might expect, the favoured model system has been the rotating hemiparkinsonian rat. These studies, whilst demonstrating the essential feasibility of expanding and transplanting precursor cells, are disappointing in terms of the relatively small numbers of neurones which express a dopaminergic phenotype in the grafts. However, a combination of gene transfer and/or trophic factor treatment of the dividing cells prior to transplantation may eventually overcome these initial problems (Ling et al., 1998; Sabaté et al., 1995, Svendsen et al., 1996).

Adult stem cells

At first it was considered that the availability of precursor cells that can be expanded by treatment with growth factors such as EGF and FGF was only a feature of the developing brain. Nevertheless, in spite of the principle derived from Cajal that all neurones in the central nervous system of mammals are born in early life (see Chapter One), there has been long-standing evidence that neurogenesis can occur throughout life. Certainly, neurogenesis in adult animals is extremely limited and restricted to a few specific locations, notably the dentate gyrus of the hippocampus and the olfactory bulb (Altman, 1963; Bayer, 1982, 1983; Bayer et al., 1992). These two areas are both implicated in learning, which raises the intriguing speculation that representations of new memories may involve not only the modification of synaptic connections but also in some cases the formation of new neurones. Indeed, Gage and colleagues have recently shown

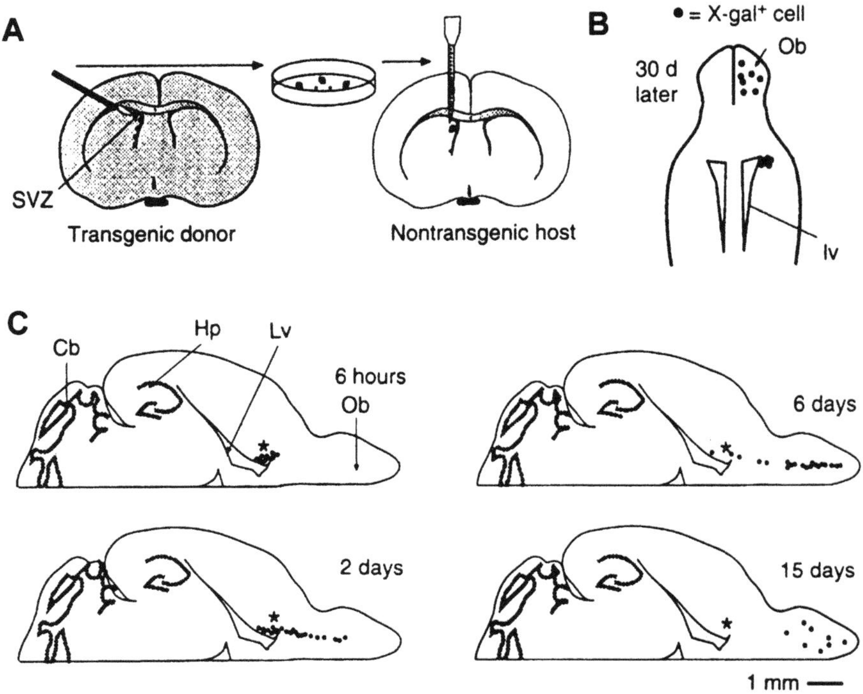

FIG. 9.4. Stem cells in the adult CNS: rostral migratory stream. (A) Cells from the subventricular zone (SVZ) of a donor mouse that carried a neuron-specific marker transgene were implanted into the SVZ of adult hosts. (B) Two weeks later donor cells were identified by staining with the X-gal reaction. Some remained in the SVZ, whereas others had migrated to the olfactory bulb (Ob). (C) Alternatively, dividing cells were labelled with [^{3}H]-thymidine and sections cut at serial time points to reveal the migratory stream of cells from the SVZ to the olfactory bulb. Cb, cerebellum; Hp, hippocampus; Lv, lateral ventricle. (Reproduced from Lois & Alvarez-Buylla, 1994, with permission © American Association for the Advancement of Science.)

that the numbers of new neurones labelled in the hippocampus is influenced by experience (Kempermann et al., 1998).

The precursor cells that give rise to these "new" neurones are not themselves resident in the areas in which the neurones end up but rather in a "subventricular zone" in the lining of the brain ventricles and a subgranular zone in the dentate gyrus. From there the cells migrate in a rostral migratory stream down to the olfactory bulb (Lois & Alavarez-Buylla, 1994) (Fig. 9.4), and over shorter distances within the hippocampus (Kuhn et al., 1997).

The discovery that precursor cells can be identified in the adult brain opens the way to seeking their expansion *in vitro*. Although the numbers of multipotent precursor cells are much lower than in the embryonic brain, precursor cells from the ventricular zone of adult rats and mice brains can similarly be expanded *in vitro* by treatment with high concentrations of EGF and/or FGF (Reynolds

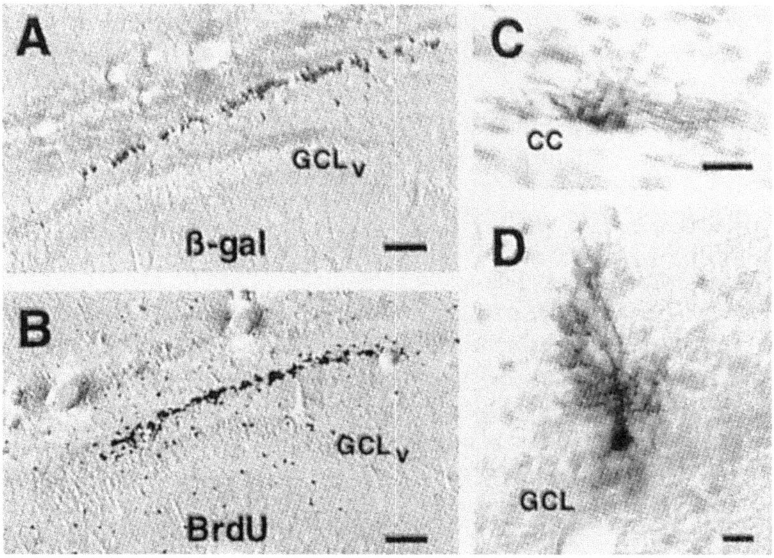

FIG. 9.5. Grafts of adult expanded precursor cells. (A) Expanded adult FGF-sensitive cells were labelled with β-galactosidase (β-Gal) and deoxybromouridine (BrdU) before implantation into the hippocampus. Labelled cells migrated to the dentate granule cell layer (A,B). At higher magnification, β-galactosidase-labelled cells are seen to adopt a neuronal morphology (C,D). CC, corpus callosum; GCLv, ventral segment of the granule cell layer. (Reproduced from Gage et al., 1995, with permission © National Academy of Sciences of the USA.)

& Weiss, 1992; Richards et al., 1992). Furthermore, these expanded adult precursor cells can not only be induced to differentiate into mature neurones and astrocytes *in vitro*, but have also been successfully transplanted into the brains of adult hosts. For example, Gage et al. (1995) expanded FGF-sensitive progenitor cells from the hippocampus of adult rats and maintained them through multiple passages for over 1 year *in vitro*. In culture, these cells could be stained both with markers of precursor cells, such as nestin, but also with markers of mature neurones and astrocytes. Moreover, they went on to transplant expanded cells into the adult host brain, specifically the hippocampus. Before implantation the cells were labelled with the marker gene for β-galactosidase that stains the cells blue and enables the fate of graft cells to be followed in the host brain. Several months after implantation the cells had migrated to take up residence in the granule cell layer of the host dentate gyrus, where they differentiated into neurones (Fig. 9.5). Thus, adult progenitor cells retain the capacity to differentiate into neurones when transplanted even after long-term isolation expansion *in vitro*; but significantly they showed no evidence of tumour formation. These cells may therefore offer another source for generating large supplies of phenotypically appropriate neurones for transplantation, and indeed this even raises the prospect of generating neuronal autografts by biopsy from the recipient's own brain. However, at this stage caution is warranted. The technology is at an early stage, and functional differentiation and incorporation of these cells is not yet demonstrated.

Immortalised cell lines

This approach involves a combination of the techniques already described to engineer precursor cells to express not only particular genes relevant to cell phenotype, but also genes that allow controlled cell proliferation. Of particular interest have been the successes associated with the temperature-sensitive Sv40 large T proto-oncogene, which induces mitosis in cells maintained at 30–33°C but which then switches off and allows the same cells to differentiate and develop into a post-mitotic phenotype when maintained at 37–39°C, either in culture or at the temperature of the host brain post-implantation. Whittemore and colleagues have found that such immortalised precursor cells derived from the embryonic brain will adopt a neuronal phenotype appropriate to the site in which they are placed following transplantation (Shihabuddin et al., 1995, 1996), allowing the hope of generating multipotential cells for implantation with the capacity to integrate fully into the host brain.

Although immortalisation using temperature-sensitive oncogenes has been applied quite widely to generate stable expansion of cells *in vitro*, the functional characterisation of the cells within these grafts is still rather limited.

However, the functional capacity of a different immortalised cell line following implantation has been evaluated by Sinden and colleagues, using a spatial learning task to characterise the deficits induced by global cerebral ischaemia in rats. The particular MHP36 cell line was derived from hippocampal neuroepithelial cells dissected from a transgenic mouse that already carried the temperature-sensitive Sv40T antigen under the control of an interferon-inducible promoter. The cells therefore exhibited a temperature-sensitive conditionally immortal phenotype when grown in permissive interferon-γ treated cultures. The cells were further transfected with the *lac Z* marker gene (so that the cells could be tracked after implantation) and a neomycin-resistant gene to enable selection for transplantation only of cells that carried the marker gene. The cells were evaluated in a global ischaemia model which results in relatively focal hippocampal damage, in particular of the CA1 cell layer. This lesion results in marked deficits in the animals' ability to navigate in a water maze task, a deficit which these authors had previously shown to be alleviated by transplants of primary embryonic neurones dissected from the homotopic area of foetal hippocampus (Hodges et al., 1996). Implants of these immortalised cells appear to have a considerable degree of phenotypic plasticity (similar to the earlier studies, described above) in that following transplantation they were seen to migrate into the neurone-depleted CA1 layer of the ischaemic hippocampus and to differentiate into mature cells with distinctive neuronal morphology. The neuronal phenotype

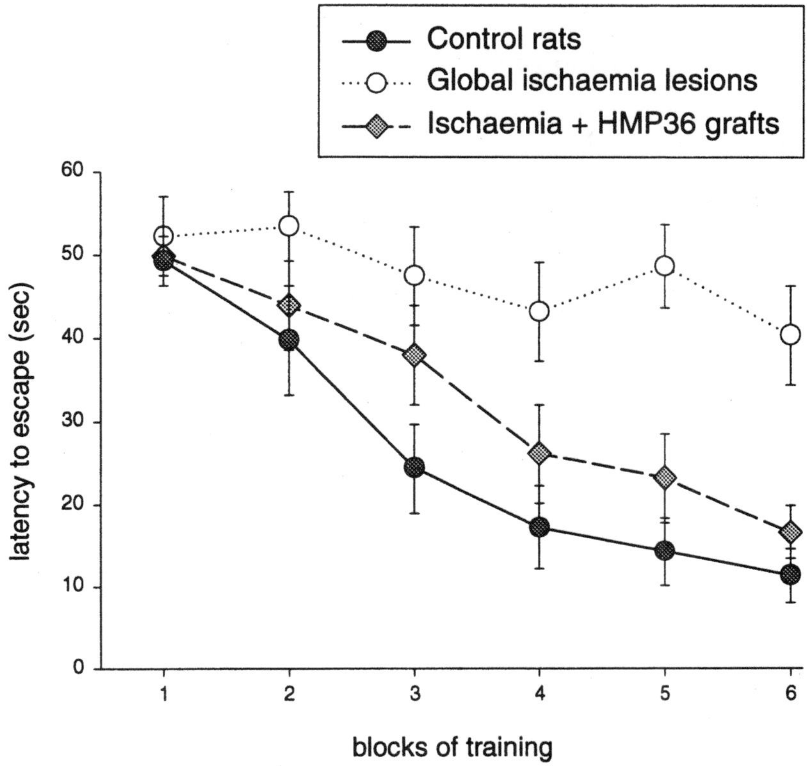

FIG. 9.6. Immortalised neurones implanted into the hippocampus reverse spatial navigation deficits associated with global ischaemic lesions in rats. (Data from Sinden et al., 1997, with permission © Elsevier Science.)

was confirmed by double labelling of β-galactosidase-labelled graft neurones with the specific neuronal marker PGP 9.5. Most dramatic of all in this study was the functional effect of the grafts. Animals were trained in the Morris water maze task and, as shown in Fig. 9.6, the profound acquisition deficit induced by the ischaemic lesion was significantly alleviated by the implants of immortalised cells, almost back to the level of performance seen in non-lesioned controls.

More recently, Martinez-Serrano, Lundberg, and colleagues have gone on to engineer a number of immortalised cell lines, first with growth factors and second with the explicit capacity to secrete tyrosine hydroxylase (TH) over prolonged time periods in the parkinsonian rat striatum (Lundberg et al., 1996; Martinez-Serano, et al., 1995a,b). These studies have yielded rather impressive functional repair and neuroprotection, a topic to which we shall return after considering the strategy and methods of engineering cells for transplantation.

EX VIVO GENE TRANSFER

Genetic engineering of cells for transplantation

Immortalisation with a temperature-sensitive gene is just one aspect of the more general principle of engineering cells with a variety of genes with the ultimate goal of designing an ideal transplant cell with a whole range of specific phenotypic features. The potential power and flexibility of this approach have attracted a great deal of recent interest in the use of genetically modified cells for the treatment of a number of neurodegenerative disorders including Parkinson's disease (reviewed in Fisher & Gage, 1993; Gage & Fisher, 1993). These therapies have variously employed cell lines derived from tumours, non-transformed immortalised cell lines such as fibroblastic NIH 3T3 and rat 208F, primary fibroblasts, myoblasts, and embryonic carcinoma cells, as well as neurones, glia, and precursor cells expanded as mitogen-stimulated neurospheres (see Fig. 9.7).

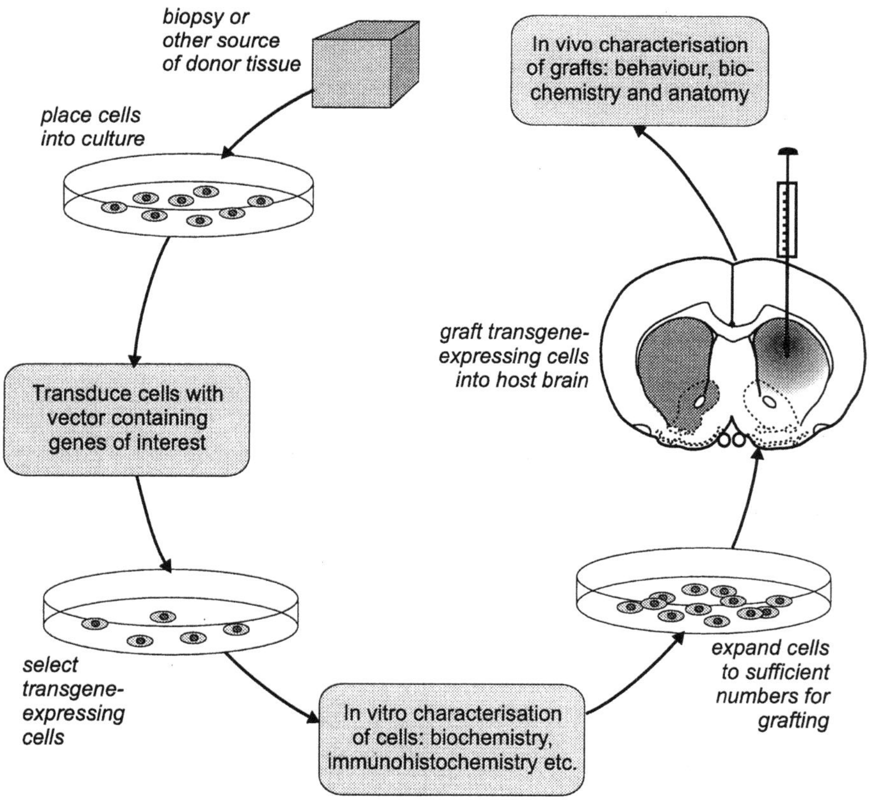

FIG. 9.7. Techniques for *ex-vivo* gene transfer to the brain. (Redrawn from Gage & Fisher, 1993, with permission © Springer-Verlag.)

Some of these therapies have the advantage that the patient's own cells can be used, which therefore avoids any immunological or practical problems in the harvesting and grafting of the tissue. Furthermore, the use of cell lines allows for the production of large quantities of donor tissue from a limited source, as is the case for neurospheres (see later). However, herein lies one of the difficulties in this approach, namely that cell lines have tumorigenic potential which may preclude their use clinically, although packing them into polymers may prove useful in this respect (Tan & Aebischer, 1996). An additional problem with this approach is that after grafting into the CNS, these cells fail to express long-term the transfected gene, namely TH in the case of animal models of Parkinson's disease (reviewed in Svendsen, 1993). Therefore, although this approach holds great promise, it is still very much in its infancy and relies on the disease being characterised by a single neurochemical deficit.

Cells suitable for transplantation. The most widely preferred choices have been fibroblasts and primary embryonic cortical astrocytes, both of which are readily available, can be expanded *in vitro*, and survive transplantation into the brain without forming tumours.

Vectors and techniques for gene transfer. A number of physical methods for gene transfer such as electroporation, lipofection and direct injection are available, but these are all relatively burdensome and inefficient. By contrast, retroviruses are considerably more efficient for transfecting large numbers of cells and have been the most widely used method to date. However, retroviral vectors only enter cells during cell division and so are dependent upon a dividing population of cells for grafting. They are of no value for gene transfer to post-mitotic neurones (but see next section on *in vivo* gene transfer).

Genes for transfer. In addition to the primary genes of interest (e.g. TH) other selection and marker genes can be combined. More recently, interest has focused on enhancing the expression of the primary genes using a variety of additional techniques, including incorporation of multiple promoters and the use of housekeeping genes which will be expressed for longer periods than viral genes. Although not yet achieved, it may be possible in the long term to insert other genes that will not only permit dopamine secretion but also alter the neuronal characteristics of the cell (e.g. specific aspects of neuronal regulation for dopamine release and re-uptake channels).

Cells to make transmitters

The most widely explored strategy has involved engineering otherwise suitable non-dopaminergic cells to express the gene for regulatory enzymes (e.g. TH) that enable the cell to synthesise dopamine from available amino acid precursors. The cells are first modified *in vitro* and then transplanted into the CNS, and research into this "*ex vivo* gene transfer" technique has focused on several key issues:

Several studies have now demonstrated the feasibility of *ex vivo* transfer of the TH gene into primary fibroblasts, astrocytes, and engineered cell lines, with the effective synthesis and secretion of dopamine *in vitro*, and their transplantation into the host brain (Fisher et al., 1991b; Horellou et al., 1991; Wolff et al., 1989). Following transplantation these grafts can down-regulate receptor supersensitivity and reduce asymmetries in apomorphine rotation, but there is generally a failure of long-term expression of the transgene once the engineered cells are implanted in the brain. Only a single study has shown long-term gene expression following CNS implantation of engineered myoblasts, for reasons that are not clear (Jiao et al., 1993).

The genes for the synthetic enzymes regulating the synthesis of many classical neurotransmitters, as well as for a large number of peptide neurotransmitters, are now known (Breakefield & Geller, 1987), which opens the way for engineering primary non-neuronal cells or cell lines to synthesise and perhaps secrete a wide variety of neurotransmitter substances. For example, fibroblasts have been transduced with the choline acetyltransferase gene to generate cells that synthesise the transmitter acetylcholine (Fisher et al., 1993). These cells, following transplantation into the neocortex, can alleviate spatial learning deficits associated with lesions of the nucleus basalis in the Morris water maze (Winkler et al., 1995; see Chapter Seven), although the specificity of these effects at both the behavioural and neurochemical level has been the subject of some discussion (Björklund & Dunnett, 1995). The opportunities for developing other transmitter-producing cell lines and their application in different models of neuronal cell loss are only beginning to be considered.

Cells to make growth factors

The second main class of functional genes for engineering has been a variety of growth factors, most notably NGF. The advantage of growth factors over transmitter-related transgenes is that functional recovery is most likely dependent upon the tonic delivery of the factor at physiological levels rather than the regulated or phasic release of a transmitter at circumscribed synapses. A variety of good neuroprotection models are available for study, and functional effects will be manifest by both protection against ongoing injury and the induction or promotion of spontaneous repair by the host neurones.

In view of the well-established role of NGF in the development, protection, and plasticity of central cholinergic neurones coupled to the long-standing problem of its central delivery (see Chapter Seven), there has been a considerable effort from several laboratories in engineering cells to express NGF for transplantation into the hippocampus. Indeed, the first successes for *ex vivo* gene

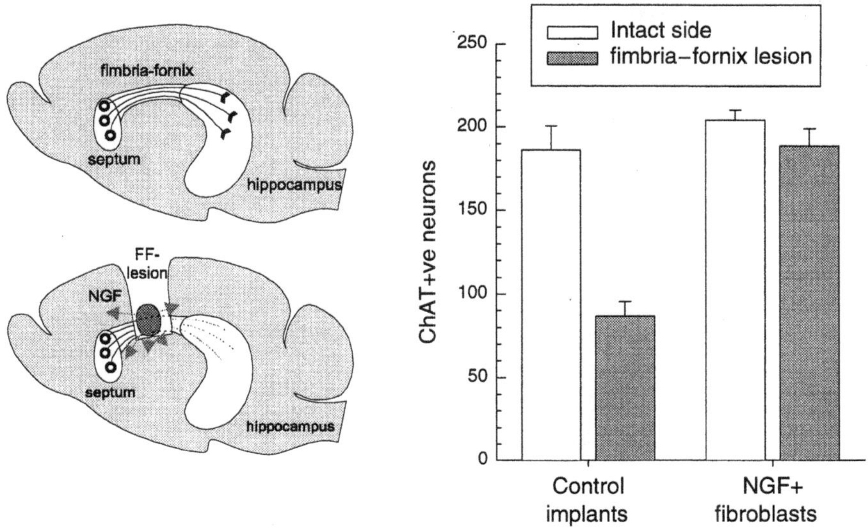

FIG. 9.8. Fibroblasts engineered to secrete NGF protect septal cholinergic neurones against retrograde degeneration following axotomy made by transection of the fimbria–fornix. (Based on data from Rosenberg et al., 1988, with permission © American Association for the Advancement of Science.)

transfer occurred in this area, and the attempts described in the previous section for engineering transmitter replacement have lagged considerably behind.

Following a speculative theoretical article by Gage and colleagues on the prospects and most likely efficient strategies for *ex vivo* gene transfer in 1987, the first clearly effective study appeared the following year. This study exploited the known observation that the retrograde degeneration of septal cholinergic neurones following transection of the fimbria–fornix projection to the hippocampus can be prevented by intraventricular administration of NGF (see Chapter Seven). Rosenberg et al. (1988) therefore implanted fibroblasts engineered to secrete NGF into the fimbria–fornix cavity in rats. The grafts of NGF-secreting fibroblasts protected the septal cholinergic neurones against retrograde cell death, whereas fibroblasts engineered with a marker gene were without effect (Fig. 9.8).

Since then there have been numerous reports with a variety of cell types engineered with NGF showing: survival after transplantation into the CNS; modification of the course of a variety of lesions in the CNS; and a beneficial impact on the behavioural deficits in such animals. Some of the most impressive of these have been the studies by Martinez-Serrano and colleagues (1995a, 1996; Martinez-Serrano & Björklund, 1997). These studies, are based on the HiB5 cell line, which is derived from multipotent neural stem cells that have been immortalised using the temperature-sensitive Sv40 large T proto-oncogene. The cell line is then engineered with the mouse NGF gene and clones that express high

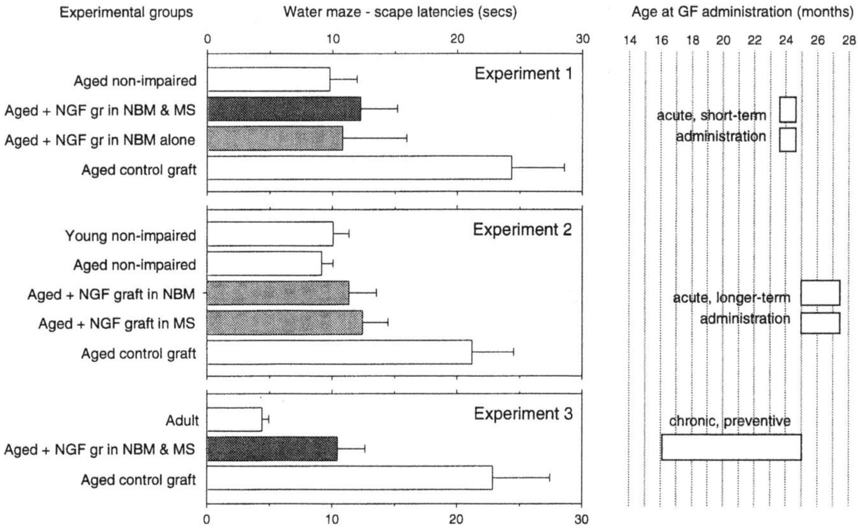

FIG. 9.9. Immortalised HiB5 progenitor cells engineered to secrete NGF alleviate spatial navigation deficits in aged animals. Each bar indicates escape latencies in the Morris water maze of each group of young, adult, or aged rats. The three experiments differ in the timing and duration of NGF administration as shown in the right panel. MS, medial septum; NBM, nucleus basalis magnocellularis; NGF, nerve growth factor. (Redrawn from Martinez-Serrano & Björklund, 1997, with permission © Elsevier Science.)

levels of NGF activity *in vitro* are selected. These engineered cells can then be maintained *in vitro* or frozen until required for transplantation. Following demonstration that the implants block the atrophy of septal neurones in response to axotomy, these authors have undertaken a series of studies to evaluate whether grafts of NGF-secreting cells can protect or reverse cholinergic deficits in ageing. As illustrated in Fig. 9.9. both strategies worked. Grafts implanted acutely into the basal forebrain or septum of aged rats reduced the age-related atrophy of cholinergic neurones and reversed the deficits in spatial navigation learning in the Morris water maze. Conversely, chronic treatments by implanting the cells in middle-aged (16-month-old) rats before the onset of either cellular atrophy or behavioural dysfunction prevented the development of either class of deficit.

Cells to promote neuroprotection

The third main class of functional genes that have been explored are those associated with neuroprotection and cell survival other than growth factors. Thus, for example, in view of the role of oxidative stress in dopamine neuronal cell death, Barkats et al. (1997) have engineered primary dopamine neurones with the gene for Cu/Zn superoxide dismutase, which acts as a free radical scavenger and is therefore important in protecting cells from the damaging effects of oxidative stress and excitotoxicity. Indeed, a deficiency of this enzyme is associated with certain forms of familial motor neurone disease. In this study they found that this manipulation served to protect the grafted cells and enhance their survival. In a similar vein, Anton et al. (1995) engineered immortalised nigral dopamine neurones with the anti-apoptotic proto-oncogene *bcl-2,* the expression of which inhibits both apoptotic and necrotic death of cells in culture. They found a marked increase in the efficacy of the grafts to alleviate apomorphine-induced rotation in the unilateral 6-hydroxydopamine (6-OHDA) lesion model. However, in this latter study the behavioural improvement was not accompanied by a significant enhancement in the numbers of cells actually surviving, so the theoretical basis of the effect remains to be elucidated.

Engineered cells may also provide improved substrates for axon growth. Thus, for example Kobayashi et al. (1995) have modified fibroblasts to express the neural cell adhesion molecule L1 for transplantation into the lesioned spinal cord with the intention of providing an improved substrate for spinal axon regeneration. The grafts were reported as massively promoting axon regeneration in the spinal cord when implanted immediately following a hemisection injury, including sprouting into and through the graft.

Each of these strategies indicates the power of genetic engineering to modify cells for transplantation. At present the technology is at an early stage of development. The most rapid progress will almost certainly be made not by designing new cells for transplantation from scratch, but by the judicious selection of cells that already exhibit many of the desired features and modifying them to produce additional factors that provide further improvement in survival, integration, and functional recovery.

IN VIVO GENE TRANSFER

Whereas the advantage of an *ex vivo* strategy is that the engineered cells can be characterised and selected *in vitro* prior to implantation, an alternative strategy may be simply to modify cells of the host brain *in situ,* if this could be achieved efficiently and safely. If we can modify cells in a culture dish by using a virus to transfer a gene into the cells, we might be able to inject the virus into the brain to transfer the desired gene directly into the living tissue—so-called *in vivo* gene therapy.

The standard techniques for gene transfer use retroviruses to transfect dividing cells. Since neurones do not divide in the mature nervous system, this approach will not work for gene therapy in the brain. However, there are a number of types of virus which will infect post-mitotic neurones which have been investigated as an alternative. These include the attenuated forms of the herpes simplex virus, the adenovirus and adeno-associated virus, and lentiviruses

TABLE 9.2
Comparison of viruses used for *in vivo* gene transfer in the CNS

	Infects non-dividing cells	*Targets neurones*	*Efficiency of infection*	*Expression*	*Cytotoxic and immunological problems*
Retrovirus	No	No	Good (dividing cells only)	Short-term	Little
Herpes simplex (HSV)	Yes	Yes	Good	Long-term	Yes
Adenovirus (AV)	Yes	No	Good	Short-term	Yes
Adeno-associated virus (AAV)	Yes	No	Modest	Long-term	Limited
Lentivirus (LV)	Yes	No	Modest	Long-term	Limited

(Verma & Somia, 1997; Wilkinson et al., 1994; see Table 9.2). Not only are these viruses efficient for infecting cells *in vitro*, but they can also be used as vectors for gene transfer directly into the brain.

Potential applications

As with *ex vivo* gene therapy, the main strategies for *in vivo* gene transfer involve either neurotransmitter-related genes or neurotrophic/neuroprotective molecules.

As an example of the first strategy, Horellou et al. (1994) have used an adenoviral vector to transfer the gene for human TH into the striatum of 6-OHDA-lesioned rats. They found that the virus infected cells in the host striatum, both astrocytes and neurones, which incorporated the transgene. Expression of TH in the infected cells was demonstrated immunohistochemically, and a functional effect was suggested by an acute reduction in apomorphine rotation. The major problem here was the limited duration of the functional effects exhibited by the virus, which may have been due to down-regulation of expression, or to the virus having induced some inflammatory or immune responses in the host brain.

Longer-term expression and behavioural recovery have been obtained using both herpes simplex viruses (HSV) and adeno-associated viruses (AAV) (During et al., 1994; Kaplitt et al., 1994). Thus, for example, During et al. (1994) inserted the human TH gene into a replication-defective HSV type 1 vector and injected the resulting construct into the striatum of rats that had previously received unilateral 6-OHDA lesions in the standard rat model. Apomorphine-induced rotation was then measured at 1 month intervals and seen to be reduced by 60–70% on the first test after injection of the TH virus vector, but not in

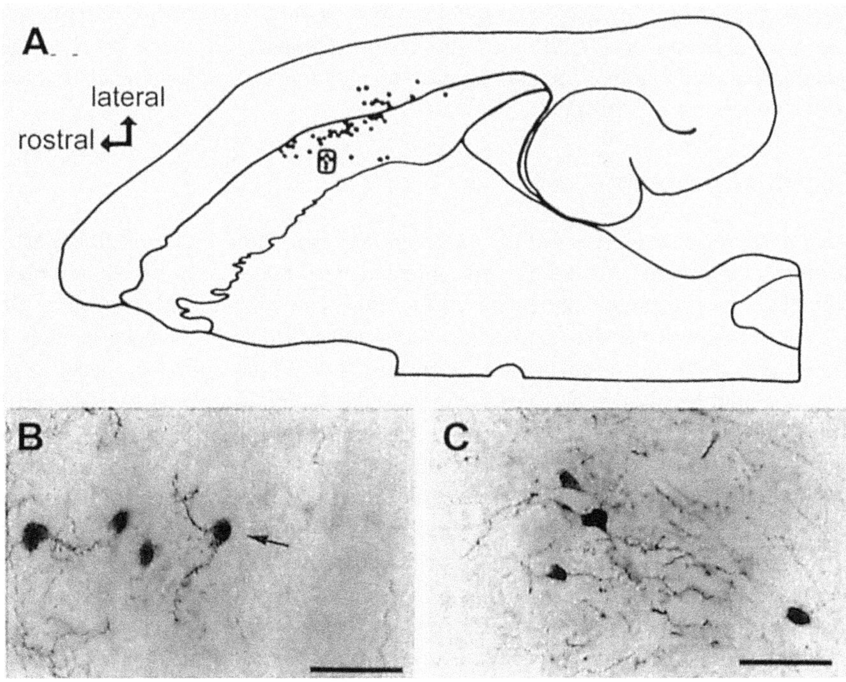

FIG. 9.10. TH-immunoreactive neurones in the striatum (A,B) and globus pallidus (C) following injection of a herpes simplex virus (HSV-1) vector carrying the human TH gene into the striatum of adult rats. Scale bars 50 μm. (Reproduced from During et al., 1994, with permission © American Association for the Advancement of Science.)

control animals injected with saline or a control virus. Moreover, the recovery on this test lasted a full 12 months after treatment. Both *in vivo* microdialysis and histology were undertaken to determine the levels of TH activity and dopamine production. The microdialysis measured L-dopa activity and the production of dopamine in the lesioned striatum 4–6 months after infection, and both were shown to be substantially increased over the level in the lesioned brain, but only partially back to control levels. At post mortem, a large number of neurones in the striatum, and a few in adjacent areas such as the globus pallidus, were seen to express high levels of TH (see Fig. 9.10), indicative of their capacity to synthesise dopamine.

Of course, the preferred alternative to replacing a lost dopamine production from degenerated nigrostriatal terminals is to block the degeneration itself. Several growth factors, and in particular GDNF, have been shown to protect nigrostriatal dopamine neurones against degeneration, using knife-cut axotomy of the nigrostriatal tract, and neurotoxic lesions using 1-methyl-4-phenyl-1,2,3,6-tetrahydropyridine (MPTP) or 6-OHDA (Gash et al., 1996; Hoffer et al., 1994; Sauer et al., 1995). In these first studies, GDNF needed to be given by repeated central injections. However, two groups have recently shown the efficient and effective delivery of GDNF into the lesioned substantia nigra by a single transfection using adenoviral and adeno-associated virus vectors (Lapchak et al., 1997; Mandel et al., 1997).

Potential problems

Such observations suggest that the basic strategy can work. However, there are a number of problems. Although cells infected with adenovirus or other viruses typically show sustained expression of the transgene when tested in culture, it is a common experience that expression shuts down within 1–2 weeks *in vivo*. It seems that there are regulatory elements in the living brain that need to be circumvented to sustain long-term expression and function in the living animal. This will most likely be achieved by the selection of appropriate promoter elements, i.e. leading segments of DNA that regulate when a gene is switched on and switched off. Indeed, there is currently extensive work being undertaken to develop "inducible promoters"; i.e. ones that can be switched on and switched off by a signal or trigger, such as a drug or hormone. Ultimately, it may not only be possible to transfer specific genes to particular areas of the brain, but also to select which cells express the gene (e.g. by linking to the promoter for glial fribrillary acidic protein, GFAP, so as to drive expression just in astrocytes).

A second problem with several classes of virus is their cytotoxicity. Several of these viruses, such as HSV, can cause substantial cell damage at the site of injection. Similarly, there has been concern that adenoviruses induce a marked immunological reaction in the host brain in the vicinity of inoculation, which can result in substantial cell loss or shrinkage at the sites of injection. It is likely that cytotoxic attributes of the viruses can be separated from their infectious capacity, and considerable effort is being directed towards elimination of the toxic components of the viral structure, leaving only those parts necessary for the transfection process.

A third major area of concern is their safety. These viruses will infect non-dividing cells of the nervous system, and some of them in their active normal state cause infective damage to the CNS, such as herpes and acquired immune deficiency virus. Consequently, rather stringent conditions are required for their safety. This usually involves making the viruses "replication defective" by removing one or several of the components in their genome necessary for them to divide and proliferate whilst allowing them to infect and insert the target gene of interest into a living cell. Typically, two or more components essential for replication are knocked out so as to eliminate even a slight chance of spontaneous mutation and recombination of the virus into an active form. Notwithstanding these manipulations, it is likely that the clinical application of *in vivo* gene therapy, at least in the brain, will confront major safety hurdles to be overcome before being allowed in the clinic.

XENOGRAFTS

We considered in an earlier chapter the special immunological privilege that facilitates transplantation in the brain and spinal cord. Thus, allografts (i.e. between unrelated animals of the same species) can be undertaken in most experimental circumstances without concern about immunological rejection. Indeed, whereas most of the clinical trials in Parkinson's disease have used immunoprotective drugs when the patients first receive transplants, these drugs can be withdrawn within a few months without compromising graft viability. We have also seen that in preparation for clinical trials in both Parkinson's disease and Huntington's disease xenotransplantation of human embryonic cells into immunosuppressed rats was used as a strategy to determine optimal age and other parameters for the preparation of human foetal donor tissues for clinical transplantation.

Porcine xenografts

Together, these observations may suggest that the immunological problems of xenotransplantation are readily overcome and that this would then provide a readily available alternative to human embryos for tissue donation. Of the variety of donor species that might be considered, pigs have received the most attention:

(1) The pig brain develops over a similar time course and reaches a similar final size to the human brain.
(2) Pigs are an established farm animal and their husbandry and welfare is well understood.
(3) Pigs breed readily in captivity and they produce large litters, increasing the yield of available donor tissues.
(4) Until recently, it was considered that, since pigs have interacted closely with man for centuries, including their use for food and tissue donation, that there would be limited safety considerations about transfer of pig diseases to a human recipient.
(5) Advances in transgenic technology suggest new strategies of overcoming hyperacute xenograft rejection, which has posed a major barrier to xenotransplantation in the past (Cozzi & White, 1995).

With these considerations in mind, pig tissues have been seen to survive cross-species transplantation into the brains of immunosuppressed rats. Thus, when the host animals have received a unilateral nigrostriatal lesion in the hemiparkinson model, the nigral grafts derived from pig embryos are seen to contain numerous TH-immunostained dopamine neurones, and to reverse the motor asymmetries in the standard tests of drug-induced rotation (Galpern et al., 1996; Huffaker et al., 1989).

These experiments provided the basis for the initiation of a clinical trial involving the approach of implanting porcine foetal nigral tissues in Parkinson's disease as well as striatal tissues in Huntington's disease. Although it is too early to determine how well such grafts function, as full neurological appraisals of these patients are not yet published, preliminary evidence from one post-mortem case suggests that pig dopamine neurones do survive in the human brain (Deacon et al., 1997).

Nevertheless, the numbers of surviving cells are probably even lower than the already low level of survival in human foetal allografts, and there remains considerable concern that the immunosuppression regimes in this first trial may not have been optimal. The development of porcine or other xenograft embryos for neural tissue transplant donation will depend on overcoming two main hurdles. First, the distinctive nature of the brain in transplantation immunology is only now beginning to receive the intensive investigation necessary to develop truly effective immunoprotection strategies for the future. Even basic issues, such as, for example, the precise nature of the rejection process with xenografts, remain unclear. Nevertheless, the immunological problems appear to be essentially soluble, and we anticipate rapid progress on this front in the coming decade.

Even when the immunological issues are fully overcome, however, there have recently been raised new safety issues, in particular concerning the possibility of transformation and cross-species transfer of porcine viruses (Butler, 1998). The at-least-theoretical risk of creation of novel human diseases has led some countries (including the UK, but notably not the USA) to introduce a moratorium on all xenotransplantation until these safety risks can be properly assessed, although exactly how that is to be achieved remains unspecified.

ENCAPSULATION

We have already encountered encapsulation of cells into semipermeable tubes in a number of contexts, notably for cellular delivery of opiates and catecholamines into the spine in terminal cancer pain, and of growth factor molecules into both brain and spinal cord for neuroprotection in several progressive neurological diseases, including Huntington's disease and amyotrophic lateral sclerosis. As a technology, encapsulation cannot be considered in isolation, but as a powerful adjunct to facilitate and promote the safety and survival of delivering different cells and molecules into the CNS.

The essential feature of encapsulation technology is that cells for implantation are packaged into a capsule or tube made of a semipermeable membrane that at one and the same time isolates the graft cells from direct physical contact with the host brain, and allows free exchange of molecules to diffuse across the capsule membrane into and out of the graft (Tan & Aebischer, 1996; see Fig. 9.11). The pore size of the capsule membrane is selected to allow passage of essential nutrients in to nourish the grafted cells, and to allow the secreted target

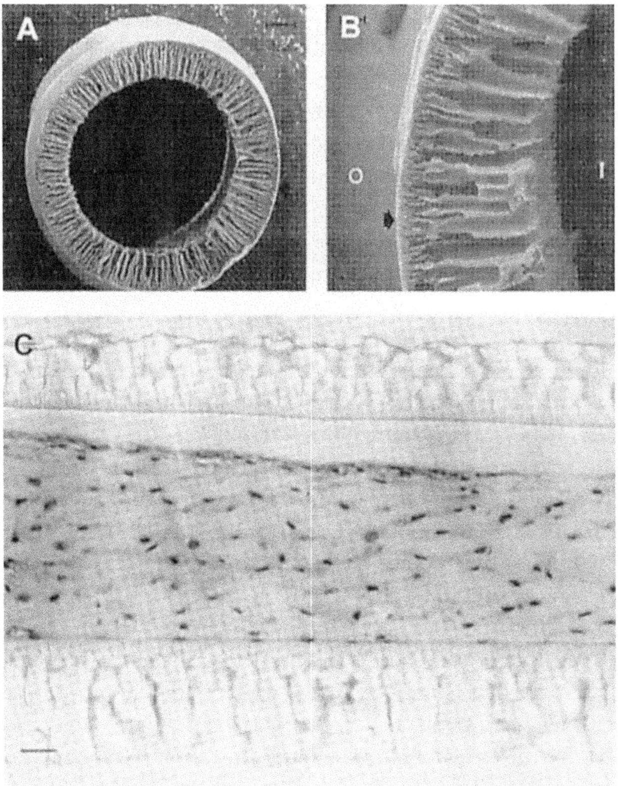

FIG. 9.11. Encapsulation of cellular grafts in semipermeable polymer tubes for implantation in the CNS. (A,B) Cross section scanning electron micrograph of the porous tube walls. (C) Longitudinal histological section of surviving chromaffin cells in a capsule. (Reproduced from Tan & Aebischer, 1996, and Hoffman et al., 1993, with permission © Wiley and Academic Press.)

products of the graft (transmitters, growth factors, hormones, drugs, etc.) to pass freely back into the host brain, while excluding passage of larger molecules (e.g. antibodies) or cells (e.g. of the immune system) that may be immunoreactive against the graft or toxic to the host.

The safety features are clearly illustrated in the case of encapsulation of cross-species grafts. Whereas a major problem for direct implantation of xenografts is how to overcome the efficient immunological mechanisms for their rejection, encapsulation protects the foreign cells both from recognition by circulating host antibodies and from the rejection response precipitated by host lymphocytes, macrophages, and microglia. In case of an adverse reaction by the host to the graft, a capsule is easily removed. Moreover, if in spite of all care in capsule preparation it were to rupture, then the implanted cells would themselves be exposed to the host immune system and be rejected.

The second safety feature of the capsules is that they can prevent the overgrowth of cell lines that would otherwise develop tumours. For example, PC12 cells that can release dopamine and alleviate rotation deficits but have limited effectiveness because of their tumorigenic potential when implanted directly into the brain, can provide more sustained effectiveness for long-term delivery of dopamine into the brain when encapsulated (Aebischer et al., 1991b, 1994; Emerich et al., 1993). In this context, using cell lines from a different species is advantageous, again because of the added safety that the grafted cell will be rejected in the case of any failure in the capsule integrity.

In our assessment, the encapsulation technology is likely to see a variety of novel applications in the next decade, in particular as a strategy to deliver a self-sustaining supply of biologically active molecules to target sites in the depths of the brain and spinal cord. The applications will be particularly potent for growth factor delivery, where these molecules do not readily cross the blood–brain barrier, and must be targeted precisely if sites in other areas of the CNS are to be avoided. It is plausible that encapsulation may also find a number of powerful applications for effective CNS delivery of drugs interacting at diffusely organised (e.g. dopaminergic or opiate) systems of the brain and spinal cord.

Conversely, encapsulation is not a sure solution for all aspects of transplant delivery. The isolation between host and graft neurones that provides the unique strength of this technology is also its major limitation: It is an essentially pharmacological strategy that is not applicable to situations requiring neuronal interaction or circuit reconstruction, as will probably be required for repair in the major neurodegenerative diseases such as Huntington's or Alzheimer's diseases, or spinal cord injury.

SUMMARY

The search for alternatives to human foetal tissues for transplantation has identified a number of possibilities. If the goal is to achieve replacement of deficient molecules or neurochemicals in the brain then a variety of naturally occurring, immortalised, or engineered cells may suffice. However, if the requirement is to repair a damaged neuronal circuit, then we need to identify alternative sources of cells with the uniquely neuronal capacity to connect and integrate with the host brain, such as stem cells or xenografts. Other advanced delivery systems include encapsulation to protect the cells from host immune responses, and *in vivo* gene transfer directly into surviving cells of the host brain in order to change or adapt their phenotypes to meet specific needs.

CHAPTER TEN

Psychological factors in graft function

Up to this point, the mechanisms of graft function have been considered in terms of the patterns of anatomical connectivity and/or neurochemical influence between the grafted cells and the host brain. However, although not yet well studied, a number of lines of evidence are accumulating to suggest that graft efficacy needs to be considered in psychological as well as structural terms, in that the training and experiences of the animal can have a substantial influence on the functional efficacy of a neural transplant.

MECHANISMS OF GRAFT FUNCTION

The first general issue to be considered relates to the mechanisms by which grafts exert functional effects on the host animal. It is well established, as has been illustrated throughout this volume, that not only do grafts survive and connect but they also exert functional effects on the behaviour of the host animals. This is most pertinent in situations where cellular transplantation is employed as a strategy to repair brain damage and alleviate the attendant functional impairments, but can also be seen where transplants influence behaviour in animals without lesions or, more critically, induce additional deficits through both specific and non-specific interactions with the host brain.

Early functional analyses observed simple structural and functional interactions and interpreted the latter, behavioural, effects as straightforward consequences of the former. Thus, for example, nigral grafts gave rise to a dopaminergic innervation of the dopamine-depleted striatum in animals that were seen to be compensated in rotation tests of motor asymmetry (see Chapter Four), and it was natural to assume that the behavioural effects were a consequence of the anatomical regrowth and re-innervation of denervated targets. Similarly, the hyperdiuresis of diabetic rats of the Brattleboro strain with a genetic deficiency in the antidiuretic hormone vasopressin is markedly decreased after implantation of hypothalamic grafts that secrete vasopressin (Gash et al., 1980), and it was natural to assume that the behavioural recovery was a simple consequence of the restoration of endocrine balance by graft-derived secretion of the deficient hormone.

With hindsight, these assumptions have turned out to be naïve in attributing effects to simple restoration of deficient neurotransmitters or neurochemicals. Rather, it has turned out that in each and every model system so far analysed in detail, graft effects could hypothetically be mediated by a wide variety of different mechanisms of greater or lesser specificity (see Table 10.1). Moreover, in any one situation, it frequently turns out that several alternative mechanisms may be acting. On the one hand, the reasons for recovery may differ from animal to animal, and graft to graft. On the other hand, several different processes may interact within the same animal, and different mechanisms may account for different aspects of the lesion syndrome or different classes of behavioural deficit. These interactions have been studied in most detail for dopaminergic grafts in the nigrostriatal system, and as was described in Chapters Four and Five many of the different mechanisms outlined in Table 10.1 can apply, depending on the particular lesion, the particular graft tissue, and the particular behaviour studied.

More detailed accounts of the different mechanisms of action of intracerebral transplants have been provided elsewhere (Björklund et al., 1987; Dunnett & Björklund, 1994). For present purposes, it suffices to emphasise that for some symptoms of some diseases functional recovery may require full reconstruction of a disconnected circuitry in the brain, whereas for other combinations of symptoms and damage or disease rather less precise restoration of pharmacological or trophic influences may suffice, and in yet other situations even quite non-specific effects of surgery may still prove beneficial.

The occasional arguments about what is *the* mechanism by which grafts work—for example, can they repair circuits in the brain or are they simply acting like fancy drug-release systems—have turned out to be sterile. A common general mechanism does not exist; rather, each specific situation needs to be analysed both theoretically and empirically to identify and describe the particular combination of circumstances that apply. Only on the basis of such an analysis, combining theoretical and empirical criteria, can we expect to develop the most effective future therapies based on rational design.

Moreover, over and above the explicit biochemical, anatomical, and physiological influences that have provided the main focus of our attempts at developing a rational strategy for brain repair, it is increasingly apparent that both psychological and physiotherapeutic factors can also influence dramatically the effectiveness (or otherwise) of neural transplantation.

TABLE 10.1
Mechanisms of graft function*

Mechanisms	*Examples*	*Author*
Non-specific or negative effects of surgery	Tumour-like overgrowth of graft tissues	Ridley et al., 1988; Dalrymple-Alford et al., 1988a Rosenstein & Brightman, 1983
	Peripheral nerve grafts have leaky blood–brain barrier, allowing drugs to penetrate the brain	
	Induction of seizure activity	Buzsaki et al., 1991
Acute trophic stimulation of recovery	Adrenal grafts stimulate sprouting response in host dopamine systems	Bohn et al., 1987
	Astrocytes stimulate recovery from frontal cortex ablation	Kesslak et al., 1986
Chronic target-derived trophic support of host projections	Cortical grafts protect basal forebrain cholinergic neurones from retrograde degeneration	Sofroniew et al., 1986
	Spinal cord grafts protect red nucleus neurones from axotomy-induced degeneration	Bregman & Reier, 1986
Diffuse release of deficient neuroactive compounds	Neurohormonal release from hypothalamic grafts	Gash et al., 1980; Krieger et al., 1982
	Catecholamine secreting polymers and encapsulated cells	Aebischer et al., 1991; McRae et al., 1991; Winn et al., 1989; Becker et al., 1990
Diffuse re-innervation of the host brain	Dopaminergic re-innervation of denervated striatum	Dunnett et al., 1981a,b,c; 1983a,b; Schmidt et al., 1983
	Cholinergic re-innervation of denervated hippocampus or cortex	Björklund & Stenevi, 1977; Björklund et al., 1983b; Nilsson et al., 1990
Passive bridges	Peripheral nerve grafts permit axonal regeneration in optic nerve and spinal cord	David & Aguayo, 1981; Vidal-Sanz et al., 1987
Active bridges	Hippocampal bridges allow regrowth of septohippocampal fibres	Buzsaki et al., 1988; Kromer et al., 1980; 1981
Reciprocal graft–host re-innervation	Striatal grafts restore cortico-striatal and striato-pallidal circuits	Sirinathsinghji et al., 1988; Dunnett, 1995
Full reconstruction of damaged circuitry	Not yet achieved in any model system	

* Table based on Björklund et al., 1987; Dunnett and Björklund, 1994, in which more detailed accounts can be found.

ENVIRONMENT

The first, and simplest, level of analysis of the role of psychological factors in the growth, connectivity, and functional efficacy of a neural graft relates to influences of the animal's environment. It has been well established that richness or poverty of an animal's environment can influence developmental processes in the neocortex, so that, for example, raising an animal in an enriched environment results in detectable increases in thickness and in the density of synaptic connections in the neocortex (Rosenzweig et al., 1972). Moreover, providing rats with an enriched environment can enhance the rate and extent of recovery after brain injury (Dalrymple-Alford et al., 1988a, b; Kelche et al., 1987; Whishaw et al., 1984). Several groups have therefore asked whether similar experiences could modify the growth, connectivity, and functional efficacy of neuronal grafts implanted in the brain. In the first such study, after making fimbria–fornix lesions followed by implants of cholinergic-rich septal grafts into the hippocampus, we housed rats either in small groups in standard laboratory rat cages ("impoverished") or as a large colony in a large wire-mesh monkey cage filled with climbing frames, branches, tubes, shelves, and other objects ("enriched") (Dunnett et al., 1986). We found that although there were no significant differences in graft survival or volume, the density of acetylcholinesterase-stained fibres in the hippocampus was significantly higher at 4 weeks after grafting. By 10 weeks, outgrowth had reached a similar high level in all animals. Thus, enrichment appeared to enhance the initial rate of fibre outgrowth, but not the final extent of re-innervation, which stabilised at a close to normal asymptotic level in all animals.

Kelche, Will, and colleagues have adopted this same fimbria–fornix lesion and septal graft paradigm to investigate further whether enriched housing conditions can lead to improved functional recovery (Kelche et al., 1988, 1995). They therefore housed control, lesion, and grafted animals in either enriched or standard environments prior to training in the Hebb–Williams series of maze learning tasks first at 2 months and then again at 10 months after surgery. Although grossly impaired in contrast to the sham-operated control animals, the lesioned and grafted rats did not differ on the short-term test. However, when retested at 10 months, there was a significant improvement in the grafted rats housed in the enriched environment. By contrast, the grafts did not by themselves yield recovery in the rats reared under standard housing conditions. As in the 10-week evaluation in the previous study, the extent of cholinergic fibre outgrowth did not differ between the two graft groups, when assessed after the 10-month tests. Thus, improved re-innervation alone is unlikely to account for the benefit provided by the enriched environment, suggesting that both regrowth and appropriate experience are required for substantial recovery in these rather complex maze tasks (see later).

CONDITIONING EFFECTS

A second area where psychological factors can influence graft effects lies in the influence of previous experience on an animal's response to training stimuli, which can in turn alter the ways grafted animals respond in tests of recovery. This issue has been most apparent in considering the extent to which changes in responsiveness of animals with nigrostriatal lesions and nigral grafts in drug tests of activity and rotation are attributable to (1) pharmacological factors (such changes in receptor sensitivity), or (2) psychological factors (such as changes due to learning and reinforcement processes).

The first concern for such processes influencing behavioural test scores came from the analysis of rotational responses in animals that had received bilateral 6-hydroxydopamine (6-OHDA) lesions and unilateral nigral grafts in infancy. Snyder-Keller and Lund (1990) found that such animals would rotate contralateral to the grafts when activated by a tail-pinch stressor only if they had previously been tested with amphetamine, whereas naïve grafted animals showed little turning response. They therefore suggested that amphetamine treatment is necessary to "prime" a graft to render it functionally effective.

The ability to modify rotational responding by associative conditioning was first demonstrated by Carey (1986a,b; 1988). He gave rats with unilateral 6-OHDA lesions repeated injections of apomorphine in one of two environments, and similar exposure to the other environment without any drug injection. As expected, the drug induced contralateral rotation, wherever tested. He then gave the same rats an injection of saline: They rotated in the contralateral direction if placed in the environment in which they had previously been given apomorphine, but did not rotate if placed in the other environment. Thus, the rats established a conditioned ("Pavlovian") association between the experience of the drug and the environment in which the drug response was tested, which would modify performance when subsequently re-exposed to that environment, even in the absence of the drug. Carey went on to demonstrate that the conditioned rotation response to the saline injection in trained animals was not blocked by antagonism of the dopamine receptors, indicating that the conditioning process was independent of changes in the receptor supersensitivity that underlie the primary rotation response to apomorphine in 6-OHDA-treated rats (Carey, 1990).

In one set of experiments designed to assess whether such conditioned associations may also influence the response of grafted animals, Reading (1994) studied the effects of conditioned hyperactivity. He first demonstrated that 6-OHDA lesions of the ventral striatum abolished both amphetamine-induced and conditioned hyperactivity in photocell cages. As in previous studies (Choulli et al., 1987; Dunnett et al., 1984; Nadaud et al., 1984), nigral grafts were found to be very effective in restoring the drug-induced response. However, the same animals showed no detectable restitution whatsoever in the conditioned response in the same apparatus. This dissociation corroborates Carey's speculation that the conditioning process is independent of primary changes in the dopamine receptors, and highlights the limitation of graft-induced restitution of conditioned behaviours.

More encouraging results were obtained by Annett et al. (1993), using the standard rotation paradigm to test rats with unilateral 6-OHDA lesions and intrastriatal nigral grafts. They gave animals injections of amphetamine in different test environments prior to treatment with saline in one. Two separate effects were identified. First, repeated injections of amphetamine produced a progressively greater response in the animals. Thus, animals with unilateral 6-OHDA nigrostriatal lesions showed greater ipsilateral rotation response on each consecutive trial. In this particular experiment, as is often the case with such grafts (Abrous et al., 1992; Dunnett et al., 1981a; Herman et al., 1985), the grafts were effective not only in completely counteracting the lesion-induced asymmetry, but also in producing an "overcompensation", i.e. turning in the contralateral direction. Moreover, the contralateral rotation in grafted animals was at progressively higher rates on each consecutive trial (Annett et al., 1993). This apparent progressive "sensitisation" of the amphetamine response is unremarkable and has been described many times before (e.g. Brown & Dunnett, 1989; Dunnett et al., 1988b). More interesting was the clear demonstration of conditioning of the rotation response (Fig. 10.1). Thus, when given saline in an environment (e.g. rotation test bowls) in which they had not received any other previous treatment, neither lesioned nor grafted animals showed any rotation, whether or not they had received amphetamine in a different environment. By contrast, parallel groups of rats that had received a series of tests with amphetamine in the rotation bowls were then injected with saline in the rotation bowls: They turned in the same direction under saline as they had previously under amphetamine—lesioned animals turned ipsilaterally under saline and graft animals turned contralaterally. Moreover, the rate of turning by the individual graft animals under saline correlated with their degree of overcompensation on the earlier amphetamine test. Most importantly, it was not previous experience of amphetamine *per se* that modified the response of lesioned or grafted animals, which would be the case if the influence was pharmacological. Rather the animals' responses were modified by experience in a discrete environment and were specific to that environment, indicative of an effect that was truly due to a conditioning process.

These studies demonstrate that an animal's response can be modified or even determined by associative conditioning to stimuli in its environment, and such a process can account for both the priming of stress-induced rotation (Snyder-Keller & Lund, 1990) and the onset of rotation in saline-treated animals (Annett et al., 1993). A similar conditioning process could equally account for the apparent "sensitisation" of rotation after repeated doses of amphetamine, and is likely to contribute to that phenomenon; but this does not rule out pharmacological

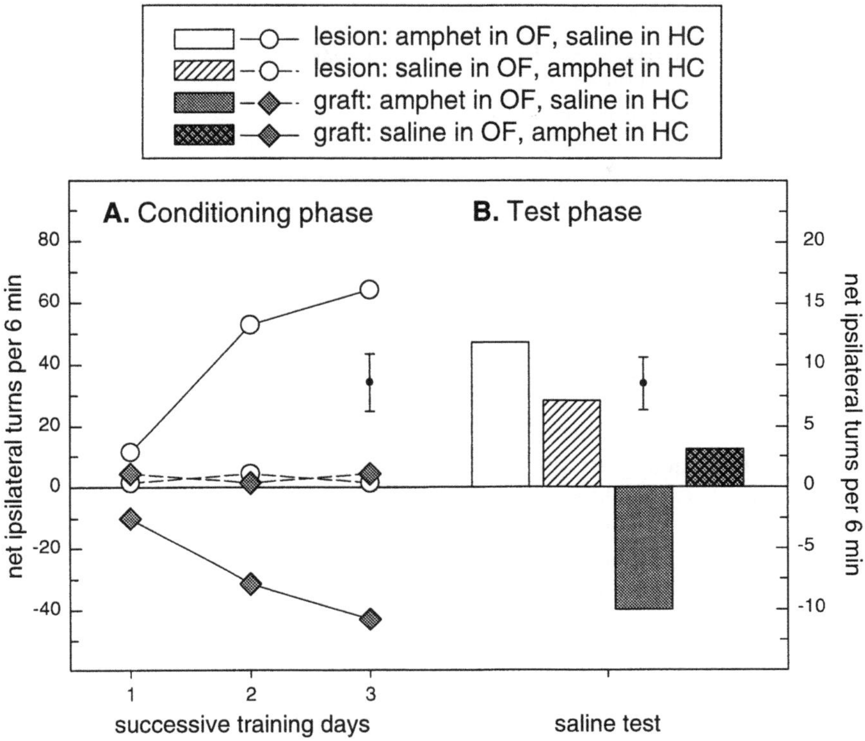

FIG. 10.1. The functional responses of animals with unilateral 6-OHDA lesions and nigral grafts is influenced by conditioning processes. (A) Sensitisation of rotation to amphetamine with repeated injections given either in an open field arena (OF) or in the home cages (HC). Saline injections were given on alternate days in the other environment. (B) Conditioned rotation under saline in the open field by rats previously given amphetamine in the OF (lesion rats to the ipsilateral side, grafted rats to the contralateral side), but not by rats previously given amphetamine in the HC and saline in the OF. (Data from Annett et al., 1993.)

changes in receptor sensitivity also playing a major role, either due to repeated receptor stimulation or simply developing with the passage of time.

LEARNING TO USE THE TRANSPLANT

The importance of training has recently become apparent in a quite different context. In a series of influential studies, Lund and colleagues have demonstrated that retinal transplants can establish connections with the host tectum to restore a functional retino–tectal projection. Thus, for example, retinal grafts placed over the tectum can detect a light stimulus and relay that information to the host brain in sufficient detail to maintain a simple reflex circuit such as the pupillary response, both in neonatal and mature rats (Klassen & Lund, 1987, 1990; Lund et al., 1991). This raised the question of whether the light stimulus was perceived and used as a visual stimulus *per se*—i.e. the input from the graft restored some aspect of "sight"—or was simply an initially neutral stimulus to which particular responses were conditioned by reinforcement, but with no intrinsic *visual* meaning to the animals?

Although the question might appear almost philosophical in nature, Coffey, Rawlins, and Lund have started to address this difficult issue in a series of elegant studies using the principles of associative conditioning and transfer of learning to identify how rats used the newly established inputs originating from light stimuli applied to retinal grafts (Coffey et al., 1990). Their experimental preparation involved removing one eye from rat pups at birth, and at the same time transplanting embryonic retinae onto the tectal surface. Once the rats had matured and the grafts had established projections to the host tectum, the overlying parietal bone was removed to expose the transplants. The viability of the graft was first confirmed by determining whether the pupil constricted to shining light onto the retinal graft, prior to fixing a Perspex window into the skull over the graft so that it could subsequently be illuminated (Coffey et al., 1989). A patch could then be put over the window so that the intact eye alone could be exposed to light stimuli, or conversely a patch could be placed over the intact eye so that the graft alone could be exposed to light stimuli.

The simplest test of visual function in the rats bearing retinal grafts was of the tendency of normal rats to avoid bright lights in an open field. Disappointingly, when placed into a large arena in which one-third was shaded, the rats would spend the majority of their time in the dark partition when the good eye was exposed but moved through all parts of the arena equally when only the retinal transplant was exposed (Coffey et al., 1990). This suggested that the rats did not use the information transduced by the grafts in the particular open field situation, but is not informative about whether that information was nevertheless present. In order to address the latter question, Coffey et al. (1989) trained rats to lever press for food reward in an operant chamber. They then trained the rats in a conditioned suppression paradigm in which they received periodic footshocks predicted by a bright light as a warning signal. Normal rats quickly learn the conditioned response to suppress lever-pressing and freeze in response to the warning signal. In this test the rats with retinal grafts could indeed learn to suppress responding on presentation of the visual stimulus, not only when trained through the good eye, but also when the eye was patched and when the only illumination detected was through the transplant. This suggests that the animals can indeed learn to use the light as a discriminable stimulus when the motivational conditions are strong, as in this test involving footshock.

Once the animals had undergone training in the conditioned suppression test, they were retested in the open field arena. Now, the grafted animals were found to spend most of the time in the shaded partition, whether tested using the normal eye or with only the retinal graft exposed (Coffey et al., 1990). This suggested that although the animals had not initially interpreted graft stimulation as light (to be avoided), they could be trained to interpret the information relayed from the graft appropriately: i.e. they had to learn to use the transplant. On the first test the visual information was relayed to the tectum, but the animal could not interpret the signal and so did not use it. After training in the conditioned suppression task, the retinal inputs acquired meaning for the animal that could then be used to guide behaviour.

Nevertheless, this does not by itself resolve what exactly training had taught the rats. On the one hand, the animal may have learned that the signal transduced by the retina was indeed light, and the animal now avoids the open area of the arena as an inbuilt response to bright visual stimuli. On the other hand, the rat may simply have learned in the course of the conditioned suppression training that the stimulus is significant, associated with aversive consequences, and to be avoided. In this second interpretation, the light stimulus transduced by the graft remains arbitrary rather than of an essentially visual nature. A preliminary indication that if animals are trained on the conditioned suppression task using the graft, learning does not transfer to the normal eye, and *vice versa* (Lund et al., 1991) suggests that the latter interpretation may be favoured; but this issue will require more detailed investigation to be resolved properly. For example, the two alternative interpretations of what the animal has learned produce opposite predictions if the animals are trained on an appetitive task with the visual information predictive of food reward prior to being tested in the open field test. In this case the light stimulus would be associated with positive rather than aversive consequences. Consequently, when tested in the open arena, the rats would still spend most of their time in the shaded partition of the arena if they have learned to interpret the neutral stimulus as a bright light in the visual modality; but they should now spend more time in the open partition if simply treating the stimulus as a positive stimulus in a not-specifically-visual modality. Preliminary data suggest that the first of these interpretations is correct: that training with positive reinforcement still results in avoidance of the dark sector of the open field, suggesting that the animals learn to treat the retinal inputs from the graft first and foremost as light stimuli (P. Coffey, personal communication); but these extended studies still await proper peer review and publication.

Further evidence of rats' need to learn how to use the transplants comes from a study of striatal grafts to alleviate rats' deficits in a visual choice reaction time task (Mayer et al., 1992). In this test, Mayer et al. trained rats to make rapid contralateral head-turn responses to brief lateralised flashes of light (i.e. turn right to a left stimulus, turn left to a right stimulus). This is a complex and rather unnatural sensorimotor response for rats; but they are nevertheless able to learn the task with extended training. The rats were then divided into three groups to remain as sham operated controls, or to receive either unilateral ibotenic acid lesions of the neostriatum alone or lesions plus additional striatal grafts. After allowing 6 months for recovery, growth, and incorporation of the grafts, the

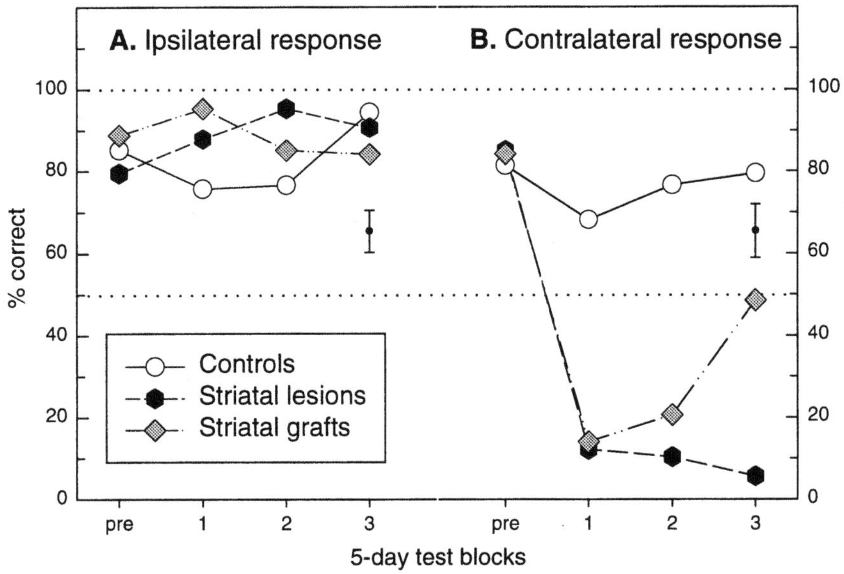

FIG. 10.2. Animals with ibotenic acid lesions and striatal transplants must "learn to use the transplant" before the functional effects are apparent. All animals were initially trained on a lateralised visual stimulus–response (S–R) association prior to lesion and graft surgery. On retest, the animals showed no impairment responding to the ipsilateral side but lesions induced marked impairment responding to the contralateral side. The grafts were initially as impaired as the lesion animals but were able to relearn the S–R association over 3 weeks, whereas the lesion rats remained permanently impaired. (Data from Mayer et al., 1992.)

animals were retested over 3 weeks on the reaction time task. Whereas the controls rapidly re-attained their initial levels of performance, the lesioned animals were seriously impaired on the task, having lasting impairments in the reaction time to initiate contralateral responses and a strong bias to respond to the ipsilateral side whatever stimulus was presented (Fig. 10.2). Although the grafted animals showed a similar impairment when first retested, their performance improved dramatically with training and by the end of three weeks of testing both the reaction time and response bias deficits converged on a normal level of performance. The 6 months survival post-transplantation was probably sufficient for anatomical reconstruction to achieve an asymptotic level of growth and reformation of connections, but was not by itself sufficient for functional recovery. Rather, the animals required additional training with relevant experience for them to be able to utilise the graft and for it to become functionally effective in this complex sensorimotor coordination task.

Subsequent studies are now under way to analyse this phenomenon in more detail. For example, Brasted et al. (1997) have used a related lateralised visual discrimination and choice reaction time task in a similar nine-hole box apparatus to train animals to discriminate stimulus presentations in near and far holes

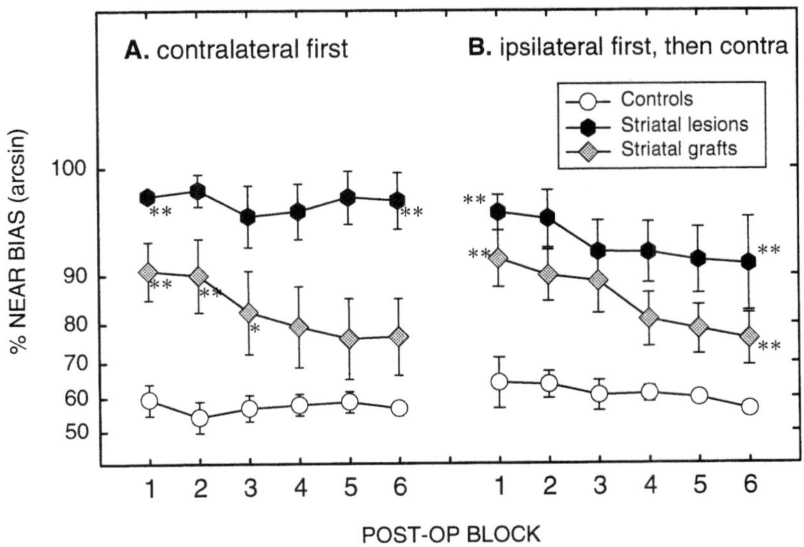

FIG. 10.3. Specificity of the "learning to use the transplant" effect. All animals were pretrained on two separate lateralised visual discriminations, on either left or right sides. The animals were retested 4 months after receiving lesions plus or minus grafts. (A) Animals with lesions were profoundly impaired on the contralateral side whether or not they bore grafts, but the transplanted animals then showed significant relearning over 30 days training. (B) Rats that first received 30 days retraining on the ipsilateral side exhibited no transfer of training: They still showed as great a lesion deficit, and the grafted animals still had to relearn the task contingencies on the contralateral side. (Data from Brasted et al., 1998.)

on either the side ipsilateral or contralateral to unilateral striatal lesions. Again, striatal lesions produced profound ipsilateral bias in responding, and impairments in the speed and accuracy in correct responding on the contralateral side.

This lateralised choice reaction time test is now providing the opportunity for using different transfer training conditions to determine the precise nature of what is retained and what needs to be relearned within the reconstructed graft–host striatal circuits. Thus, in one study (Brasted et al., 1998), animals were first trained to make the lateralised discrimination on both sides, between two stimulus–response (S–R) locations on the left side on every other day, and between two different S–R locations on the right side on the alternate days. They then received lesions and grafts, and waited 4 months before retesting. One subgroup was retested on the contralateral side. As shown in Fig. 10.3A, these animals all showed a marked lesion deficit, whether or not they bore grafts, but whereas the deficit remained stable in the lesion alone group, the grafted animals exhibited substantial relearning over 30 days of training. This replicates the basic "learning to use the transplant" phenomenon. The other subgroup of animals first received 30 days retesting on the less affected ipsilateral side before being tested on the contralateral side. The lesioned groups showed absolutely no benefit of the ipsilateral training, and grafted animals had to relearn the S–R association from exactly the same baseline as the subgroup of animals not given this extra training. This indicates that the functions that must be relearned are not related to the general task demands, but require specific training of the affected striatum (and its new graft-derived circuit) on the specific lateralised S–R associations represented in contralateral space.

Another aspect of these data was of interest. The specific relearning appeared to be required for associative aspects of task performance, such as are represented by accuracy, bias and errors in task performance. Measures of more basic motor aspects of task performance, such as simple reaction times and the movement times to execute the lateralised response, were also impaired by the lesions and alleviated by the grafts, but in these measures no relearning was required: the grafted animals were simply improved at all test points. Thus, the "relearning to use the transplant" appears to apply specifically to behavioural measures involving the neostriatum in the formation of S–R associations, i.e. "habits" (Mishkin et al., 1984; White, 1989). We hypothesise that these functions may be dependent upon the reformation of cortico-striatal circuits through the grafts (see Chapter Six). When such behaviours are lost following the lesion, they have to be re-acquired through specific relevant experience (i.e. retraining). Conversely, behavioural measures that are primarily motoric (e.g. reaction time and the speed of movement) are not associative and do not require explicit retraining. Such behaviours reflect the generalised activation of motor outputs from the grafted striatum, and may be dependent simply upon the regrowth of inhibitory striato-pallidal projections.

REHABILITATION OF TRANSPLANT PATIENTS?

The essential feature of the "learning to use the transplant" effect is that it is most apparent when the tasks involve discriminations, responses, or habits. These involve specific S–R associations that had been learned explicitly prior to injury and on which there is no recovery without explicit retraining. Behaviours such as general locomotion, paw use, and co-ordinated turning are part of the animal's normal repertoire of behaviour, feeding, and social interactions in the home cage, and so new motor habits and reflexes have ample opportunity for establishment within the circuitries of the grafted striatum.

These observations, although first observed in theoretical studies of graft integration and function, should have profound implications for patient care and rehabilitation of transplant patients, although what they are is only now beginning to be considered. Thus, as in the case of surgical treatment for congenital blindness, where the individual has to learn to see and interpret a complex and deeply confusing visual world, so also must we consider how to enable transplant patients to make best use of the repaired circuits of the brain. It will not be sufficient to focus only on the practical issues of how to achieve optimal graft survival and connectivity. If, from the initial clinical trials of neural transplantation, this new surgery is most likely to continue to develop applications in the basal ganglia, in diseases such as Parkinson's, Huntington's and, perhaps next, multiple system atrophy (Wenning et al., 1996), then we need to consider not only the anatomical connectivity needed to reconstruct the damaged circuitry but also the relearning and retraining of the normal adult's rich repertoire of motor skills and habits. This is the realm of the rehabilitation specialists, who have to this point not been active participants in existing transplantation programmes. We might expect, though, that they (you) have much to offer, and the marriage of rehabilitation and neurobiological disciplines may pave the way to marked improvements in present strategies for therapy.

SUMMARY AND CONCLUSIONS

The extent and pattern of interaction between the graft and host brain depends not just on such obvious structural or "anatomical" factors as the nature of the underlying deficit, the tissue that is implanted, and the extent of reciprocal connections that happen to be formed between the graft and the host brain, but also on more subtle aspects such as the total glial, vascular, pharmacological, and growth factor environment of the grafted tissue. Moreover, the extent and limitations of functional recovery substantially depend on the selection of tests to characterise the animals' deficits. Finally, it is increasingly becoming clear that "psychological" factors, including the role of the sensory environment, and the opportunities for relearning knowledge, acquiring experience, and re-acquiring motor skills, also play an important role in graft-derived recovery, even though such factors are even less tangible and more difficult to characterise than the anatomical incorporation of the grafts.

Striatal disease is the first area for major development of neural transplantation to clinical application. With the striatum envisaged as a system for the initiation of goal-directed action and the formation of motor habits, the identification of the specific associations that need to be re-established if we are to achieve a return of normal function highlights the fact that effective clinical trials of transplantation for basal ganglia disease are not just a matter of optimising the neurobiology but emphasise the critical role for additional psychological and physiotherapeutic expertise in the design of postoperative rehabilitation protocols.

References

Abrous, D.N., Torres, E.M., Annett, L.E., Reading, P.J., & Dunnett, S.B. (1992). Intrastriatal dopamine-rich grafts induce a hyperexpression of Fos protein when challenged with amphetamine. *Experimental Brain Research, 91*, 181–190.

Adams, C.E., Hoffman, A.F., Hudson, J.L., Hoffer, B.J., & Boyson, S.J. (1994). Chronic treatment with levodopa and/or selegiline does not affect behavioral recovery induced by fetal ventral mesencephalic grafts in unilaterally 6-hydroxydopamine-lesioned rats. *Experimental Neurology, 130*, 261–268.

Aebischer, P., Tresco, P.A., Sagen, J., & Winn, S.R. (1991). Transplantation of microencapsulated bovine chromaffin cells reduces lesion-induced rotational asymmetry in rats. *Brain Research, 560*, 43–49.

Aebischer, P., Tresco, P.A., Winn, S.R., Greene, L.A., & Jaeger, C.B. (1991). Long-term cross-species brain transplantation of a polymer-encapsulated dopamine-secreting cell line. *Experimental Neurology, 111*, 269–275.

Aebischer, P., Goddard, M., Signore, A.P., & Timpson, R.L. (1994). Functional recovery in hemiparkinsonian primates transplanted with polymer-encapsulated PC12 cells. *Experimental Neurology, 126*, 151–158.

Aebischer, P., Schluep, M., Deglon, N., Joseph, J.M., Hirt, L., Heyd, B., Goddard, M., Hammang, J.P., Zurn, A.D., Kato, A.C., Regli, F., & Baetge, E.E. (1996). Intrathecal delivery of CNTF using encapsulated genetically-modified xenogeneic cells in amyotrophic lateral sclerosis patients. *Nature Medicine, 2*, 696–699.

Agid, Y. (1991). Parkinson's disease: pathophysiology. *Lancet, 337*, 1321–1324.

Agid, Y. (1998). Levodopa: Is toxicity a myth? *Neurology, 50*, 858–863.

Agid, Y., Cervera, P., Hirsch, E., Javoy-Agid, F., Lehericy, S., Raisman, R., & Ruberg, M. (1989). Biochemistry of Parkinson's disease 28 years later—a critical review. *Movement Disorders, 4*, S12b–144S.

Aguayo, A.J., Björklund, A., Stenevi, U., & Carlstedt, T. (1984). Fetal mesencephalic neurons survive and extend long axons across peripheral nervous system grafts inserted into the adult rat striatum. *Neuroscience Letters, 45*, 53–58.

Ahlskog, J.E., Tyce, G.M., Kelly, P.J., Van Heerden, J.A., Stoddard, S.L., & Carmichael, S.W. (1989). Cerebrospinal fluid indices of blood–brain barrier permeability following adrenal–brain transplantation in patients with Parkinson's disease. *Experimental Neurology, 105*, 152–161.

Ahlskog, J.E., Kelly, P.J., Van Heerden, J.A., Stoddard, S.L., Tyce, G.M., Windebank, A.J., Bailey, P.A., Bell, G.N., Blexrud, M.D., & Carmichael, S.W. (1990). Adrenal medullary transplantation into the brain for treatment of Parkinson's disease: clinical outcome and neurochemical studies. *Mayo Clinic Proceedings, 65*, 305–328.

Alexander, G.E., DeLong, M.R., & Strick, P.L. (1986). Parallel organization of functionally segregated circuits linking basal ganglia and cortex. *Annual Review of Neuroscience, 9*, 357–381.

Alexander, G.E., Crutcher, M.D., & DeLong, M.R. (1990). Basal ganglia-thalamocortical circuits: parallel substrates for motor, oculomotor, prefrontal and limbic functions. *Progress in Brain Research, 85*, 119–146.

Allen, G.S., Burns, R.S., Tulipan, N.B., & Parker, R.A. (1989). Adrenal medullary transplantation to the caudate nucleus in Parkinson's disease: initial clinical results in 18 patients. *Archives of Neurology, 46*, 487–491.

Altman, J. (1963). Autoradiographic investigation of cell proliferation in the brains of rats and cats. *Anatomical Record, 145*, 573–592.

Anderson, D.J. (1993). Molecular control of cell fate in the neural crest: the sympathoadrenal lineage. *Annual Review of Neuroscience, 16*, 129–158.

Annett, L.E., Reading, P.J., Tharumaratnam, D., Abrous, D.N., Torres, E.M., & Dunnett, S.B. (1993). Conditioning versus priming of dopaminergic grafts by amphetamine. *Experimental Brain Research, 93*, 46–54.

Anton, R., Kordower, J.H., Kane, D.J., Markham, C.H., & Bredesen, D.E. (1995). Neural transplantation of cells expressing the anti-apoptotic gene *bcl-2*. *Cell Transplantation, 4*, 49–54.

Apostolides, C., Sanford, E., Hong, M., & Mendez, I. (1998). Glial cell line-derived neurotrophic factor improves intrastriatal graft survival of stored dopaminergic cells. *Neuroscience, 83*, 363–372.

Apuzzo, M.L.J., Neal, J.H., Waters, C.H., Appley, A.J., Boyd, S.D., Couldwell, W.T., Wheelock, V.H., & Weiner, L.P. (1990). Utilization of unilateral and bilateral stereotaxically placed adrenomedullary-striatal autografts in parkinsonian humans: rationale, techniques, and observations. *Neurosurgery, 26*, 746–757.

Arbuthnott, G.W., Dunnett, S.B., & MacLeod, N. (1985). The electrophysiological properties of single units in mesencephalic transplants in rat brain. *Neuroscience Letters, 57*, 205–210.

Åkesson, E., Kjaeldgaard, A., & Seiger, Å. (1998). Human embryonic spinal cord grafts in adult rat spinal cord cavities: Survival, growth, and interactions with the host. *Experimental Neurology, 149*, 262–276.

Backlund, E.O., Granberg, P.O., Hamberger, B., Knutsson, E., Mårtensson, A., Sedvall, G., Seiger, Å., & Olson, L. (1985). Transplantation of adrenal medullary tissue to striatum in parkinsonism. *Journal of Neurosurgery, 62*, 169–173.

Baird, A. (1993). Fibroblast growth factors: what's in a name? *Endocrinology, 132*, 487–488.

Bakay, R.A.E., Watts, R.L., Freeman, A., Iuvone, P.M., Watts, N., & Graham, S.D. (1990). Preliminary report on adrenal–brain transplantation for parkinsonism in man. *Stereotactic and Functional Neurosurgery, 54*, 312–323.

Bandtlow, C.E., Zachleder, T., & Schwab, M.E. (1990). Oligodendrocytes arrest neurite growth by contact inhibition. *Journal of Neuroscience, 10*, 3837–3848.

Bankiewicz, K.S., Oldfield, E.H., Chiueh, C.C., Doppman, J.L., Jacobowitz, D.M., & Kopin, I.J. (1986). Hemiparkinsonism in monkeys after unilateral internal carotid artery infusion of 1-methyl-4-phenyl-1,2,3,6-tetrahydropyridine (MPTP). *Life Sciences, 39*, 7–16.

Bankiewicz, K.S., Plunkett, R.J., Kopin, I.J., Jacobowitz, D.M., London, W.T., & Oldfield, E.H. (1988). Transient behavioral recovery in hemiparkinsonian primates after adrenal medullary autografts. *Progress in Brain Research, 78*, 543–550.

Bankiewicz, K.S., Plunkett, R.J., Jacobowitz, D.M., Kopin, I.J., & Oldfield, E.H. (1991). Fetal nondopaminergic neural implants in parkinsonian primates—histochemical and behavioral studies. *Journal of Neurosurgery, 74*, 97–104.

Barde, Y.A. (1988). What, if anything, is a neurotrophic factor? *Trends in Neurosciences, 11*, 343–346.

Barkats, M., Nakao, N., Grasbon-Frodl, E.M., Bilang-Bleuel, A., Revah, F., Mallet, J., & Brundin, P. (1997). Intrastriatal grafts of embryonic mesencephalic rat neurons genetically modified using an adenovirus encoding human Cu/Zn superoxide dismutase. *Neuroscience, 78*, 703–713.

Barker, R.A., & Dunnett, S.B. (1993). The biology and behaviour of intracere-bral adrenal transplants in animals and man. *Reviews in the Neurosciences, 4*, 113–146.

Barker, R.A., Fricker, R.A., & Dunnett, S.B. (1994). Factors important in the survival of dopamine neurons in intracerebral grafts of embryonic substantia nigra. In T.R. Flanagan, D.F. Emerich & S.R. Winn (Eds.), *Providing pharmacological access to the brain* (pp. 237–252). New York: Academic Press.

Barker, R.A., Fricker, R.A., Abrous, D.N., Fawcett, J.W., & Dunnett, S.B. (1995). A comparative study of the preparation techniques for improving the viability of nigral grafts using vital stain, *in vitro* cultures and *in vivo* grafts. *Cell Transplantation, 4*, 173–200.

Bartlett, P.F., Rosenfeld, J.V., Bailey, K.A., Cheesman, H., Harvey, A.R., & Kerr, R.S.C. (1990). Allograft rejection overcome by immunoselection of neuronal precursor cells. *Progress in Brain Research, 82*, 153–160.

Bartus, R.T., Dean, R.L., Beer, B., & Lippa, A.S. (1982). The cholinergic hypothesis of geriatric memory dysfunction. *Science, 217*, 408–417.

Bayer, S.A. (1982). Changes in total number of dentate granule cells in juvenile and adult rats: a correlated volumetric and ^{3}H-thymidine autoradiographic study. *Experimental Brain Research, 46*, 315–323.

Bayer, S.A. (1983). ^{3}H-thymidine-radiographic studies of neurogenesis in the rat olfactory bulb. *Experimental Brain Research, 50*, 329–340.

Bayer, S.A., Yackel, J.W., & Puri, P.S. (1982). Neurons in the rat dentate gyrus granular layer substantially increase during juvenile and adult life. *Science, 216*, 890–892.

Beal, M.F. (1994). Huntington's disease, energy, and excitotoxicity. *Neurobiology of Aging, 15*, 275–276.

Beal, M.F., Brouillet, E.P., Jenkins, B.G., Ferrante, R.J., Kowall, N.W., Miller, J.M., Storey, E., Srivastava, R., Rosen, B.R., & Hyman, B.T. (1993a). Neurochemical and histologic characterisation of striatal excitotoxic lesions produced by the mitochondrial toxin 3-nitropropionic acid. *Journal of Neuroscience, 13*, 4181–4192.

Beal, M.F., Hyman, B.T., & Koroshetz, W. (1993b). Do defects in mitochondrial energy metabolism underlie the pathology of neurodegenerative diseases? *Trends in Neurosciences, 16*, 125–131.

Becker, J.B., & Freed, W.J. (1988). Adrenal medulla grafts enhance functional activity of the striatal dopamine system following substantia nigra lesions. *Brain Research, 462*, 401–406.

Becker, J.B., Robinson, T.E., Barton, P., Sintov, A., Siden, R., & Levy, R.J. (1990). Sustained behavioral recovery from unilateral nigrostriatal damage produced by the controlled release of dopamine from a silicone polymer pellet placed into the denervated striatum. *Brain Research, 508*, 60–64.

Beckstead, R.M., & Cruz, C.J. (1986). Striatal axons to the globus pallidus, entopeduncular nucleus and substantia nigra come mainly from separate cell populations in cat. *Neuroscience, 19*, 147–158.

Berry, M., & Henry, J. (1975). Response of neonatal CNS to injury. *Neuropathology and Applied Neurobiology, 2*, 166.

Berry, M., Maxwell, W.L., Logan, A., Mathewson, A., McConnell, P., Ashurst, D.E., & Thomas, G.H. (1983). Deposition of scar tissue in the central nervous system. *Acta Neurochirurgica, Supplementum, 32*, 31–53.

Bès, J.C., Tkaczuk, J., Czech, K.A., Tafani, M., Bastide, R., Caratero, C., Pappas, G.D., & Lazorthes, Y. (1998). One-year chromaffin cell allograft survival in cancer patients with chronic pain: morphological and functional evidence. *Cell Transplantation, 7*, 227–238.

Bing, G., Notter, M.F.D., Hansen, J.T., & Gash, D.M. (1988). Comparison of adrenal medullary, carotid body and PC12 cell grafts in 6-OHDA lesioned rats. *Brain Research Bulletin, 20*, 399–406.

Bing, G., Notter, M.F.D., Hansen, J.T., Kellogg, C., Kordower, J.H., & Gash, D.M. (1990). Cografts of adrenal medulla with C6 glioma cells in rats with 6-hydroxydopamine-induced lesions. *Neuroscience, 34*, 687–697.

Björklund, A., & Dunnett, S.B. (1995). Acetylcholine revisited (News & Views). *Nature, 375*, 446.

Björklund, A., & Lindvall, O. (1986). Catecholamine brain stem regulatory systems. In Anonymous, *Handbook of physiology. Section I. The nervous system. Volume IV. Intrinsic regulatory systems of the brain* (pp. 155–235). Washington: American Physiological Society.

Björklund, A., & Stenevi, U. (1971). Growth of central catecholamine neurones into smooth muscle grafts in the rat mesencephalon. *Brain Research, 31*, 1–20.

Björklund, A., & Stenevi, U. (1977). Reformation of the severed septohippocampal cholinergic pathway in the adult rat by transplanted septal neurons. *Cell and Tissue Research, 185*, 289–302.

Björklund, A., & Stenevi, U. (1979). Reconstruction of the nigrostriatal dopamine pathway by intracerebral transplants. *Brain Research, 177*, 555–560.

Björklund, A., Dunnett, S.B., Stenevi, U., Lewis, M.E., & Iversen, S.D. (1980a). Reinnervation of the denervated striatum by substantia nigra transplants: functional consequences as revealed by pharmacological and sensorimotor testing. *Brain Research, 199*, 307–333.

Björklund, A., Schmidt, R.H., & Stenevi, U. (1980b). Functional reinnervation of the neostriatum in the adult rat by use of intraparenchymal grafting of dissociated cell suspensions from the substantia nigra. *Cell and Tissue Research, 212*, 39–45.

Björklund, A., Stenevi, U., Schmidt, R.H., Dunnett, S.B., & Gage, F.H. (1983a). Intracerebral grafting of neuronal cell-suspensions. I. Introduction and general methods of preparation. *Acta Physiologica Scandinavica, Supplementum, 522*, 1–7.

Björklund, A., Gage, F.H., Stenevi, U., & Dunnett, S.B. (1983b). Intracerebral grafting of neuronal cell suspensions. VI. Survival and growth of intrahippocampal implants of septal cell suspensions. *Acta Physiologica Scandinavica, Supplementum, 522*, 49–58.

Björklund, A., Lindvall, O., Isacson, O., Brundin, P., Wictorin, K., Strecker, R.E., Clarke, D.J., & Dunnett, S.B. (1987). Mechanisms of action of intracerebral neural implants—studies on nigral and striatal grafts to the lesioned striatum. *Trends in Neurosciences, 10*, 509–516.

Björklund, A., Campbell, K., Sirinathsinghji, D.J.S., Fricker, R.A., & Dunnett, S.B. (1994). Functional capacity of striatal transplants in the rat Huntington model. In S.B. Dunnett & A. Björklund (Eds.), *Functional Neural Transplantation* (pp. 157–195). New York: Raven Press.

Blakemore, W.F., & Franklin, R.J.M. (1991). Transplantation of glial cells into the CNS. *Trends in Neurosciences, 14*, 323–327.

Blunt, S.B., Jenner, P., & Marsden, C.D. (1991). The effect of L-dopa and carbidopa treatment on the survival of rat fetal dopamine grafts assessed by tyrosine hydroxylase immunohistochemistry and [H-3] mazindol autoradiography. *Neuroscience, 43*, 95–110.

Blunt, S.B., Jenner, P., & Marsden, C.D. (1992). Motor function, graft survival and gliosis in rats with 6-OHDA lesions and fetal ventral mesencephalic grafts chronically treated with L-dopa and carbidopa. *Experimental Brain Research, 88*, 326–340.

Boer, G.J. (1994). Ethical guidelines for the use of human embryonic or fetal tissue for experimental and clinical neurotransplantation and research. *Journal of Neurology, 242*, 1–13.

Bohn, M.C., Cupit, L., Marciano, F., & Gash, D.M. (1987). Adrenal grafts enhance recovery of striatal dopaminergic fibers. *Science, 237*, 913–916.

Bohn, M.C., & Kanuicki, M. (1990). Bilateral recovery of striatal dopamine after unilateral adrenal grafting into the striatum of the 1-methyl-4-(2′methylphenyl)-1,2,3,6-tetrahydropyridine (2′CH3-MPTP)-treated mice. *Journal of Neuroscience Research, 25*, 281–286.

Bracken, M.B., Shepard, M.J., Holford, T.R., LeoSummers, L., Aldrich, E.F., Fazl, M., Fehlings, M., Herr, D.L., Hitchon, P.W., Marshall, L.F., Nockels, R.P., Pascale, V., Perot, P.L., Piepmeier, J.,

Sonntag, V.K.H., Wagner, F., Wilberger, J.E., Winn, H.R., & Young, W. (1997). Administration of methyl-prednisolone for 24 or 48 hours or tirilazad mesylate for 48 hours in the treatment of acute spinal cord injury: Results of the Third National Acute Spinal Cord Injury Randomised Controlled Trial. *Journal of the American Medical Association, 277*, 1597–1604.

Brasted, P., Humby, T., Dunnett, S.B., & Robbins, T.W. (1997). Response space deficits following unilateral excitotoxic lesions of the dorsal striatum in the rat. *Journal of Neuroscience, 17*, 8919–8926.

Brasted, P.J., Döbrössy, M.D., Eagle, D.M., Nathwani, F., Robbins, T.W., & Dunnett, S.B. (1998). Operant analysis of striatal dysfunction. In D.W. Emerich, R.L. Dean & P.R. Sanberg (Eds.), *Innovative models of CNS diseases: From molecules to therapy,* Totowa, NJ: Humana.

Brasted, P.J., Watts, C., Robbins, T.W., & Dunnett, S.B. (1999). Associative plasticity in striatal transplants. Submitted. *Proceedings of the National Academy of Science*, USA.

Breakefield, X.O., & Geller, A.I. (1987). Gene transfer into the nervous system. *Molecular Neurobiology, 1*, 339–371.

Brecknell, J.E., Haque, N.S.K., Du, J.-S., Muir, E.M., Hlavin, M.-L., Fawcett, J.W., & Dunnett, S.B. (1996). Functional and anatomical reconstruction of the 6-OHDA lesioned nigrostriatal system of the adult rats by RN22 nigrostriatal bridge grafts. *Neuroscience, 71*, 913–925.

Bregman, B.S. (1987). Spinal cord transplants permit the growth of serotonergic axons across the site of neonatal spinal cord transection. *Developmental Brain Research, 34*, 265–279.

Bregman, B.S. (1994). Recovery of function after spinal cord injury: transplantation strategies. In S.B. Dunnett & A. Björklund (Eds.), *Functional neural transplantation* (pp. 489–529). New York: Raven Press.

Bregman, B.S., & Reier, P.J. (1986). Neural tissue transplants rescue axotomized rubrospinal cells from retrograde death. *Journal of Comparative Neurology, 244*, 86–95.

Bregman, B.S., Kunkel-Bagden, E., Reier, P.J., Dai, H.N., McAtee, M., & Gao, D. (1993). Recovery of function after spinal cord injury: Mechanisms underlying transplant-mediated recovery of function differ after spinal cord injury in newborn and adult rats. *Experimental Neurology, 123*, 3–16.

Bregman, B.S., Kunkel-Bagden, E., Schnell, L., Dai, H.N., Gao, D., & Schwab, M.E. (1995). Recovery from spinal cord injury mediated by antibodies to neurite growth inhibitors. *Nature, 378*, 498–501.

Broggi, G., Pluchino, F., Gennari, L., Geminiani, S., Tamma, F., & Caraceni, T. (1989). Adrenal medulla autograft in caudate nucleus as treatment for Parkinson's disease. *Acta Neurochirurgica, Supplementum, 52*, 45–47.

Brooks, D.J., Ibanez, V., Sawle, G.V., Quinn, N.P., Lees, A.J., Mathias, C.J., Bannister, R., Marsden, C.D., & Frackowiak, R.S.J. (1990). Differing patterns of striatal 18F-dopa uptake in Parkinson's disease, multiple system atrophy, and progressive supranuclear palsy. *Annals of Neurology, 28*, 547–555.

Broseta, J., Diaz-Cascajo, P., Garcia-March, G., & Sanchez-Ledesma, M.J. (1989). Critical approach to intrastriatal medullary adrenal implants via open surgery in parkinsonism: a case report. *Acta Neurochirurgica, Supplementum, 52*, 46–47.

Brown, V.J., & Dunnett, S.B. (1989). Comparison of adrenal and fetal nigral grafts on drug-induced rotation in rats with 6-OHDA lesions. *Experimental Brain Research, 78*, 214–218.

Brown, V.J., & Robbins, T.W. (1989). Elementary processes of response selection mediated by distinct regions of the striatum. *Journal of Neuroscience, 9*, 3760–3765.

Brundin, P. (1992). Dissection, preparation, and implantation of human embryonic brain tissue. In S.B. Dunnett & A. Björklund (Eds.), *Neural transplantation: A practical approach* (pp. 139–160). Oxford: IRL Press.

Brundin, P., Isacson, O., & Björklund, A. (1985). Monitoring of cell viability in suspensions of embryonic CNS tissue and its use as a criterion for intracerebral graft survival. *Brain Research, 331*, 251–259.

Brundin, P., Nilsson, O.G., Strecker, R.E., Lindvall, O., Åstedt, B., & Björklund, A. (1986). Behavioral effects of human fetal dopamine neurons grafted in a rat model of Parkinson's disease. *Experimental Brain Research, 65*, 235–240.

Bruno, J.P., Jackson, D., Zigmond, M.J., & Stricker, E.M. (1987). Effect of dopamine-depleting brain lesions in rat pups: role of striatal serotonergic neurons in behavior. *Behavioral Neuroscience, 101*, 806–811.

Buchanan, J.T., & Nornes, H.O. (1986). Transplants of embryonic brainstem containing the locus coeruleus into spinal cord enhance the hindlimb flexion reflex in adult rats. *Brain Research, 381*, 225–236.

Buck, P.S. (1962). *A bridge for passing.* New York: John Day Co.

Burns, R.S. (1991). Subclinical damage to the nigrostriatal dopamine system by MPTP as a model of preclinical Parkinson's disease—a review. *Acta Neurologica Scandinavica, 84*, 29–36.

Butler, D. (1998). Last chance to stop and think on risks of xenotransplants. *Nature, 391*, 320–324.

Cahill, D.W., & Olanow, C.W. (1990). Autologous adrenal medulla to caudate nucleus transplantation in advanced Parkinson's disease: 18 month results. *Progress in Brain Research, 82*, 637–642.

Cajal, S.R.Y. (1928). *Degeneration and regeneration of the nervous system.* Oxford: Oxford University Press.

Calne, D.B., & McGeer, P.L. (1988). Tissue transplantation for Parkinson's disease. *Canadian Journal of Neurological Sciences, 15*, 364–365.

Campbell, K., Wictorin, K., & Björklund, A. (1992). Differential regulation of neuropeptide mRNA expression in intrastriatal striatal transplants by host dopaminergic afferents. *Proceedings of the National Academy of Sciences of the United States of America, 89*, 10489–10493.

Carey, R.J. (1986a). Conditioned rotational behaviour in rats with unilateral 6-hydroxydopamine lesions of the substantia nigra. *Brain Research, 365*, 379–382.

Carey, R.J. (1986b). A conditioned anti-parkinsonian drug effect in the hemiparkinsonian rat. *Psychopharmacology, 89*, 269–272.

Carey, R.J. (1988). Application of the unilateral 6-hydroxydopamine rat model of rotational behavior to the study of conditioned drug effects. *Journal of Neuroscience Methods, 22*, 253–261.

Carey, R.J. (1990). Dopamine receptors mediate drug-induced but not Pavlovian conditioned contralateral rotation in the unilateral 6-OHDA animal model. *Brain Research, 515*, 292–298.

Carli, M., Evenden, J.L., & Robbins, T.W. (1985). Depletion of unilateral striatal dopamine impairs initiation of contralateral actions and not sensory attention. *Nature, 313*, 679–682.

Carlstedt, T., Cullheim, S., Risling, M., & Ulfhake, B. (1989). Nerve fibre regeneration across the PNS–CNS interface at the root–spinal cord junction. *Brain Research Bulletin, 22*, 93–102.

Carmichael, S.W., Wilson, R.J., Brimijoin, W.S., Melton, L.J., Okazaki, H., Yaksh, T.L., Ahlskog, J.E., Stoddard, S.L., & Tyce, G.M. (1988). Decreased catecholamines in the adrenal medulla of patients with parkinsonism. *New England Journal of Medicine, 318*, 254.

Cassel, J.C., Kelche, C., Peterson, G.M., Ballough, G.P., Goepp, I., & Will, B. (1991). Graft-induced behavioral recovery from subcallosal septohippocampal damage in rats depends on maturity stage of donor tissue. *Neuroscience, 45*, 571–586.

Cenci, M.A., Campbell, K., Wictorin, K., & Björklund, A. (1992). Striatal c-fos induction by cocaine or apomorphine occurs preferentially in output neurons projecting to the substantia nigra in the rat. *European Journal of Neuroscience, 4*, 376–380.

Cervera, P., Rascol, O., Ploska, A., Gaillard, G., Raisman, R., Duyckaerts, C., Hauw, J.J., Scherman, D., Montastruc, J.L., Javoy-Agid, F., & Agid, Y. (1988). Noradrenaline, adrenaline and tyrosine hydroxylase in adrenal medulla from parkinsonian patients. *Journal of Neurology, Neurosurgery and Psychiatry, 51*, 1104–1105.

Cheng, H., Cao, Y.H., & Olson, L. (1996). Spinal cord repair in adult paraplegic rats—partial restoration of hind-limb function. *Science, 273*, 510–513.

Chéramy, A., Leviel, V., & Glowinski, J. (1981). Dendritic release of dopamine in the substantia nigra. *Nature, 289*, 537–542.

Choi, C.R., Lee, J.S., Sung, K.W., & Song, J.U. (1990). Adrenal medullary transplantation for Parkinson's disease. *Stereotactic and Functional Neurosurgery, 54–5*, 324–327.

Choi, D.W. (1990). Cerebral hypoxia: some new approaches and unanswered questions. *Journal of Neuroscience, 10*, 2493–2501.

Choi, D.W. (1992). Excitotoxic cell death. *Journal of Neurobiology, 23*, 1261–1276.

Choulli, K., Herman, J.P., Rivet, J.M., Simon, H., & Le Moal, M. (1987). Spontaneous and graft-induced behavioral recovery after 6-hydroxydopamine lesions of the nucleus accumbens in the rat. *Brain Research, 407*, 376–380.

Chung, S.S., Kim, S.H., & Yoon, D.H. (1990). Stereotaxic transplantation of adrenal medullary tissue in Parkinson's disease. *Stereotactic and Functional Neurosurgery, 54–5*, 272–276.

Clarke, D.J., & Dunnett, S.B. (1993). Synaptic relationships between cortical and dopaminergic inputs and intrinsic GABAergic systems within intrastriatal striatal grafts. *Journal of Chemical Neuroanatomy, 6*, 147–158.

Clarke, D.J., Brundin, P., Strecker, R.E., Nilsson, O.G., Björklund, A., & Lindvall, O. (1988a). Human fetal dopamine neurons grafted in a rat model of Parkinson's disease: ultrastructural evidence for synapse formation using tyrosine hydroxylase immunocytochemistry. *Experimental Brain Research, 73*, 115–126.

Clarke, D.J., Dunnett, S.B., Isacson, O., Sirinathsinghji, D.J.S., & Björklund, A. (1988b). Striatal grafts in rats with unilateral neostriatal lesions. I. Ultra-structural evidence of afferent synaptic inputs from the host nigrostriatal pathway. *Neuroscience, 24*, 791–801.

Clarke, D.J., Wictorin, K., Dunnett, S.B., & Bolam, J.P. (1994). Internal composition of striatal grafts: light and electron microscopy. In G. Percheron, J.S. McKenzie & J. Féger (Eds.), *The basal ganglia IV. New ideas on structure and function* (pp. 189–196). New York: Plenum Press.

Clarke, P.G.H. (1990). Developmental cell-death—morphological diversity and multiple mechanisms. *Anatomy and Embryology, 181*, 195–213.

Clowry, G.J., & Vrbová, G. (1992). Observations on the development of transplanted embryonic ventral horn neurones grafted into adult spinal cord and connected to skeletal muscle implants via peripheral nerve. *Experimental Brain Research, 91*, 249–258.

Coffey, P.J., Lund, R.D., & Rawlins, J.N.P. (1989). Retinal transplant-mediated learning in a conditioned suppression task in rats. *Proceedings of the National Academy of Sciences of the United States of America, 86*, 7248–7249.

Coffey, P.J., Lund, R.D., & Rawlins, J.N.P. (1990). Detecting the world through a retinal implant. *Progress in Brain Research, 82*, 269–275.

Collier, T.J., Gash, D.M., & Sladek, J.R. (1988). Transplantation of norepinephrine neurons into aged rats improves performance in a learned task. *Brain Research, 448*, 77–87.

Collier, T.J., Gallagher, M.J., & Sladek, C.D. (1993). Cryopreservation and storage of embryonic rat mesencephalic dopamine neurons for one year: Comparison to fresh tissue in culture and neural grafts. *Brain Research, 623*, 249–256.

Condé, H. (1992). Organization and physiology of the substantia nigra. *Experimental Brain Research, 88*, 233–248.

Coyle, J.T., & Schwarcz, R. (1976). Lesions of striatal neurones with kainic acid provide a model for Huntington's chorea. *Nature, 263*, 244–246.

Coyle, J.T., Price, D.L., & DeLong, M.R. (1983). Alzheimer's disease: a disorder of cortical cholinergic innervation. *Science, 219*, 1184–1190.

Cozzi, E., & White, D.J.G. (1995). The generation of transgenic pigs as potential organ donors for humans. *Nature Medicine, 1*, 964–966.

Cummings, J.L. (1992). Depression and Parkinson's disease: a review. *American Journal of Psychiatry, 149*, 443–454.

Cunningham, L.A., Hansen, J.T., Short, M.P., & Bohn, M.C. (1991). The use of genetically altered astrocytes to provide nerve growth factor to adrenal chromaffin cells grafted into the striatum. *Brain Research, 561*, 192–202.

Cunningham, L.A., Short, M.P., Breakefield, X.O., & Bohn, M.C. (1994). Nerve growth factor released by transgenic astrocytes enhances the function of adrenal chromaffin cell grafts in a rat model of Parkinson's disease. *Brain Research, 658*, 219–231.

Curran, E.J., & Becker, J.B. (1991). Changes in blood–brain barrier permeability are associated with behavioral and neurochemical indexes of recovery following intraventricular adrenal medulla grafts in an animal model of Parkinson's disease. *Experimental Neurology, 114*, 184–192.

Czech, K.A., & Sagen, J. (1995). Update on cellular transplantation into the CNS as a novel therapy for chronic pain. *Progress in Neurobiology, 46*, 507–529.

Dahlström, A., & Fuxe, K. (1974). Evidence for the existence of monoamine-containing neurons in the central nervous system. I. Demonstration of monoamines in the cell bodies of brain stem neurons. *Acta Physiologica Scandinavica, Supplementum, 232*, 1–55.

Dalrymple-Alford, J.C., Kelche, C., Cassel, J.C., Toniolo, G., Pallage, V., & Will, B.E. (1988a). Behavioral deficits after intrahippocampal fetal septal grafts in rats with selective fimbria–fornix lesions. *Experimental Brain Research, 69*, 545–558.

Dalrymple-Alford, J.C., Kelche, C., Eclancher, F., & Will, B. (1988b). Pre-operative enrichment and behavioral recovery in rats with septal lesions. *Behavioral and Neural Biology, 49*, 361–373.

Das, G.D., & Altman, J. (1971). Transplanted precursors of nerve cells: their fate in the cerebellums of young rats. *Science, 173*, 637–638.

Date, I., Felten, S.Y., Olschowka, J.A., & Felten, D.L. (1990). Limited recovery of striatal dopaminergic fibers by adrenal medullary grafts in MPTP-treated aging mice. *Experimental Neurology, 107*, 197–207.

Date, I., Asari, S., & Ohmoto, T. (1995). Two-year follow-up study of a patient with Parkinson's disease and severe motor fluctuations treated by co-grafts of adrenal medulla and peripheral nerve into bilateral caudate nuclei: Case report. *Neurosurgery, 37*, 515–518.

Date, I., Yoshimoto, Y., Imaoka, T., Miyoshi, Y., Furuta, T., Asari, S., & Ohmoto, T. (1994). Cografts of adrenal medulla with peripheral nerve for Parkinson's disease. *Cell Transplatation, 3*, S47–S49.

David, S., & Aguayo, A.J. (1981). Axonal elongation into peripheral nervous system "bridges" after central nervous system injury in adult rats. *Science, 214*, 931–933.

Davie, C.A., Barker, G.J., Webb, S., Tofts, P.S., Thompson, A.J., Harding, A.E., McDonald, W.I., & Miller, D.H. (1995). Persistent functional deficit in multiple sclerosis and autosomal dominant cerebellar ataxia is associated with axon loss. *Brain, 118*, 1583–1592.

Davies, S.J.A., Fitch, M.T., Memberg, S.P., Hall, A.K., Raisman, G., & Silver, J. (1997). Regeneration of adult axons in white matter tracts of the central nervous system. *Nature, 390*, 680–683.

Davies, S.W., Turmaine, M., Cozens, B.A., DiFiglia, M., Sharp, A.H., Ross, C.A., Scherzinger, E., Wanker, E.E., Mangiarini, L., & Bates, G.P. (1997). Formation of neuronal intranuclear inclusions (NII) underlies the neurological dysfunction in mice transgenic for the HD mutation. *Cell, 90*, 537–548.

Dawson, T.M., Dawson, V.L., Gage, F.H., Fisher, L.J., Hunt, M.A., & Wamsley, J.K. (1991a). Down-regulation of muscarinic receptors in the rat caudateputamen after lesioning of the ipsilateral nigrostriatal dopamine pathway with 6-hydroxydopamine (6-OHDA)—normalization by fetal mesencephalic transplants. *Brain Research, 540*, 145–152.

Dawson, T.M., Dawson, V.L., Gage, F.H., Fisher, L.J., Hunt, M.A., & Wamsley, J.K. (1991b). Functional recovery of supersensitive dopamine receptors after intrastriatal grafts of fetal substantia nigra. *Experimental Neurology, 111*, 282–292.

Deacon, T., Schumacher, J., Dinsmore, J., Thomas, C., Palmer, P., Kott, S., Edge, A., Penney, D., Kassissieh, S., Dempsey, P., & Isacson, O. (1997). Histological evidence of fetal pig neural cell survival after transplantation into a patient with Parkinson's disease. *Nature Medicine, 3*, 350–353.

Deckel, A.W., Robinson, R.G., Coyle, J.T., & Sanberg, P.R. (1983). Reversal of long-term locomotor abnormalities in the kainic acid model of Huntington's disease by day 18 fetal striatal implants. *European Journal of Pharmacology, 92*, 287–288.

Diamond, M.E., Armstrong-James, M., & Ebner, F.F. (1993). Experience-dependent plasticity in adult rat barrel cortex. *Proceedings of the National Academy of Sciences of the United States of America, 90*, 2082–2086.

Diener, P.S., & Bregman, B.S. (1998). Fetal spinal cord transplants support the development of target reaching and coordinated postural adjustments after neonatal cervical spinal cord injury. *Journal of Neuroscience, 18*, 763–778.

DiFiglia, M., Sapp, E., Chase, K.O., Davies, S.W., Bates, G.P., Vonsattel, J.-P., & Aronin, N. (1997). Aggregation of huntingtin in neuronal intranuclear inclusions and dystrophic neurites in brain. *Science, 277*, 1990–1993.

Ding, Y.J., Zhang, W.C., Jiao, S.S., Cao, J.K., Meng, J.M., Ding, M.C., Sun, J.B., Zhang, Z.M., & Shi, M.T. (1988). Functional improvement by transplanting auto-adrenal medulla grafts into caudate in patients with parkinsonism. *Chinese Medical Journal, 101*, 631–636.

Divac, I., Rosvold, H.E., & Szwarcbart, M.K. (1967). Behavioral effects of selective ablation of the caudate nucleus. *Journal of Comparative and Physiological Psychology, 63*, 184–190.

Doering, L.C., & Aguayo, A.J. (1987). Hirano bodies and other cytoskeletal abnormalities develop in fetal rat CNS grafts isolated for long periods in peripheral nerve. *Brain Research, 401*, 178–184.

Doering, L.C. (1992). Peripheral nerve segments promote consistent long-term survival of adrenal medulla transplants in the brain. *Experimental Neurology, 118*, 253–260.

Dohan, F.C., Robertson, J.T., Feler, C., Schweltzer, J., Hall, C., & Robertson, J.H. (1988). Autopsy findings in a Parkinson's disease patient treated with adrenal medullary to caudate nucleus transplant. *Society for Neuroscience Abstracts, 14*, 8.

Doucet, G., Murata, Y., Brundin, P., Bosler, O., Mons, N., Geffard, M., Ouimet, C.C., & Björklund, A. (1989). Host afferents into intrastriatal transplants of fetal ventral mesencephalon. *Experimental Neurology, 106*, 1–9.

Doucet, G., Brundin, P., Descarries, L., & Björklund, A. (1990). Effect of prior dopamine denervation on survival and fiber outgrowth from intrastriatal fetal mesencephalic grafts. *European Journal of Neuroscience, 2*, 279–290.

Doupé, A.J., Landis, S.C., & Patterson, P.H. (1985). Environmental influences in the development of neural crest derivatives: glucocorticoids, growth factors, and chromaffin cell plasticity. *Journal of Neuroscience, 5*, 2119–2142.

Drucker-Colín, R., Madrazo, I., Ostrosky-Solis, F., Shkurovich, M., Franco, R., & Torres, C. (1988). Adrenal medullary tissue transplants in the caudate nucleus of Parkinson's patients. *Progress in Brain Research, 78*, 567–574.

Drucker-Colín, R., García-Hernández, F., Mendoza-Ramirez, J.L., Pacheco-Cano, M.T., & Komisurak, B.R. (1990). Possible mechanisms of action of adrenal transplants in Parkinson's disease. *Progress in Brain Research, 82*, 509–514.

Duff, K., Eckman, C., Zehr, C., Yu, X., Prada, C.M., Pereztur, J., Hutton, M., Buee, L., Harigaya, Y., Yager, D., Morgan, D., Gordon, M.N., Holcomb, L., Refolo, L., Zenk, B., Hardy, J., & Younkin, S. (1996). Increased amyloid-beta-42(43) in brains of mice expressing mutant presenilin-1. *Nature, 383*, 710–713.

Dunn, E.H. (1917). Primary and secondary findings in a series of attempts to transplant cerebral cortex in the albino rat. *Journal of Comparative Neurology, 27*, 565–582.

Dunnett, S.B. (1990a). Neural transplantation in animal models of dementia. *European Journal of Neuroscience, 2*, 567–587.

Dunnett, S.B. (1990b). Is it possible to repair the damaged prefrontal cortex by neural tissue transplantation? *Progress in Brain Research, 85*, 285–297.

Dunnett, S.B. (1991). Cholinergic grafts, memory and ageing. *Trends in Neurosciences, 14*, 371–376.

Dunnett, S.B. (1995). Functional repair of striatal systems by neural transplants: evidence for circuit reconstruction. *Behavioural Brain Research, 66*, 133–142.

Dunnett, S.B., & Barth, T.M. (1991). Animal models of Alzheimer's disease and dementia (with an emphasis on cortical cholinergic systems). In P. Willner (Ed.), *Behavioural models in psychopharmacology* (pp. 359–418). Cambridge: Cambridge University Press.

Dunnett, S.B., & Björklund, A. (1987). Mechanisms of function of neural grafts in the adult mammalian brain. *Journal of Experimental Biology, 132*, 265–289.

Dunnett, S.B., & Björklund, A. (1992). Staging and dissection of rat embryos. In S.B. Dunnett & A. Björklund (Eds.), *Neural transplantation: A practical approach* (pp. 1–19). Oxford: IRL Press.

Dunnett, S.B., & Björklund, A. (1994). Mechanisms of function of neural grafts in the injured brain. In S.B. Dunnett & A.Björklund (Eds.), *Functional neural transplantation* (pp. 531–567). New York: Raven Press.

Dunnett, S.B., & Everitt, B.J. (1998). Topographic factors affecting the functional viability of dopamine-rich grafts in the neostriatum. In T.B. Freeman & J.H. Kordower (Eds.), *Cell transplantation for neurological disorders* (pp. 135–169). Totowa, NJ: Humana Press.

Dunnett, S.B., & Mayer, E. (1992). Neural grafts, growth factors and trophic mechanisms of recovery. In A.J. Hunter & M. Clarke (Eds.), *Neurodegeneration* (pp. 183–217). New York: Academic Press.

Dunnett, S.B., Björklund, A., Stenevi, U., & Iversen, S.D. (1981a). Behavioral recovery following transplantation of substantia nigra in rats subjected to 6–OHDA lesions of the nigrostriatal pathway. 1. Unilateral lesions. *Brain Research, 215*, 147–161.

Dunnett, S.B., Björklund, A., Stenevi, U., & Iversen, S.D. (1981b). Grafts of embryonic substantia nigra reinnervating the ventrolateral striatum ameliorate sensorimotor impairments and akinesia in rats with 6-OHDA lesions of the nigrostriatal pathway. *Brain Research, 229*, 209–217.

Dunnett, S.B., Björklund, A., Stenevi, U., & Iversen, S.D. (1981c). Behavioral recovery following transplantation of substantia nigra in rats subjected to 6-OHDA lesions of the nigrostriatal pathway. 2. Bilateral lesions. *Brain Research, 229*, 457–470.

Dunnett, S.B., Low, W.C., Iversen, S.D., Stenevi, U., & Björklund, A. (1982). Septal transplants restore maze learning in rats with fornix–fimbria lesions. *Brain Research, 251*, 335–348.

Dunnett, S.B., Björklund, A., Schmidt, R.H., Stenevi, U., & Iversen, S.D. (1983a). Intracerebral grafting of neuronal cell suspensions. IV. Behavioral recovery in rats with unilateral 6-OHDA lesions following implantation of nigral cell suspensions in different forebrain sites. *Acta Physiologica Scandinavica, Supplementum, 522*, 29–37.

Dunnett, S.B., Björklund, A., Schmidt, R.H., Stenevi, U., & Iversen, S.D. (1983b). Intracerebral grafting of neuronal cell suspensions. V. Behavioral recovery in rats with bilateral 6-OHDA lesions following implantation of nigral cell suspensions. *Acta Physiologica Scandinavica, Supplementum, 522*, 39–47.

Dunnett, S.B., Bunch, S.T., Gage, F.H., & Björklund, A. (1984). Dopamine-rich transplants in rats with 6-OHDA lesions of the ventral tegmental area. 1. Effects on spontaneous and drug-induced locomotor activity. *Behavioural Brain Research, 13*, 71–82.

Dunnett, S.B., Whishaw, I.Q., Bunch, S.T., & Fine, A. (1986). Acetylcholine-rich neuronal grafts in the forebrain of rats: effects of environmental enrichment, neonatal noradrenaline depletion, host transplantation site and regional source of embryonic donor cells on graft size and acetylcholinesterase-positive fiber outgrowth. *Brain Research, 378*, 357–373.

Dunnett, S.B., Whishaw, I.Q., Rogers, D.C., & Jones, G.H. (1987). Dopamine-rich grafts ameliorate whole body motor asymmetry and sensory neglect but not independent limb use in rats with 6-hydroxydopamine lesions. *Brain Research, 415*, 63–78.

Dunnett, S.B., Badman, F., Rogers, D.C., Evenden, J.L., & Iversen, S.D. (1988a). Cholinergic grafts in the neocortex or hippocampus of aged rats: reduction of delay-dependent deficits in the delayed non-matching to position task. *Experimental Neurology, 102*, 57–64.

Dunnett, S.B., Hernandez, T.D., Summerfield, A., Jones, G.H., & Arbuthnott, G.W. (1988b). Graft-derived recovery from 6-OHDA lesions: specificity of ventral mesencephalic graft tissues. *Experimental Brain Research, 71*, 411–424.

Dunnett, S.B., Isacson, O., Sirinathsinghji, D.J.S., Clarke, D.J., & Björklund, A. (1988c). Striatal grafts in rats with unilateral neostriatal lesions. III. Recovery from dopamine-dependent motor asymmetry and deficits in skilled paw reaching. *Neuroscience, 24*, 813–820.

Dunnett, S.B., Martel, F.L., Rogers, D.C., & Finger, S. (1989a). Factors affecting septal graft amelioration of differential reinforcement of low rates (DRL) and activity deficits after fimbria–fornix lesions. *Restorative Neurology and Neuroscience, 1*, 83–92.

Dunnett, S.B., Rogers, D.C., & Richards, S.J. (1989b). Nigrostriatal reconstruction after 6-OHDA lesions in rats: combination of dopamine-rich nigral grafts and nigrostriatal bridge grafts. *Experimental Brain Research, 75*, 523–535.

Dunnett, S.B., Everitt, B.J., & Robbins, T.W. (1991). The basal forebrain cortical cholinergic system: interpreting the functional consequences of excitotoxic lesions. *Trends in Neurosciences, 14*, 494–501.

Dunnett, S.B., Kendall, A.L., Watts, C., & Torres, E.M. (1997). Neuronal cell transplantation for Parkinson's and Huntington's diseases. *British Medical Bulletin, 53*, 757–776.

Dunnett, S.B., Torres, E.M., & Annett, L.E. (1998). A lateralised grip strength test to evaluate unilateral nigrostriatal lesions in rats. *Neuroscience Letters, 245*, 1–4.

During, M.J., Naegele, J.R., O'Malley, K.L., & Geller, A.I. (1994). Long-term behavioral recovery in parkinsonian rats by an HSV vector expressing tyrosine hydroxylase. *Science, 266*, 1399–1402.

Duyao, M.P., Auerbach, A.B., Ryan, A., Persichetti, F., Barnes, G.T., McNeil, S.M., Ge, P., Vonsattel, J.-P., Gusella, J.F., Joyner, A.L., & MacDonald, M.E. (1995). Inactivation of the mouse Huntington's disease gene homolog *Hdh. Science, 269*, 407–410.

Dwork, A.J., Pezzoli, G., Silani, V., Fahn, S., & Hill, R. (1988). Transplantation of fetal substantia nigra and adrenal medulla to the caudate nucleus in 2 patients with Parkinson's disease. *New England Journal of Medicine, 319*, 370–371.

Eddleston, M., & Mucke, L. (1993). Molecular profile of reactive astrocytes—implications for their role in neurologic disease. *Neuroscience, 54*, 15–36.

Emerich, D.F., McDermott, P.E., Krueger, P.M., Frydel, B., Sanberg, P.R., & Winn, S.R. (1993). Polymer-encapsulated PC12 cells promote recovery of motor function in aged rats. *Experimental Neurology, 122*, 37–47.

Eriksdotter-Nilsson, M., Gerhardt, G.A., Seiger, Å., Hoffer, B.J., & Granholm, A.-C. (1989a). Multiple changes in noradrenergic mechanisms in the coeruleohippocampal pathway during aging. Structural and functional correlates in intraocular double grafts. *Neurobiology of Aging, 10*, 117–124.

Eriksdotter-Nilsson, M., Gerhardt, G.A., Seiger, Å., Olson, L., Hoffer, B.J., & Granholm, A.-C. (1989b). Age-related alterations in noradrenergic input to the hippocampal formation: structural and functional studies in intraocular transplants. *Brain Research, 478*, 269–280.

Eriksson, P.S., Perfilieva, E., Björk-Eriksson, T., Alborn, A.M., Nordborg, C., Peterson, D.A., & Gage, F.H. (1998). Neurogenesis in the adult human hippocampus. *Nature Medicine, 4*, 1313–1317.

Espejo, E.F., Montoro, R.J., Armengol, J.A., & López-Barneo, J. (1998). Cellular and functional recovery of parkinsonian rats after intrastriatal transplantation of carotid body cell aggregates. *Neuron, 20*, 197–206.

Ewing, S.E., Weber, R.J., Zauner, A., & Plunkett, R.J. (1992). Recovery in hemiparkinsonian rats following intrastriatal implantation of activated leukocytes. *Brain Research, 576*, 42–48.

Factor, S.A., & Weiner, W.J. (1993). Early combination therapy with bromocriptine and levodopa in Parkinson's disease. *Movement Disorders, 8*, 257–262.

Fawcett, J.W., & Geller, H.M. (1998). Regeneration in the CNS: optimism mounts. *Trends in Neuroscience, 21*, 179–180,

Fawcett, J.W., & Keynes, R.J. (1990). Peripheral nerve regeneration. *Annual Review of Neuroscience, 13*, 43–60.

Fawcett, J.W., Housden, E., Smith-Thomas, L., & Meyer, R.L. (1989). The growth of axons in three-dimensional astrocyte cultures. *Developmental Biology, 133*, 140–147.

Fawcett, J.W., Barker, R.A., & Dunnett, S.B. (1995). Dopaminergic neuronal survival and the effects of bFGF in explant, three-dimensional and monolayer cultures of embryonic rat ventral mesencephalon. *Experimental Brain Research, 106*, 275–282.

Fazzini, E., Dwork, A.J., Blum, C., Burke, R., Cote, L., Goodman, R.R., Jacobs, T.P., Naini, A.B., Pezzoli, G., Pullman, S., Solomon, R.A., Truong, D., Weber, C.J., & Fahn, S. (1991). Stereotaxic implantation of autologous adrenal medulla into caudate nucleus in 4 patients with parkinsonism: one-year follow-up. *Archives of Neurology, 48*, 813–820.

Fearnley, J., & Lees, A.J. (1996). Parkinson's disease: neuropathology. In R.L.Watts & W.C. Koller (Eds.), *Movement disorders: Neurologic principles and practice* (pp. 263–278). New York: McGraw-Hill.

Ferguson, B., Matyszak, M.K., Esiri, M.M., & Perry, V.H. (1997). Axonal damage in acute multiple sclerosis lesions. *Brain, 120*, 393–399.

Fiandaca, M.S., Kordower, J.H., Hansen, J.T., Jiao, S.S., & Gash, D.M. (1988). Adrenal medullary autografts into the basal ganglia of cebus monkeys: injury-induced regeneration. *Experimental Neurology, 102*, 76–91.

Filoteo, J.V., Delis, D.C., Roman, M.J., Demadura, T., Ford, E., Butters, N., Salmon, D.P., Paulsen, J., Shults, C.W., Swenson, M., & Swerdlow, N. (1995). Visual attention and perception in patients with Huntington's disease: Comparisons with other subcortical and cortical dementias. *Journal of Clinical and Experimental Neuropsychology, 17*, 654–667.

Fischer, W., Wictorin, K., Björklund, A., Williams, L.R., Varon, S., & Gage, F.H. (1987). Amelioration of cholinergic neuron atrophy and spatial memory impairment in aged rats by nerve growth factor. *Nature, 329*, 65–68.

Fischer, W., Wictorin, K., Isacson, O., & Björklund, A. (1988). Trophic effects on cholinergic striatal interneurons by submaxillary gland transplants. *Progress in Brain Research, 78*, 409–412.

Fisher, L.J., & Gage, F.H. (1993). Grafting in the mammalian central nervous system. *Physiological Reviews, 73*, 583–616.

Fisher, L.J., Young, S.J., Tepper, J.M., Groves, P.M., & Gage, F.H. (1991a). Electrophysiological characteristics of cells within mesencephalon suspension grafts. *Neuroscience, 40*, 109–122.

Fisher, L.J., Jinnah, H.A., Kale, L.C., Higgins, G.A., & Gage, F.H. (1991b). Survival and function of intrastriatally grafted primary fibroblasts genetically modified to produce L-dopa. *Neuron, 6*, 371–380.

Fisher, L.J., Raymon, H.K., & Gage, F.H. (1993). Cells engineered to produce acetylcholine: Therapeutic potential for Alzheimer's disease. *Annals of the New York Academy of Sciences, 695*, 278–284.

Flores, E.G., Decanini, H.L., Salazar, M.F., Morales, E.L., Zuniga, M.D., & Campos, A.M. (1990). Is autologous transplant of adrenal medulla into the striatum an effective therapy for Parkinson's disease? *Progress in Brain Research, 82*, 643–655.

Folkerth, R.D., & Durso, R. (1996). Survival and proliferation of non-neural tissues, with obstruction of cerebral ventricles, in a parkinsonian patient treated with fetal allografts. *Neurology, 46*, 1219–1225.

Forno, L.S. (1990). Pathology of Parkinson's disease: the importance of the substantia nigra and Lewy bodies. In G. Stern (Ed.), *Parkinson's disease* (pp. 185–238). London: Chapman and Hall.

Forno, L.S., & Langston, J.W. (1989). Adrenal medullary transplant to the brain for Parkinson's disease: neuropathology of an unsuccessful case. *Journal of Neuropathology and Experimental Neurology, 48*, 339–339.

Forno, L.S., & Langston, J.W. (1991). Unfavorable outcome of adrenal medullary transplant for Parkinson's disease. *Acta Neuropathologica, 81*, 691–694.

Foster, A.C., Gill, R., & Woodruff, G.N. (1988). Neuroprotective effects of MK-801 *in vivo*: selectivity and evidence for delayed degeneration mediated by NMDA receptor activation. *Journal of Neuroscience, 8*, 4745–4754.

Foster, G.A., Brodin, E., Gage, F.H., Maxwell, D.J., Roberts, M.H.T., & Sharp, T. (1990). Restoration of function to the denervated spinal cord after implantation of embryonic 5HT-containing and substance P-containing raphe neurons. *Progress in Brain Research, 82*, 247–259.

Fox, M.W., Ahlskog, J.E., & Kelly, P.J. (1991). Stereotaxic ventrolateralis thalamotomy for medically refractory tremor in post levodopa era Parkinson's disease patients. *Journal of Neurosurgery, 75*, 723–730.

Fray, P.J., Dunnett, S.B., Iversen, S.D., Björklund, A., & Stenevi, U. (1983). Nigral transplants reinnervating the dopamine-depleted neostriatum can sustain intracranial self stimulation. *Science, 219*, 416–419.

Freed, C.R., Breeze, R.E., Rosenberg, N.L., Schneck, S.A., Wells, T.H., Barrett, J.N., Grafton, S.T., Huang, S.C., Eidelberg, D., & Rottenberg, D.A. (1990). Transplantation of human fetal dopamine cells for Parkinson's disease. Results at 1 year. *Archives of Neurology, 47*, 505–512.

Freed, C.R., Breeze, R.E., Rosenberg, N.L., Schneck, S.A., Kriek, E., Qi, J., Lone, T., Zhang, L., Snyder, J.A., Wells, T.H., Ramig, L.O., Thompson, L., Mazziotta, J.C., Huang, S.C., Grafton, S.T., Brooks, D., Sawle, G., Schroter, G., & Ansari, A.A. (1992). Survival of implanted fetal dopamine cells and neurologic improvement 12 to 46 months after transplantation for Parkinson's disease. *New England Journal of Medicine, 327*, 1549–1555.

Freed, W.J. (1983). Functional brain tissue transplantation: reversal of lesion-induced rotation by intraventricular substantia nigra and adrenal medulla grafts, with a note on intracranial retinal grafts. *Biological Psychiatry, 18*, 1205–1267.

Freed, W.J., Perlow, M.J., Karoum, F., Seiger, Å., Olson, L., Hoffer, B.J., & Wyatt, R.J. (1980). Restoration of dopaminergic function by grafting of fetal rat substantia nigra to the caudate nucleus: long term behavioral, biochemical, and histochemical studies. *Annals of Neurology, 8*, 510–519.

Freed, W.J., Morihisa, J.M., Spoor, E., Hoffer, B.J., Olson, L., Seiger, Å., & Wyatt, R.J. (1981). Transplanted adrenal chromaffin cells in rat brain reduce lesion-induced rotational behavior. *Nature, 292*, 351–352.

Freed, W.J., Karoum, F., Spoor, H.E., Morihisa, J.M., Olson, L., & Wyatt, R.J. (1983). Catecholamine content of intracerebral adrenal medulla grafts. *Brain Research, 269*, 184–189.

Freed, W.J., Cannon-Spoor, H.E., & Krauthamer, E. (1986a). Intrastriatal adrenal medulla grafts in rats: long-term survival and behavioral effects. *Journal of Neurosurgery, 65*, 664–670.

Freed, W.J., Patel-Vaidya, U., & Geller, H.M. (1986b). Properties of PC12 pheochromocytoma cells transplanted to the adult rat brain. *Experimental Brain Research, 63*, 557–566.

Freed, W.J., Poltorak, M., & Becker, J.B. (1990). Intracerebral adrenal medulla grafts: a review. *Experimental Neurology, 110*, 139–166.

Freeman, T.B., Spence, M.S., Boss, B.D., Spector, D.H., Strecker, R.E., Olanow, C.W., & Kordower, J.H. (1991). Development of dopaminergic neurons in the human substantia nigra. *Experimental Neurology, 113*, 344–355.

Freeman, T.B., Olanow, C.W., Hauser, R.A., Nauert, G.M., Smith, D.A., Borlongan, C.V., Sanberg, P.R., Holt, D.A., Kordower, J.H., Vingerhoets, F.J.G., Snow, B.J., Calne, D.B., & Gauger, L.I. (1995a). Bilateral fetal nigral transplantation into the postcommissural putamen in Parkinson's disease. *Annals of Neurology, 38*, 379–388.

Freeman, T.B., Sanberg, P.R., Nauert, G.M., Boss, B.D., Spector, D., Olanow, C.W., & Kordower, J.H. (1995b). The influence of donor age on the survival of solid and suspension intraparenchymal human embryonic nigral grafts. *Cell Transplantation, 4*, 141–154.

Freund, T.F., Bolam, J.P., Björklund, A., Stenevi, U., Dunnett, S.B., Powell, J.F., & Smith, A.D. (1985). Efferent synaptic connections of grafted dopaminergic-neurons reinnervating the host neostriatum: a tyrosine hydro-xylase immunocytochemical study. *Journal of Neuroscience, 5*, 603–616.

Fricker, R.A., Barker, R.A., Fawcett, J.W., & Dunnett, S.B. (1996). A comparative study of preparation techniques for improving the viability of striatal grafts using vital stains, *in vitro* cultures and *in vivo* grafts. *Cell Transplantation, 5*, 599–611.

Fricker, R.A., Torres, E.M., Hume, S.P., Myers, R., Opacka-Juffry, J., Ashworth, S., & Dunnett, S.B. (1997). The effects of donor stage on the survival and function of embryonic striatal grafts. II. Correlation between positron emission tomography and reaching behaviour. *Neuroscience, 79*, 711–722.

Friedman, E., Nilaver, G., Carmel, P., Perlow, M.J., Spatz, L., & Latov, N. (1986). Myelination by transplanted fetal and neonatal oligodendrocytes in a dysmyelinating mutant. *Brain Research, 378*, 142–146.

Frim, D.M., Uhler, T.A., Short, M.P., Ezzedine, Z.D., Klagsbrun, M., Breakefield, X.O., & Isacson, O. (1993). Effects of biologically delivered NGF, BDNF and bFGF on striatal excitotoxic lesions. *NeuroReport, 4*, 367–370.

Gage, F.H., & Björklund, A. (1986). Cholinergic septal grafts into the hippocampal formation improve spatial learning and memory in aged rats by an atropine-sensitive mechanism. *Journal of Neuroscience, 6*, 2837–2847.

Gage, F.H., & Fisher, L.J. (1993). Genetically modified cells for intracerebral transplantation. In O. Lindvall (Ed.), *Restoration of brain function by tissue transplantation* (pp. 51–61). Berlin, Heidelberg, New York: Springer-Verlag.

Gage, F.H., Dunnett, S.B., Björklund, A., & Stenevi, U. (1982). Functional recovery following brain damage: conceptual frameworks and biological mechanisms. *Scandinavian Journal of Psychology, S1*, 112–120.

Gage, F.H., Dunnett, S.B., Stenevi, U., & Björklund, A. (1983). Aged rats: recovery of motor impairments by intrastriatal nigral grafts. *Science, 221*, 966–969.

Gage, F.H., Björklund, A., Stenevi, U., Dunnett, S.B., & Kelly, P.A.T. (1984). Intrahippocampal septal grafts ameliorate learning impairments in aged rats. *Science, 225*, 533–536.

Gage, F.H., Wolff, J.A., Rosenberg, M.B., Xu, L., Yee, J.K., Shults, C., & Friedmann, T. (1987). Grafting genetically modified cells to the brain: possibilities for the future. *Neuroscience, 23*, 795–807.

Gage, F.H., Coates, P.W., Palmer, T.D., Kuhn, H.G., Fisher, L.J., Suhonen, J.O., Peterson, D.A., Suhr, S.T., & Ray, J. (1995). Survival and differentiation of adult neuronal progenitor cells transplanted to the adult brain. *Proceedings of the National Academy of Sciences of the United States of America, 92*, 11879–11883.

Galpern, W.R., Burns, L.H., Deacon, T.W., Dinsmore, J., & Isacson, O. (1996). Xenotransplantation of porcine fetal ventral mesencephalon in a rat model of Parkinson's disease: Functional recovery and graft morphology. *Experimental Neurology, 140*, 1–13.

Games, D., Adams, D., Alessandrini, R., Barbour, R., Berthelette, P., Blackwell, C., Carr, T., Clemens, J., Donaldson, T., Gillespie, F., Guido, T., Hagoplan, S., Johnson-Wood, K., Khan, K., Lee, M., Leibowitz, P., Lieberberg, I., Little, S., Masliah, E., McConlogue, L., Montoya-Zavala, M., Mucke, L., Paganini, L., Penniman, E., Power, M., Schenk, D., Seubert, P., Snyder, B., Soriano, F., Tan, H., Vitale, J., Wadsworth, S., Wolozin, B., & Zhao, J. (1995). Alzheimer-type neuropathology in transgenic mice overexpressing V71F b-amyloid precursor protein. *Nature, 373*, 523–527.

Garraghty, P.E., & Kaas, J.H. (1991a). Functional reorganization in adult monkey thalamus after peripheral nerve injury. *NeuroReport, 2*, 747–750.

Garraghty, P.E., & Kaas, J.H. (1991b). Large-scale functional reorganization in adult monkey cortex after peripheral-nerve injury. *Proceedings of the National Academy of Sciences of the United States of America, 88*, 6976–6980.

Garry, D.J., Caplan, A.L., Vawter, D.E., & Kearney, W. (1992). Are there really alternatives to the use of fetal tissue from elective abortions in transplantation research? *New England Journal of Medicine, 327*, 1592–1595.

Gash, D.M., Sladek, J.R., & Sladek, C.D. (1980). Functional development of grafted vasopressin neurons. *Science, 210*, 1367–1369.

Gash, D.M., Zhang, Z., Ovadia, A., Cass, W.A., Yi, A., Simmerman, L., Russell, D., Martin, D., Lapchak, P.A., Collins, F., Hoffer, B.J., & Gerhardt, G.A. (1996). Functional recovery in parkinsonian monkeys treated with GDNF. *Nature, 380*, 252–255.

Geist, M.J., Maris, D.O., & Grady, M.S. (1991). Blood–brain barrier permeability is not altered by allograft or xenograft fetal neural cell suspension grafts. *Experimental Neurology, 111*, 166–174.

Gerlach, M., Riederer, P., Przuntek, H., & Youdim, M.B.H. (1991). MPTP mechanisms of neurotoxicity and their implications for Parkinson's disease. *European Journal of Pharmacology: Molecular Pharmacology, 208*, 273–286.

German, D.C., & Manaye, K.F. (1993). Midbrain dopaminergic-neurons (Nuclei A8, A9, and A10): 3-dimensional reconstruction in the rat. *Journal of Comparative Neurology, 331*, 297–309.

Geschwind, N. (1965a). Disconnexion syndromes in animals and man. Part I. *Brain, 88*, 237–294.

Geschwind, N. (1965b). Disconnexion syndromes in animals and man. Part II. *Brain, 88*, 585–644.

Gibb, W.R.G. (1989). The pathology of Parkinson's disease. In N.P. Quinn (Ed.), *Disorders of movement* (pp. 32–57). London and San Diego: Academic Press.

Gilbert, C.D., & Wiesel, T.N. (1992). Receptive field dynamics in adult primary visual cortex. *Nature, 356*, 150–152.

Gildenberg, P.L., Pettigrew, L.C., Merrell, R., Butler, I., Conklin, R., Katz, J., & Defrance, J. (1990). Transplantation of adrenal medullary tissue to caudate nucleus using stereotaxic techniques. *Stereotactic and Functional Neurosurgery, 54–5*, 268–271.

Ginzburg, R., & Seltzer, Z. (1990). Subarachnoid spinal cord transplantation of adrenal medulla suppresses chronic neuropathic pain behavior in rats. *Brain Research, 523*, 147–150.

Glass, D.J., & Yancopoulos, G.D. (1993). The neurotrophins and their receptors. *Trends in Cell Biology, 3*, 262–268.

Glees, P. (1940). The differentiation of the brain and other tissues in an implanted portion of embryonic head. *Journal of Anatomy, 75*, 239–247.

Glees, P. (1955). Studies of cortical regeneration with special reference to cerebral implants. In W.E. Windle (Ed.), *Regeneration in the central nervous system* (pp. 94–111). Springfield, IL: Charles C. Thomas.

Goedert, M. (1993). Tau protein and the neurofibrillary pathology of Alzheimer's disease. *Trends in Neurosciences, 16*, 460–465.

Goedert, M., Wischik, C.M., Crowther, R.A., Walker, J.E., & Klug, A. (1988). Cloning and sequencing of the cDNA-encoding a core protein of the paired helical filament of Alzheimer's disease—identification as the microtubule-associated protein tau. *Proceedings of the National Academy of Sciences of the United States of America, 85*, 4051–4055.

Goetz, C.G., Olanow, C.W., Koller, W.C., Penn, R.D., Cahill, D.W., Morantz, R., Stebbins, G., Tanner, C.M., Klawans, H.L., Shannon, K.M., Comella, C.L., Witt, T., Cox, C., Waxman, M., & Gauger, L. (1989). Multicenter study of autologous adrenal medullary transplantation to the corpus striatum in patients with advanced Parkinson's disease. *New England Journal of Medicine, 320*, 337–341.

Goetz, C.G., Tanner, C.M., Penn, R.D., Stebbins, G.T., Gilley, D.W., Shannon, K.M., Klawans, H.L., Comella, C.L., Wilson, R.S., & Witt, T. (1990). Adrenal medullary transplant to the striatum of patients with advanced Parkinson's disease: 1-year motor and psychomotor data. *Neurology, 40*, 273–276.

Goetz, C.G., Stebbins, G.T., Klawans, H.L., Koller, W.C., Grossman, R.G., Bakay, R.A.E., & Penn, R.D. (1991). United Parkinson Foundation neurotransplantation registry on adrenal medullary transplants: presurgical, and 1-year and 2-year follow up. *Neurology, 41*, 1719–1722.

Goldberg, Y.P., Kalchman, M.A., Metzler, M., Nasir, J., Zeisler, J., Graham, R., Koide, K., O'Kusky, J.R., Sharp, A.H., Ross, C.A., Jirik, F., & Hayden, M.R. (1996). Absence of disease phenotype and intergenerational stability of the CAG repeat in transgenic mice expressing the human Huntington disease transcript. *Human Molecular Genetics, 5*, 177–185.

Gout, O., Gansmuller, A., Baumann, N., & Gumpel, M. (1988). Remyelination by transplanted oligodendrocytes of a demyelinated lesion in the spinal cord of the adult shiverer mouse. *Neuroscience Letters, 87*, 195–199.

Grasbon-Frodl, E.M., Nakao, N., & Brundin, P. (1996). The lazaroid U-83836E improves the survival of rat embryonic mesencephalic tissue stored at 4°C and subsequently used for cultures or intracerebral transplantation. *Brain Research Bulletin, 39*, 341–347.

Graybiel, A.M., Liu, F.C., & Dunnett, S.B. (1989). Intrastriatal grafts derived from fetal striatal primordia. 1. Phenotypy and modular organization. *Journal of Neuroscience, 9*, 3250–3271.

Groves, A.K., Barnett, S.C., Franklin, R.J.M., Crang, A.J., Mayer, M., Blakemore, W.F., & Noble, M. (1993). Repair of demyelinated lesions by transplantation of purified O-2A progenitor cells. *Nature, 362*, 453–455.

Guest, J.D., Hesse, D., Schnell, L., Schwab, M.E., Bunge, M.B., & Bunge, R.P. (1997). Influence of IN-1 antibody and acidic FGF-fibrin glue on the response of injured corticospinal tract axons to human Schwann cell grafts. *Journal of Neuroscience Research, 50*, 888–905.

Gumpel, M., Baumann, N., Raoul, M., & Jacque, C. (1993). Survival and differentiation of oligodendrocytes from neural tissue transplanted into new-born mouse brain. *Neuroscience Letters, 37*, 307–311.

Guttman, M., Burns, R.S., Martin, W.R.W., Peppard, R.F., Adam, N.J., Ruth, T.J., Allen, G.S., Parker, R.A., Tulipan, N.B., & Calne, D.B. (1989). PET studies of parkinsonian patients treated with autologous adrenal implants. *Canadian Journal of Neurological Sciences, 16*, 305–309.

Hall, S.M., & Kent, A.P. (1987). The response of regenerating peripheral neurites to a grafted optic nerve. *Journal of Neurocytology, 16*, 317–331.

Hansen, J.T., Kordower, J.H., Fiandaca, M.S., Jiao, S.S., Notter, M.F.D., & Gash, D.M. (1988). Adrenal medullary autografts into the basal ganglia of cebus monkeys: graft viability and fine structure. *Experimental Neurology, 102*, 65–75.

Hansen, J.T., Fiandaca, M.S., Kordower, J.H., Notter, M.F.D., & Gash, D.M. (1990). Striatal adrenal medulla/sural nerve co-grafts in hemiparkinsonian monkeys. *Progress in Brain Research, 82*, 573–580.

Hantraye, P., Riche, D., Mazière, M., & Isacson, O. (1992). Intrastriatal transplantation of cross-species fetal striatal cells reduces abnormal movements in a primate model of Huntington disease. *Proceedings of the National Academy of Sciences of the United States of America, 89*, 4187–4191.

Haque, N.S.K., Hlavin, M.-L., Fawcett, J.W., & Dunnett, S.B. (1996). The neurotrophin NT-4/5, but not NT-3, enhances the efficacy of nigral grafts in a rat model of Parkinson's disease. *Brain Research, 712*, 45–52.

Hardy, J. (1997). Amyloid, the presenilins and Alzheimer's disease. *Trends in Neurosciences, 20*, 154–159.

Hargraves, R.W., & Freed, W.J. (1987). Chronic intrastriatal dopamine infusions in rats with unilateral lesions of the substantia nigra. *Life Sciences, 40*, 959–966.

Harper, P.S. (1996). *Huntington's disease* (2nd ed.). London: W.B. Saunders.

Hauser, R.A., Olanow, C.W., Snow, B.J., & Freeman, T.B. (1998). Fetal nigral transplantation in Parkinson's disease: the USF pilot program (12 to 24 month evaluation). In T.B. Freeman & H. Widner (Eds.), *Cell transplantation in neurological disease* (pp. 19–30). Totowa, NJ: Humana Press.

Hefti, F. (1983). Is Alzheimer's disease caused by a lack of nerve growth factor? *Annals of Neurology, 13*, 109–110.

Hefti, F. (1986). Nerve growth factor promotes survival of septal cholinergic neurons after fimbrial transections. *Journal of Neuroscience, 6*, 2155–2162.

Hefti, F., Hartikka, J., & Schlumpf, M. (1985). Implantation of PC12 cells into the corpus striatum of rats with lesions of the dopaminergic nigrostriatal neurons. *Brain Research, 348*, 283–288.

Henderson, B.T.H., Clough, C.G., Hughes, R.C., Hitchcock, E.R., & Kenny, B.G. (1991). Implantation of human fetal ventral mesencephalon to the right caudate nucleus in advanced Parkinson's disease. *Archives of Neurology, 48*, 822–827.

Henderson, J.M., & Dunnett, S.B. (1998). Targeting the subthalamic nucleus in the treatment of Parkinson's disease. *Brain Research Bulletin, 46*, 467–474.

Herman, J.P., & Abrous, D.N. (1994). Dopaminergic neural grafts after fifteen years: Results and perspectives. *Progress in Neurobiology, 44*, 1–35.

Herman, J.P., Choulli, K., & Le Moal, M. (1985). Hyper-reactivity to amphetamine in rats with dopaminergic grafts. *Experimental Brain Research, 60*, 521–526.

Herman, J.P., Choulli, K., Geffard, M., Nadaud, D., Taghzouti, K., & Le Moal, M. (1986). Reinnervation of the nucleus accumbens and frontal cortex of the rat by dopaminergic grafts and effects on hoarding behavior. *Brain Research, 372*, 210–216.

Herrera-Marschitz, M., Strömberg, I., Olsson, D., Ungerstedt, U., & Olson, L. (1984). Adrenal medullary implants in the dopamine-denervated rat striatum. 2. Acute behavior as a function of graft amount and location and its modulation by neuroleptics. *Brain Research, 297*, 53–61.

Himes, B.T., Goldberger, M.E., & Tessler, A. (1994). Grafts of fetal central nervous system tissue rescue axotomized Clarke's nucleus neurons in adult and neonatal operates. *Journal of Comparative Neurology, 339*, 117–131.

Hirsch, E.C., Duyckaerts, C., Javoy-Agid, F., Hauw, J.J., & Agid, Y. (1990). Does adrenal graft enhance recovery of dopaminergic neurons in Parkinson's disease? *Annals of Neurology, 27*, 676–682.

Hitchcock, E.R., Clough, C.G., Hughes, R.C., & Kenny, B.G. (1989). Transplantation in Parkinson's disease: stereotactic implantation of adrenal medulla and foetal mesencephalon. *Acta Neurochirurgica, 46*, 48–50.

Hitchcock, E.R., Kenny, B.G., Clough, C.G., Hughes, R.C., Henderson, B.T.H., & Detta, A. (1990). Stereotactic implantation of foetal mesencephalon (STIM): the UK experience. *Progress in Brain Research, 82*, 723–728.

Hodges, H., Allen, Y.S., Kershaw, T., Lantos, P.L., Gray, J.A., & Sinden, J. (1991a). Effects of cholinergic-rich neural grafts on radial maze performance of rats after excitotoxic lesions of the forebrain cholinergic projection system. 1. Amelioration of cognitive deficits by transplants into cortex and hippocampus but not into basal forebrain. *Neuroscience, 45*, 587–607.

Hodges, H., Allen, Y.S., Sinden, J., Lantos, P.L., & Gray, J.A. (1991b). Effects of cholinergic-rich neural grafts on radial maze performance of rats after excitotoxic lesions of the forebrain cholinergic projection system. 2. Cholinergic drugs as probes to investigate lesion-induced deficits and transplant-induced functional recovery. *Neuroscience, 45*, 609–623.

Hodges, H., Sowinski, P., Fleming, P., Kershaw, T.R., Sinden, J.D., Meldrum, B.S., & Gray, J.A. (1996). Contrasting effects of fetal CA1 and CA3 hippocampal grafts on deficits in spatial learning and working memory induced by global cerebral ischaemia in rats. *Neuroscience, 72*, 959–988.

Hoffer, B.J., & Olson, L. (1991). Ethical issues in brain cell transplantation. *Trends in Neurosciences, 14*, 384–388.

Hoffer, B.J., Hoffman, A., Bowenkamp, K., Huettl, P., Hudson, J., Martin, D., Lin, L.-F.H., & Gerhardt, G.A. (1994). Glial cell line-derived neurotrophic factor reverses toxin-induced injury to midbrain dopaminergic neurons *in vivo*. *Neuroscience Letters, 182*, 107–111.

Hoffman, D., Breakefield, X.O., Short, M.P., & Aebischer, P. (1993). Transplantation of a polymer-encapsulated cell line genetically engineered to release NGF. *Experimental Neurology, 122*, 100–106.

Horellou, P., Lundberg, C., Lebourdelles, B., Wictorin, K., Brundin, P., Kalén, P., Björklund, A., & Mallet, J. (1991). Behavioural effects of genetically engineered cells releasing DOPA and dopamine after intracerebral grafting in a rat model of Parkinson's disease. *Journal de Physiologie, 85*, 158–170.

Horellou, P., Vigne, E., Castel, M.-N., Barnéoud, P., Colin, P., Perricaudet, M., Delaere, P., & Mallet, J. (1994). Direct intracerebral gene transfer of an adenoviral vector expressing tyrosine hydroxylase in a rat model of Parkinson's disease. *NeuroReport, 6*, 49–53.

Hori, Y., Kageyama, H., Kihara, T., Ikeda, M., Nakano, A., & Kurosawa, A. (1993). Transient improvement of amphetamine-induced rotational behavior by PC12 cell grafts: Studies with microdialysis. *Restorative Neurology and Neuroscience, 6*, 49–55.

Houle, J.D., & Reier, P.J. (1988). Transplantation of fetal spinal cord tissue into the chronically injured adult rat spinal cord. *Journal of Comparative Neurology, 269*, 535–547.

Hubel, D.H. (1995). *Eye, brain and vision.* New York: W.H. Freeman.

Hubel, D.H., Wiesel, T.N., & LeVay, S. (1977). Plasticity of ocular dominance columns in monkey striate cortex. *Philosophical Transactions of the Royal Society of London, Series B, 277*, 377–409.

Huffaker, T.K., Boss, B.D., Morgan, A.S., Neff, N.T., Strecker, R.E., Spence, M.S., & Miao, R. (1989). Xenografting of fetal pig ventral mesencephalon corrects motor asymmetry in the rat model of Parkinson's disease. *Experimental Brain Research, 77*, 329–336.

Hughes, A.J., Daniel, S.E., Kilford, L., & Lees, A.J. (1992). Accuracy of clinical diagnosis of idiopathic Parkinson's disease: a clinicopathological study of 100 cases. *Journal of Neurology, Neurosurgery and Psychiatry, 55*, 181–184.

Huntington, G. (1872). On chorea. *Advances in Neurology, 1*, 33–35.

Huntington's Disease Collaborative Research Group (1993). A novel gene containing a trinucleotide repeat that is expanded and unstable on Huntington's disease chromosomes. *Cell, 72*, 971–983.

Hurtig, H., Joyce, J., Sladek, J.R., & Trojanowski, J.Q. (1989). Post mortem analysis of adrenal-medulla-to-caudate autograft in a patient with Parkinson's disease. *Annals of Neurology, 25*, 607–614.

Hutchison, W.D., Lozano, A.M., Davis, K.D., St. Cyr, J.A., Lang, A.E., & Dostrovsky, J.O. (1994). Differential neuronal activity in segments of globus pallidus in Parkinson's disease patients. *NeuroReport, 5*, 1533–1537.

Isacson, O., Brundin, P., Kelly, P.A.T., Gage, F.H., & Björklund, A. (1984). Functional neuronal replacement by grafted striatal neurons in the ibotenic acid lesioned rat striatum. *Nature, 311*, 458–460.

Isacson, O., Dunnett, S.B., & Björklund, A. (1986). Graft-induced behavioral recovery in an animal model of Huntington disease. *Proceedings of the National Academy of Sciences of the United States of America, 83*, 2728–2732.

Isacson, O., Riche, D., Hantraye, P., Sofroniew, M.V., & Mazière, M. (1989). A primate model of Huntington's disease: cross-species implantation of striatal precursor cells to the excitotoxically lesioned baboon caudate-putamen. *Experimental Brain Research, 75*, 213–220.

Itakura, T., Kamei, I., Nakai, K., Naka, Y., Nakakita, K., Imai, H., & Komai, N. (1988). Autotransplantation of the superior cervical ganglion into the brain: a possible therapy for Parkinson's disease. *Journal of Neurosurgery, 68*, 955–959.

Itakura, T., Nakai, M., Nakao, N., Ooiwa, Y., Uematsu, Y., & Komai, N. (1994). Transplantation of autologous cervical sympathetic ganglion into the brain with Parkinson's disease: experimental and clinical studies. *Cell Transplantation, 3*, S43–S45.

Itoh, Y., Sugawara, T., Kowada, M., & Tessler, A. (1993). Time course of dorsal root axon regeneration into transplants of fetal spinal cord: An electron microscopic study. *Experimental Neurology, 123*, 133–146.

Janec, E., & Burke, R.E. (1993). Naturally occurring cell death during postnatal development of the substantia nigra pars compacta of the rat. *Molecular and Cellular Neuroscience, 4*, 30–35.

Jankovic, J., Grossman, R., Goodman, C., Pirozzolo, F., Schneider, L., Zhu, Z., Scardino, P., Garber, A.J., Jhingran, S.G., & Martin, S. (1989). Clinical, biochemical, and neuropathologic findings following transplantation of adrenal medulla to the caudate nucleus for treatment of Parkinson's disease. *Neurology, 39*, 1227–1234.

Jeffery, N.D., & Blakemore, W.F. (1997). Locomotor deficits induced by experimental spinal cord demyelination are abolished by spontaneous remyelination. *Brain, 120*, 27–37.

Jenkins, W.M., & Merzenich, M.M. (1987). Reorganisation of neocortical representations after brain injury: a neurophysiological model of the bases of recovery from stroke. *Progress in Brain Research, 71*, 249–266.

Jenkins, W.M., Merzenich, M.M., Ochs, M.T., Allard, T., & Guic-Robles, E. (1990). Functional reorganization of primary somatosensory cortex in adult owl monkeys after behaviorally controlled tactile stimulation. *Journal of Neurophysiology, 63*, 82–104.

Jenner, P., & Olanow, C.W. (1996). Oxidative stress and the pathogenesis of Parkinson's disease. *Neurology, 47*, S161–S170.

Jensen, S., Sorensen, T., & Zimmer, J. (1987). Cryopreservation of fetal rat brain tissue later used for intracerebral transplantation. *Cryobiology, 24*, 120–134.

Jiao, S., Zhang, W.C., Cao, J.K., Zhang, Z.M., Wang, H., Ding, M.C., Zhang, Z., Sun, J.B., Sun, Y.C., & Shi, M.T. (1988). Study of adrenal medullary tissue transplantation to striatum in parkinsonism. *Progress in Brain Research, 78*, 575–580.

Jiao, S.S., Ding, Y.J., Zhang, W.C., Cao, J.K., Zhang, G.F., Zhang, Z.M., Ding, M.C., Zhang, Z., & Meng, J.M. (1989). Adrenal medullary autografts in patients with Parkinson's disease. *New England Journal of Medicine, 321*, 324–325.

Jiao, S.S., Gurevich, V., & Wolff, J.A. (1993). Long-term correction of rat model of Parkinson's disease by gene therapy. *Nature, 362*, 450–453.

Kamo, H., Kim, S., McGeer, P.L., & Shin, D. (1986). Functional recovery in a rat model of Parkinson's disease following transplantation of cultured human sympathetic neurons. *Brain Research, 397*, 372–376.

Kang, J., Lemaire, H.-G., Unterbeck, A., Salbaum, J.M., Masters, C.L., Grzeschik, K.-H., Multhaup, G., Beyreuther, K., & Müller-Hill, B. (1987). The precursor of Alzheimer's disease amyloid A4 protein resembles a cell-surface receptor. *Nature, 325*, 733–736.

Kaplitt, M.G., Leone, P., Samulski, R.J., Xiao, X., Pfaff, D.W., O'Malley, K.L., & During, M.J. (1994). Long-term gene expression and phenotypic correction using adeno-associated virus vectors in the mammalian brain. *Nature Genetics, 8*, 148–154.

Kelche, C., Dalrymple-Alford, J.C., & Will, B. (1987). Effects of postoperative environment on recovery of function after fimbria–fornix transection in the rat. *Physiology and Behavior, 40*, 731–736.

Kelche, C., Dalrymple-Alford, J.C., & Will, B. (1988). Housing conditions modulate the effects of intracerebral grafts in rats with brain lesions. *Behavioural Brain Research, 28*, 287–295.

Kelche, C., Roeser, C., Jeltsch, H., Cassel, J.C., & Will, B. (1995). The effects of intrahippocampal grafts, training, and postoperative housing on behavioral recovery after septohippocampal damage in the rat. *Behavioral and Neural Biology, 63*, 155–166.

Kempermann, G., Kuhn, H.G., & Gage, F.H. (1998). More hippocampal neurons in adult mice living in an enriched environment. *Nature, 386*, 493–495.

Kendall, A.L., Rayment, F.D., Torres, E.M., Baker, H.F., Ridley, R.M., & Dunnett, S.B. (1998). Functional integration of striatal allografts in a primate model of Huntington's disease. *Nature Medicine, 4*, 727–729.

Kerr, J.F.R., & Harmon, B.V. (1991). Definition and incidence of apoptosis: An historical perspective. In L.D. Tomei & F.O. Cope (Eds.), *Apoptosis: The molecular basis of cell death* (pp. 5–29). Cold Spring Harbor: Cold Spring Harbor Laboratory Press.

Kish, S.J., Shannak, J.K., & Hornykiewicz, O. (1988). Uneven pattern of dopamine loss in the striatum of patients with idiopathic Parkinson's disease: Pathophysiologic and clinical implications. *New England Journal of Medicine, 318*, 876–881.

Klassen, H., & Lund, R.D. (1987). Retinal transplants can drive a pupillary reflex in host rat brains. *Proceedings of the National Academy of Sciences of the United States of America, 84*, 6958–6960.

Klassen, H., & Lund, R.D. (1990). Retinal graft-mediated pupillary responses in rats: restoration of a reflex function in the mature mammalian brain. *Journal of Neuroscience, 10*, 578–587.

Kobayashi, S., Miura, M., Asou, H., Inoue, H.K., Ohye, C., & Uyemura, K. (1995). Grafts of genetically modified fibroblasts expressing neural cell adhesion molecule L1 into transected spinal cord of adult rats. *Neuroscience Letters, 188*, 191–194.

Kolb, B., & Fantie, B. (1994). Cortical graft function in adult and neonatal rats. In S.B. Dunnett & A. Björklund (Eds.), *Functional neural transplantation* (pp. 415–435). New York: Raven Press.

Kolb, B., & Whishaw, I.Q. (1990). *Fundamentals of human neuropsychology.* New York: W.H. Freeman.

Koller, W.C., Waxman, M., & Morantz, R. (1990). Adrenal neural transplants in Parkinson's disease. *Advances in Neurology, 53*, 559–565.

Kondoh, T., & Low, W.C. (1994). Glutamate uptake blockade induces striatal dopamine release in 6-hydroxydopamine rats with intrastriatal grafts: Evidence for host modulation of transplanted dopamine neurons. *Experimental Neurology, 127*, 191–198.

Kopyov, O.V., Jacques, D., Lieberman, A., Duma, C.M., & Rogers, R.L. (1996). Clinical study of fetal mesencephalic intracerebral transplants for the treatment of Parkinson's disease. *Cell Transplantation, 5*, 327–337.

Kopyov, O.V., Jacques, S., Lieberman, A., Duma, C.M., & Eagle, K.S. (1998). Safety of intrastriatal neurotransplantation for Huntington's disease patients. *Experimental Neurology, 119*, 97–108.

Kordower, J.H., Cochran, E., Penn, R.D., & Goetz, C.G. (1990). NGF-like trophic support from peripheral nerve for grafted rhesus adrenal chromaffin cells. *Journal of Neurosurgery, 73*, 418–428.

Kordower, J.H., Cochran, E., Penn, R.D., & Goetz, C.G. (1991). Putative chromaffin cell survival and enhanced host-derived TH-fiber innervation following a functional adrenal medulla autograft for Parkinson's disease. *Annals of Neurology, 29*, 405–412.

Kordower, J.H., Freeman, T.B., Snow, B.J., Vingerhoets, F.J.G., Mufson, E.J., Sanberg, P.R., Hauser, R.A., Smith, D.A., Nauert, G.M., Perl, D.P., & Olanow, C.W. (1995). Neuropathological evidence of graft survival and striatal reinnervation after the transplantation of fetal mesencephalic tissue in a patient with Parkinson's disease. *New England Journal of Medicine, 332*, 1118–1124.

Kordower, J.H., Freeman, T.B., & Olanow, C.W. (1998). Neuropathology of fetal nigral grafts in patients with Parkinson's disease. *Movement Disorders, 13*, 88–95.

Krack, P., Pollak, P., Limousin, P., Hoffmann, D., Xie, J., Benazzouz, A., & Benabid, A.L. (1998). Subthalamic nucleus or internal pallidal stimulation in young onset Parkinson's disease. *Brain, 121*, 451–457.

Krieger, D.T., Perlow, M.J., Gibson, M.J., Davies, T.F., Zimmerman, E.A., Ferin, M., & Charlton, H.M. (1982). Brain grafts reverse hypogonadism of gonadotropin releasing hormone deficiency. *Nature, 298*, 468–471.

Kromer, L.F., Björklund, A., & Stenevi, U. (1980). Innervation of embryonic hippocampal implants by regenerating axons of cholinergic septal neurons in the adult rat. *Brain Research, 210*, 153–171.

Kromer, L.F., Björklund, A., & Stenevi, U. (1981). Regeneration of the septohippocampal pathway in adult rats is promoted by utilizing embryonic hippocampal implants as bridges. *Brain Research, 210*, 173–200.

Kuhn, H.G., Dickinson-Anson, H., & Gage, F.H. (1997). Neurogenesis in the dentate gyrus of the adult rat: age-related decrease of neuronal progenitor proliferation. *Journal of Neuroscience, 16*, 2027–2033.

Kunkel-Bagden, E., Dai, H.N., & Bregman, B.S. (1993). Methods to assess the development and recovery of locomotor function after spinal cord injury in rats. *Experimental Neurology, 119*, 153–164.

Lange, K.W., Sahakian, B.J., Quinn, N.P., Marsden, C.D., & Robbins, T.W. (1995). Comparison of executive and visuospatial memory function in Huntington's disease and dementia of Alzheimer-type matched for degree of dementia. *Journal of Neurology, Neurosurgery and Psychiatry, 58*, 598–606.

Langston, J.W., Ballard, P., Tetrud, J.W., & Irwin, I. (1983). Chronic parkinsonism in humans due to a product of meperidine-analog synthesis. *Science, 219*, 979–980.

Langston, J.W., Widner, H., & Goetz, C.G. (1992). Core assessment program for intracerebral transplantation (CAPIT). *Movement Disorders, 7*, 2–13.

Lapchak, P.A., Araujo, D.M., Hilt, D.C., Sheng, J., & Jiao, S.S. (1997). Adenoviral vector-mediated GDNF gene therapy in a rodent lesion model of late stage Parkinson's disease. *Brain Research, 777*, 153–160.

Lauder, J.M., & Bloom, F.E. (1974). Ontogeny of monoamine neurons in the locus coeruleus, raphe nuclei and substantia nigra of the rat. *Journal of Comparative Neurology, 155*, 469–482.

Laursen, A.M. (1963). Corpus striatum. *Acta Physiologica Scandinavica, supplementum, 211*, 1–106.

Le Gros Clark, W.E. (1940). Neuronal differentiation in implanted foetal cortical tissue. *Journal of Neurology and Psychiatry, 3*, 263–284.

Le Gros Clark, W.E. (1942). The problem of neuronal regeneration in the central nervous system. I. The influence of spinal ganglia and nerve fragments grafted in the brain. *Journal of Anatomy, 77*, 20–48.

LeVay, S., Wiesel, T.N., & Hubel, D.H. (1980). The development of ocular dominance columns in normal and visually deprived monkeys. *Journal of Comparative Neurology, 191*, 1–51.

LeVere, T.E., & LeVere, N.D. (1985). Transplants to the central nervous system as a therapy for brain pathology. *Neurobiology of Aging, 6*, 151–152.

Li, Y., Field, P.M., & Raisman, G. (1997). Repair of adult rat corticospinal tract by transplants of olfactory ensheathing cells. *Science, 277*, 2000–2002.

Lieb, K., Andersen, C., Lazarov, N., Zienecker, R., Urban, I., Reisert, I., & Pilgrim, C. (1996). Prenatal development and postnatal development of dopaminergic neuron numbers in the male and female mouse midbrain. *Developmental Brain Research, 94*, 37–43.

Lieberman, A., Ransohoff, J., Berczeiler, P., Brous, P., Eng, K., Goldstein, M., Kaufman, B., Koslow, M., & Lieberman, I. (1990a). Adrenal medullary transplants as a treatment for Parkinson's disease. *Advances in Neurology, 53*, 567–570.

Lieberman, A., Ransohoff, J., Berczeiler, P., & Goldstein, M. (1990b). Adrenal medullary transplants as a treatment for advanced Parkinson's disease. *Progress in Brain Research, 82*, 665–669.

Lillien, L.E., & Claude, P. (1985). Nerve growth factor is a mitogen for cultured chromaffin cells. *Nature, 317*, 632–634.

Lindsey, R.M., Wiegand, S.J., Altar, C.A., & DiStefano, P.S. (1994). Neurotrophic factors: from molecule to man. *Trends in Neuroscience, 17*, 182–190.

Lindvall, O. (1997). Neural transplantation: a hope for patients with Parkinson's disease? *NeuroReport, 8*, iii–x.

Lindvall, O., Backlund, E.O., Farde, L., Sedvall, G., Freedman, R., Hoffer, B., Nobin, A., Seiger, A., & Olson, L. (1987). Transplantation in Parkinson's disease: 2 cases of adrenal medullary grafts to the putamen. *Annals of Neurology, 22*, 457–468.

Lindvall, O., Gustavii, B., Åstedt, B., Lindholm, T., Rehncrona, S., Brundin, P., Widner, H., Björklund, A., Leenders, K.L., Frackowiak, R., Rothwell, J.C., Marsden, C.D., Johnels, B., Steg, G., Freedman, R., Hoffer, B.J., Seiger, Å., Strömberg, I., & Bygdeman, M. (1988). Fetal dopamine-rich mesencephalic grafts in Parkinson's disease. *Lancet, 2*, 1483–1484.

Lindvall, O., Rehncrona, S., Brundin, P., Gustavii, B., Åstedt, B., Widner, H., Lindholm, T., Björklund, A., Leenders, K.L., Rothwell, J.C., Frackowiak, R., Marsden, C.D., Johnels, B., Steg, G., Freedman, R., Hoffer, B.J., Seiger, Å., Bygdeman, M., Strömberg, I., & Olson, L. (1989). Human fetal dopamine neurons grafted into the striatum in 2 patients with severe Parkinson's disease: a detailed account of methodology and a 6-month follow-up. *Archives of Neurology, 46*, 615–631.

Lindvall, O., Brundin, P., Widner, H., Rehncrona, S., Gustavii, B., Frackowiak, R., Leenders, K.L., Sawle, G., Rothwell, J.C., Marsden, C.D., & Björklund, A. (1990). Grafts of fetal dopamine neurons survive and improve motor function in Parkinson's disease. *Science, 247*, 574–577.

Lindvall, O., Widner, H., Rehncrona, S., Brundin, P., Odin, P., Gustavii, B., Frackowiak, R., Leenders, K.L., Sawle, G., Rothwell, J.C., Björklund, A., & Marsden, C.D. (1992). Transplantation of fetal dopamine neurons in Parkinson's disease: one year clinical and neurophysiological observations in 2 patients with putaminal implants. *Annals of Neurology, 31*, 155–165.

Lindvall, O., Sawle, G., Widner, H., Rothwell, J.C., Björklund, A., Brooks, D., Brundin, P., Frackowiak, R., Marsden, C.D., Odin, P., & Rehncrona, S. (1994). Evidence for long-term survival and function of dopaminergic grafts in progressive Parkinson's disease. *Annals of Neurology, 35*, 172–180.

Ling, Z.D., Potter, E.D., Lipton, J.W., & Carvey, P.M. (1998). Differentiation of mesencephalic progenitor cells into dopaminergic neurons by cytokines. *Experimental Neurology, 149*, 411–423.

Lipton, S.A. (1989). Growth factors for neuronal survival and process regeneration: implications in the mammalian central nervous system. *Archives of Neurology, 46*, 1241–1248.

Liuzzi, F.J., & Lasek, R.J. (1987). Astrocytes block axonal regeneration in mammals by activating the physiological stop pathway. *Science, 237*, 642–645.

Lois, C., & Alvarez-Buylla, A. (1994). Long-distance neuronal migration in the adult mammalian brain. *Science, 264*, 1145–1148.

López-Lozano, J.J., Bravo, G., & Abascal, J. (1990). A long-term study of Parkinson's patients subjected to autoimplants of perfused adrenal medulla into the caudate nucleus. *Transplantation Proceedings, 22*, 2243–2246.

López-Lozano, J.J., Bravo, G., & Abascal, J. (1991). Grafting of perfused adrenal medullary tissue into the caudate nucleus of patients with Parkinson's disease. *Journal of Neurosurgery, 75*, 234–243.

López-Lozano, J.J., Bravo, G., Brera, B., Dargallo, J., Salmean, J., Uria, J., Insausti, J., Millan, I., Aragones, P., Martinez, R., de la Torre, C., & Moreno, R. (1995). Long-term follow-up in 10 Parkinson's disease patients subjected to fetal brain grafting into a cavity in the caudate nucleus: the Clinica-Puerta-de-Hierro experience. *Transplantation Proceedings, 27*, 1395–1400.

Lund, R.D., & Bannerjee, R. (1992). Immunological considerations in neural transplantation. In S.B. Dunnett & A. Björklund (Eds.), *Neural transplantation: A practical approach* (pp. 161–176). Oxford: IRL Press.

Lund, R.D., & Hauschka, S.D. (1976). Transplanted neural tissue develops connections with host rat brain. *Science, 193*, 582–585.

Lund, R.D., Radel, J.D., & Coffey, P.J. (1991). The impact of intracerebral retinal transplants on types of behavior exhibited by host rats. *Trends in Neurosciences, 14*, 358–362.

Lundberg, C., Horellou, P., Mallet, J., & Björklund, A. (1996). Generation of DOPA-producing astrocytes by retroviral transduction of the human tyrosine hydroxylase gene: *in vitro* characterisation and *in vivo* effects in the rat Parkinson model. *Experimental Neurology, 139*, 39–53.

Machado-Salas, J., Cornejo, A., Ibarra, O., Aceves, J., Fong, D.M., Huerta, G., & Kuri, J. (1990). Multidisciplinary analysis of the effectiveness of autologous neural transplant (adrenal-medulla) as treatment of Parkinson's disease. *Stereotactic and Functional Neurosurgery, 54–5*, 306–311.

Madrazo, I., Drucker-Colín, R., Díaz, V., Martínez-Mata, J., Torres, C., & Becerril, J.J. (1987). Open microsurgical autograft of adrenal medulla to the right caudate nucleus in two patients with intractable Parkinson's disease. *New England Journal of Medicine, 316*, 831–834.

Madrazo, I., Leon, V., Torres, C., Aguilera, M.C., Varela, G., Alvarez, F., Fraga, A., Drucker-Colín, R., Ostrosky, F., Skurovich, M., & Franco, R. (1988). Transplantation of fetal substantia nigra and adrenal medulla to the caudate nucleus in two patients with Parkinson's disease. *New England Journal of Medicine, 318*, 51.

Madrazo, I., Franco-Bourland, R., Ostrosky-Solis, F., Aguilera, M., Cuevas, C., Zamorano, C., Morelos, A., Magallon, E., & Guizar-Sahagun, G. (1990). Fetal homotransplants (ventral mesencephalon and adrenal tissue) to the striatum of parkinsonian subjects. *Archives of Neurology, 47*, 1281–1285.

Madrazo, I., Franco-Bourland, R.E., Castrejon, H., Cuevas, C., & Ostrosky-Solis, F. (1995). Fetal striatal homotransplantation for Huntington's disease: First two case reports. *Neurological Research, 17*, 312–315.

Mahalik, T.J., Finger, T.E., Strömberg, I., & Olson, L. (1985). Substantia nigra transplants into denervated striatum of the rat: ultrastructure of graft and host interconnections. *Journal of Comparative Neurology, 240*, 60–70.

Mahalik, T.J., & Clayton, G.H. (1991). Specific outgrowth from neurons of ventral mesencephalic grafts to the catecholamine-depleted striatum of adult hosts. *Experimental Neurology, 113*, 18–27.

Mandel, R.J., Brundin, P., & Björklund, A. (1990). The importance of graft placement and task complexity for transplant induced recovery of simple and complex sensorimotor deficits in dopamine denervated rats. *European Journal of Neuroscience, 2*, 888–894.

Mandel, R.J., Spratt, S.K., Snyder, R.O., & Leff, S.E. (1997). Midbrain injection of recombinant adeno-associated virus encoding rat glial cell line-derived neurotrophic factor protects nigral neurons in a progressive 6-hydroxydopamine-induced degeneration model of Parkinson's disease in rats. *Proceedings of the National Academy of Sciences of the United States of America, 94*, 14083–14088.

Mangiarini, L., Sathasivam, K., Seller, M., Cozens, B., Harper, A., Hetherington, C., Lawton, M., Trottier, Y., Lehrach, H., Davies, S.W., & Bates, G.P. (1996). Exon 1 of the *HD* gene with an expanded CAG repeat is sufficient to cause a progressive neurological phenotype in transgenic mice. *Cell, 87*, 493–506.

Mann, D.M.A. (1985). The neuropathology of Alzheimer's disease: a review with pathogenetic, aetiological and therapeutic considerations. *Mechanisms of Ageing and Development, 31*, 213–255.

Mann, D.M.A. (1997). *Sense and senility: The neuropathy of the aged human brain.* Austin: R.G. Landes.

Marder, K., Tang, M.-X., Cote, L., Stern, Y., & Mayeux, R. (1995). The frequency and associated risk factors for dementia in patients with Parkinson's disease. *Archives of Neurology, 52*, 695–701.

Marshall, J.F., Richardson, J.S., & Teitelbaum, P. (1974). Nigrostriatal bundle damage and the lateral hypothalamic syndrome. *Journal of Comparative and Physiological Psychology, 87*, 808–830.

Martinez-Serrano, A., & Björklund, A. (1997). Immortalized neural progenitor cells for CNS gene transfer and repair. *Trends in Neurosciences, 20*, 530–538.

Martinez-Serrano, A., Fischer, W., & Björklund, A. (1995a). Reversal of age-dependent cognitive impairments and cholinergic neuron atrophy by NGF-secreting neural progenitors grafted to the basal forebrain. *Neuron, 15*, 473–484.

Martinez-Serrano, A., Lundberg, C., Horellou, P., Fischer, W., Bentlage, C., Campbell, K., McKay, R.D.G., Mallet, J., & Björklund, A. (1995b). CNS-derived neural progenitor cells for gene transfer of nerve growth factor to the adult rat brain: Complete rescue of axotomized cholinergic neurons after transplantation into the septum. *Journal of Neuroscience, 15*, 5668–5680.

Martinez-Serrano, A., Fischer, W., Söderström, S., Ebendal, T., & Björklund, A. (1996). Long-term functional recovery from age-induced spatial memory impairments by nerve growth factor gene transfer to the rat basal forebrain. *Proceedings of the National Academy of Sciences of the United States of America, 93*, 6355–6360.

Mason, D.W., Charlton, H.M., Jones, A.J., Lavy, C.B.D., Puklavec, M., & Simmonds, S.J. (1986). The fate of allogeneic and xenogeneic neuronal tissue transplanted into the third ventricle of rodents. *Neuroscience, 19*, 685–694.

Mason, S.T., Sanberg, P.R., & Fibiger, H.C. (1978). Kainic acid lesions of the striatum dissociate amphetamine and apomorphine stereotypy: similarities to Huntington's chorea. *Science, 201*, 352–355.

Mason, S.T., & Fibiger, H.C. (1979). Kainic acid lesions of the striatum mimic the spontaneous locomotor abnormalities of Huntington's disease. *Neuropharmacology, 18*, 403.

Mayer, E., Brown, V.J., Dunnett, S.B., & Robbins, T.W. (1992). Striatal graft-associated recovery of a lesion-induced performance deficit in the rat requires learning to use the transplant. *European Journal of Neuroscience, 4*, 119–126.

Mayer, E., Fawcett, J.W., & Dunnett, S.B. (1993). Basic fibroblast growth factor promotes the survival of embryonic ventral mesencephalic dopaminergic neurons. II. Effects on neural transplants *in vivo*. *Neuroscience, 56*, 389–398.

McDonald, W.I., Miller, D.H., & Barnes, D. (1992). The pathological evolution of multiple sclerosis. *Neuropathology and Applied Neurobiology, 18*, 319–334.

McKay, R., Valtz, N., Cunningham, M., & Hayes, T. (1990). Mechanisms regulating cell number and type in the mammalian central nervous system. *Cold Spring Harbor Symposia on Quantitative Biology, 55*, 291–301.

McKeon, R.J., Schreiber, R.C., Rudge, J.S., & Silver, J. (1991). Reduction of neurite outgrowth in a model of glial scarring following CNS injury is correlated with the expression of inhibitory molecules on reactive astrocytes. *Journal of Neuroscience, 11*, 3398–3411.

McRae, A., Hjorth, S., Mason, D.W., Dillon, L., & Tice, T.R. (1991). Microencapsulated dopamine (DA)-induced restitution of function in 6-OHDA denervated rat striatum *in vivo*: comparison between two microsphere excipients. *Journal of Neural Transplantation and Plasticity, 2*, 165–173.

McRae, A., Ling, E.A., Hjorth, S., Dahlström, A., Mason, D., & Tice, T. (1994). Catecholamine-containing biodegradable microsphere implants as a novel approach in the treatment of CNS neurodegenerative disease: A review of experimental studies in DA-lesioned rats. *Molecular Neurobiology, 9*, 191–205.

Meldrum, B., & Garthwaite, J. (1990). Excitatory amino acid neurotoxicity and neurodegenerative disease. *Trends in Pharmacological Sciences, 11*, 379–387.

Mena, M.A., Pardo, B., Paíno, C.L., & Garcia De Yebenes, J. (1993). Levodopa toxicity in foetal rat midbrain neurones in culture: Modulation by ascorbic acid. *NeuroReport, 4*, 438–440.

Mendez, I., Elisevich, K., & Flumerfelt, B. (1991). Dopaminergic innervation of substance p-containing striatal neurons by fetal nigral grafts — an ultrastructural double-labeling immunocytochemical study. *Journal of Comparative Neurology, 308*, 66–78.

Mendez, I.M., Naus, C.C.G., Elisevich, K., & Flumerfelt, B.A. (1993). Normalization of striatal proenkephalin and preprotachykinin mRNA expression by fetal substantia nigra grafts. *Experimental Neurology, 119*, 1–10.

Mennicken, F., Savasta, M., Chritin, M., Feuerstein, C., Le Moal, M., Herman, J.P., & Abrous, D.N. (1995). The neonatal lesion of the meso-telencephalic dopaminergic pathway increases intrastriatal D2 receptor levels and synthesis and this effect is reversed by neonatal dopaminergic rich graft. *Molecular Brain Research, 28*, 211–221.

Messersmith, D.J., Fabrazzo, M., Mochetti, I., & Kromer, L.F. (1991). Effects of sciatic nerve transplants after fimbria–fornix lesion: examination of the role of nerve growth factor. *Brain Research, 557*, 293–297.

Mishkin, M., Malamut, B., & Bachevalier, J. (1984). Memories and habits: two neural systems. In G. Lynch, J.L. McGaugh, & N.M. Weinberger (Eds.), *Neurobiology of learning and memory* (pp. 65–77). New York: Guilford Press.

Molina, H., Quiñones, R., Alvarez, L., Ortega, I., Muñoz, J.L., González, C., De la Cuétara, K., Torres, O., Suárez, C., León, M., Rojas, M.J., Rachid, M., Macías, R., García, J.C., Lorigados, L., Castellanos, O., & Hernández, O. (1992). Stereotactic transplantation of fetal ventral mesencephalic cells: Cuban experience with five patients with idiopathic Parkinson's disease. *Journal of Neural Transplantation and Plasticity, 3*, 338–339.

Molina, H., Quiñones, R., Alvarez, L., Suárez, C., Ortega, I., Muñoz, J.L., Rachid, M., Torres, O., Rojas, M.J., León, M., García, J.C., González, G., Lorigados, L., Perry, T., Piedra, J., González, C., Araújo, F., & Hernández, O. (1992). Transplantation of human fetal mesencephalic tissue in caudate nucleus as a treatment for Parkinson's disease: long-term follow up. *Journal of Neural Transplantation and Plasticity, 3*, 323–324.

Montoya, C.P., Astell, S., & Dunnett, S.B. (1990). Effects of nigral and striatal grafts on skilled forelimb use in the rat. *Progress in Brain Research, 82*, 459–466.

Moore, R.Y., & Bloom, F.E. (1978). Central catecholamine neuron systems: Anatomy and physiology of the dopamine systems. *Annual Review of Neuroscience, 1*, 129–169.

Moorman, S.J., Whalen, L.R., & Nornes, H.O. (1990). A neurotransmitter specific functional recovery mediated by fetal implants in the lesioned spinal cord of the rat. *Brain Research, 508*, 194–198.

Moreau, T., Coles, A., Wing, M., Thorpe, J.W., Miller, D.H., Moseley, I.F., Isaacs, J., Hale, G., Clayton, D., Scolding, N.J., Waldmann, H., & Compston, D.A.S. (1996). CAMPATH-1H in multiple sclerosis. *Multiple Sclerosis, 1*, 357–365.

Mori, F., Himes, B.T., Kowada, M., Murray, M., & Tessler, A. (1997). Fetal spinal cord transplants rescue some axotomized rubrospinal neurons from retrograde cell death in adult rats. *Experimental Neurology, 143*, 45–60.

Morihisa, J.M., Nakamura, R.K., Freed, W.J., Mishkin, M., & Wyatt, R.J. (1984). Adrenal medulla grafts survive and exhibit catecholamine specific fluorescence in the primate brain. *Experimental Neurology, 84*, 643–653.

Motti, E.D.F., Pezzoli, G., Silani, V., & Scarlato, G. (1988). Surgical lesions, parkinsonism, and brain graft operations. *Lancet, 2*, 346.

Muller, T.H., & Unsicker, K. (1981). High-performance liquid chromatography with electrochemical detection as a highly efficient tool for studying catecholaminergic systems. 1. Quantification of noradrenaline, adrenaline and dopamine in cultured adrenal medullary cells. *Journal of Neuroscience Methods, 4*, 39–52.

Murer, M.G., Dziewczapolski, G., Menalled, L.B., Garcia, M.C., Agid, Y., Gershanik, O., & Raisman-Vozari, R. (1998). Chronic levodopa is not toxic for remaining dopamine neurons, but instead promotes their recovery, in rats with moderate nigrostriatal lesions. *Annals of Neurology, 43*, 561–575.

Nadaud, D., Herman, J.P., Simon, H., & Le Moal, M. (1984). Functional recovery following transplantation of ventral mesencephalic cells in rats subjected to 6-OHDA lesions of the mesolimbic dopaminergic neurons. *Brain Research, 304*, 137–141.

Nakai, M., Itakura, T., Kamei, I., Nakai, K., Naka, Y., Imai, H., & Komai, N. (1990). Autologous transplantation of the superior cervical ganglion into the brain of parkinsonian monkeys. *Journal of Neurosurgery, 72*, 91–95.

Nakao, N., Frodl, E.M., Duan, W.-M., Widner, H., & Brundin, P. (1994). Lazaroids improve the survival of grafted rat embryonic dopamine neurons. *Proceedings of the National Academy of Sciences of the United States of America, 91*, 12408–12412.

Nappi, G., Petraglia, F., Martignoni, E., Facchinetti, F., Bono, G., & Genazzani, A.R. (1985). Beta-endorphin cerebrospinal fluid decrease in untreated Parkinsonian patients. *Neurology, 35*, 1371–1374.

Naujoks, K.W., Korsching, S., Rohrer, H., & Thoenen, H. (1982). Nerve growth factor-mediated induction of tyrosine hydroxylase and of neurite outgrowth in cultures of bovine adrenal chromaffin cells—dependence on developmental stage. *Developmental Biology, 92*, 365–379.

Nieto-Sampedro, M., Manthrope, M., Barbin, G., Varon, S., & Cotman, C.W. (1983). Injury-induced neuronotrophic activity in adult rat brain: correlation with survival of delayed implants in the wound cavity. *Journal of Neuroscience, 3*, 2219–2229.

Nieto-Sampedro, M., Whittemore, S.R., Needels, D.L., Larson, J., & Cotman, C.W. (1984). The survival of brain transplants is enhanced by extracts from injured brain. *Proceedings of the National Academy of Sciences of the United States of America, 81*, 6250–6254.

Nikkhah, G., Odin, P., Smits, A., Tingström, A., Othberg, A., Brundin, P., Funa, K., & Lindvall, O. (1992). Platelet-derived growth factor promotes survival of rat and human mesencephalic dopaminergic neurons in culture. *Experimental Brain Research, 92*, 516–523.

Nilsson, O.G., Shapiro, M.L., Gage, F.H., Olton, D.S., & Björklund, A. (1987). Spatial learning and memory following fimbria–fornix transection and grafting of fetal septal neurons to the hippocampus. *Experimental Brain Research, 67*, 195–215.

Nilsson, O.G., Brundin, P., & Björklund, A. (1990). Amelioration of spatial memory impairment by intrahippocampal grafts of mixed septal and raphe tissue in rats with combined cholinergic and serotonergic denervation of the forebrain. *Brain Research, 515*, 193–206.

Nishino, H., Ono, T., Shibata, R., Kawamata, S., Watanabe, H., Shiosaka, S., Tohyama, M., & Karadi, Z. (1988). Adrenal medullary cells transmute into dopaminergic neurons in dopamine-depleted rat caudate and ameliorate motor disturbances. *Brain Research, 445*, 325–337.

Nornes, H., Björklund, A., & Stenevi, U. (1983). Reinnervation of the denervated adult spinal cord of rats by intraspinal transplants of embryonic brain stem neurons. *Cell and Tissue Research, 230*, 15–35.

Nógrádi, A., & Vrbová, G. (1994). The use of embryonic spinal cord grafts to replace identified motoneuron pools depleted by a neurotoxic lectin, volkensin. *Experimental Neurology, 129*, 130–141.

Nógrádi, A., & Vrbová, G. (1996). Improved motor function of denervated rat hindlimb muscles induced by embryonic spinal cord grafts. *European Journal of Neuroscience, 8*, 2198–2203.

Obeso, J.A., Guridi, J., & DeLong, M.R. (1997). Surgery for Parkinson's disease. *Journal of Neurology, Neurosurgery and Psychiatry, 62*, 2–8.

Okuda, O., Bressler, J., Chang, L., & Brightman, M. (1991). Viral Kirsten ras infection differentiates PC12 cells and enhances their survival upon implantation into brain. *Experimental Neurology, 113*, 330–337.

Olanow, C.W., Koller, W., Goetz, C.G., Stebbins, G.T., Cahill, D.W., Gauger, L.L., Morantz, R., Penn, R.D., Tanner, C.M., Klawans, H.L., Shannon, K.M., Comella, C.L., & Witt, T. (1990). Autologous transplantation of adrenal medulla in Parkinson's disease: 18-month results. *Archives of Neurology, 47*, 1286–1289.

Olanow, C.W. (1996). GPi pallidotomy—have we made a dent in Parkinson's disease? *Annals of Neurology, 40*, 341–343.

Olanow, C.W., Kordower, J.H., & Freeman, T.B. (1996). Fetal nigral transplantation as a therapy for Parkinson's disease. *Trends in Neurosciences, 19*, 102–109.

Oliver, C., & Holland, A.J. (1986). Down's syndrome and Alzheimer's disease. *Psychological Medicine, 16*, 307–322.

Olson, L. (1970). Fluorescence histochemical evidence for axonal growth and secretion from transplanted adrenal medullary tissue. *Histochemie, 22*, 1–7.

Olson, L., & Malmfors, T. (1970). Growth characteristics of adrenergic nerves in the adult rat. Fluorescence histochemical and 3H-noradrenaline uptake studies using tissue transplantation to the anterior chamber of the eye. *Acta Physiologica Scandinavica, Supplementum, 348*, 1–112.

Olson, L., & Seiger, Å. (1972). Brain tissue transplanted to the anterior chamber of the eye. I. Fluorescence histochemistry of immature catecholamine and 5-hydroxytryptamine neurons innervating the iris. *Zeitung Zellforschung, 195*, 175–194.

Olson, L., Seiger, Å., Friedman, R., & Hoffer, B.J. (1980). Chromaffin cells can innervate brain tissue: evidence from intra-ocular double grafts. *Experimental Neurology, 70*, 414–426.

Olson, L., Seiger, Å., & Strömberg, I. (1983). Intraocular transplantation in rodents: a detailed account of the procedure and examples of its use in neurobiology with special reference to brain tissue grafting. *Advances in Cellular Neurobiology, 4*, 407–442.

Olson, L., Backlund, E.O., Ebendal, T., Freedman, R., Hamberger, B., Hansson, P., Hoffer, B.J., Lindblom, U., Meyerson, B., Strömberg, I., Sydow, O., & Seiger, Å. (1991). Intraputaminal infusion of nerve growth factor to support adrenal medullary autografts in Parkinson's disease: one year follow-up of first clinical trial. *Archives of Neurology, 48*, 373–381.

Olson, L., Hoffer, B.J., Backlund, E.O., Ebendal, T., Freedman, R., Hamberger, B., Hansson, P., Lindblom, U., Meyerson, B., Strömberg, I., Sydow, O., & Seiger, Å. (1992). Intraputaminal infusion of nerve growth factor to support adrenal medullary autografts in Parkinson's disease (Abstract). *Restorative Neurology and Neuroscience, 4*, 194.

Olsson, M., Nikkhah, G., Bentlage, C., & Björklund, A. (1995). Forelimb akinesia in the rat Parkinson model: differential effects of dopamine agonists and nigral transplants as assessed by a new stepping test. *Journal of Neuroscience, 15*, 3863–3875.

Ostrosky-Solis, F., Quintanar, L., Madrazo, I., Drucker-Colín, R., Franco-Bourland, R., & Leonmeza, V. (1988). Neuropsychological effects of brain autograft of adrenal medullary tissue for the treatment of Parkinson's disease. *Neurology, 38*, 1442–1450.

Paíno, C.L., & Bunge, M.B. (1991). Induction of axon growth into Schwann cell implants grafted into lesioned adult rat spinal cord. *Experimental Neurology, 114*, 254–257.

Paíno, C.L., Fernandez-Valle, C., Bates, M.L., & Bunge, M.B. (1994). Regrowth of axons in lesioned adult rat spinal cord—promotion by implants of cultured Schwann cells. *Journal of Neurocytology, 23*, 433–452.

Palfi, S., Nguyen, J.P., Brugieres, P., LeGuerinel, C., Hantraye, P., Rémy, P., Rostaing, S., Defer, G.L., Césaro, P., Keravel, Y., & Peschanski, M. (1998). MRI-stereotactical approach for neural grafting in basal ganglia disorders. *Experimental Neurology, 150*, 272–281.

Palfi, S.P., Ferrante, R.J., Brouillet, E., Beal, M.F., Dolan, R., Guyot, M.C., Peschanski, M., & Hantraye, P. (1996). Chronic 3-nitropropionic acid treatment in baboons replicates the cognitive and motor deficits of Huntington's disease. *Journal of Neuroscience, 16*, 3019–3025.

Pappas, G.D., Lazorthes, Y., Bès, J.C., Tafani, M., & Winnie, A.P. (1997). Relief of intractable cancer pain by human chromaffin cell transplants: Experience at two medical centers. *Neurological Research, 19*, 71–77.

Pappas, G.D., & Sagen, J. (1988). Fine structural correlates of vascular permeability of chromaffin cell transplants in CNS pain modulatory regions. *Experimental Neurology, 102*, 280–289.

Patel-Vaidya, U., Wells, M.R., & Freed, W.J. (1985). Survival of dissociated adrenal chromaffin cells of rat and monkey transplanted into rat brain. *Cell and Tissue Research, 240,* 281–285.

Patterson, P.H., & Nawa, H. (1993). Neuronal differentiation factors, cytokines and synaptic plasticity. *Cell, 72*, 123–137.

Pearson, R.C.A., & Powell, T.P.S. (1989). The neuroanatomy of Alzheimer's disease. *Reviews in the Neurosciences, 2*, 101–122.

Penn, R.D., Kroin, J.S., Kroin, S.A., Tanner, C.M., Shannon, K.M., Comella, C.L., Carvey, P.M., Zhang, T.J., Witt, T., Wilson, R., Stebbins, G.T., Gilley, D.W., Yaksh, T., O'Dorisio, T., & McRae-Degueurce, A. (1990). The adrenal medullary transplant operation: the Chicago experience. *Progress in Brain Research, 82*, 627–635.

Perlow, M.J., Freed, W.J., Hoffer, B.J., Seiger, Å., Olson, L., & Wyatt, R.J. (1979). Brain grafts reduce motor abnormalities produced by destruction of nigrostriatal dopamine system. *Science, 204*, 643–647.

Perlow, M.J., Kumakura, K., & Guidotti, A. (1980). Prolonged survival of bovine adrenal chromaffin cells in rat cerebral ventricles. *Proceedings of the National Academy of Sciences of the United States of America, 77*, 5278–5281.

Perry, E.K., Tomlinson, B.E., Blessed, G., Bergmann, K., Gibson, P.H., & Perry, R.H. (1978). Correlation of cholinergic abnormalities with senile plaques and mental test scores in senile dementia. *British Medical Journal, ii*, 1457–1459.

Peschanski, M., Defer, G., N'Guyen, J.P., Ricolfi, F., Montfort, J.C., Rémy, P., Geny, C., Samson, Y., Hantraye, P., Jeny, R., Gaston, A., Kéravel, Y., Degos, J.D., & Cesaro, P. (1994). Bilateral motor improvement and alteration of L-dopa effect in two patients with Parkinson's disease following intrastriatal transplantation of foetal ventral mesencephalon. *Brain, 117*, 487–499.

Peschanski, M., Cesaro, P., & Hantraye, P. (1995). Rationale for intrastriatal grafting of striatal neuroblasts in patients with Huntington's disease. *Neuroscience, 68*, 273–285.

Peterson, D.I., Price, L., & Small, C.S. (1989). Autopsy findings in a patient who had an adrenal-to-brain transplant for Parkinson's disease. *Neurology, 39*, 235–238.

Petruk, K.C., Wilson, A.F., Schindel, D.R., Witt, N.J., Mclean, D.R., Mcfarland, P.A., Johnston, R.G., Mcphee, M.S., Martin, W.R., & Calne, D.B. (1990). Treatment of refractory Parkinson's disease with adrenal medullary autografts utilizing 2–stage surgery. *Progress in Brain Research, 82*, 671–676.

Pezzoli, G., Fahn, S., Dwork, A., Truong, D.D., de Yebenes, J.G., Jackson-Lewis, V., Herbert, J., & Cadet, J.L. (1988). Nonchromaffin tissue plus nerve growth factor reduces experimental parkinsonism in aged rats. *Brain Research, 459*, 398–403.

Pezzoli, G., Motti, E., Zechinelli, A., Ferrante, C., Silani, V., Falini, A., Pizzuti, A., Mulazzi, D., Baratta, P., Vegato, A., Villani, R., & Scarlato, G. (1990). Adrenal medulla autograft in 3 parkinsonian patients: results using two different approaches. *Progress in Brain Research, 82*, 677–682.

Pifl, C., Schingnitz, G., & Hornykiewicz, O. (1991). Effect of 1-methyl-4-phenyl-1,2,3,6-tetrahydropyridine on the regional distribution of brain mono-amines in the rhesus monkey. *Neuroscience, 44*, 591–605.

Plunkett, R.J., Bankiewicz, K.S., Cummins, A.C., Miletich, R.S., Schwartz, J.P., & Oldfield, E.H. (1990). Long-term evaluation of hemiparkinsonian monkeys after adrenal autografting or cavitation alone. *Journal of Neurosurgery, 73*, 918–926.

Polkinghorne, J. (1989). *Review of the guidance on the research use of fetuses and fetal material.* London: HMSO.

Pons, T.P., Garraghty, P.E., Ommaya, A.K., Kaas, J.H., Taub, E., & Mishkin, M. (1991). Massive cortical reorganization after sensory deafferentation in adult macaques. *Science, 252*, 1857–1860.

Privat, A., Mansour, H., & Geffard, M. (1988). Transplantation of fetal serotonin neurons into the transected spinal cord of adult rats: morphological development and functional influence. *Progress in Brain Research, 78*, 155–166.

Privat, A., Mansour, H., Rajaofetra, N., & Geffard, M. (1989). Intraspinal transplants of serotonergic neurons in the adult rats. *Brain Research Bulletin, 22*, 123–129.

Quinn, N.P. (1990). The clinical application of cell grafting techniques in patients with Parkinson's disease. *Progress in Brain Research, 82*, 619–625.

Quinn, N.P., Parkes, J.D., Janota, I., & Marsden, C.D. (1986). Preservation of the substantia nigra and locus coeruleus in a patient receiving levodopa (2kg) plus decarboxylase inhibitor over a four year period. *Movement Disorders, 1*, 65–68.

Quinn, N.P., Brown, R., Craufurd, D., Goldman, S., Hodges, J.R., Kieburtz, K., Lindvall, O., MacMillan, J.C., & Roos, R.A.C. (1996). Core assessment programme for intracerebral transplantation in Huntington's disease (CAPIT-HD). *Movement Disorders, 11*, 143–150.

Quon, D., Wang, Y., Catalano, R., Scardina, J.M., Murakami, K., & Cordell, B. (1991). Formation of β-amyloid protein deposits in brains of transgenic mice. *Nature, 352*, 239–241.

Raisman, G. (1969). Neuronal plasticity in the septal nuclei of the adult brain. *Brain Research, 14*, 25–48.

Rajput, A.H. (1992). Frequency and cause of Parkinson's disease. *Canadian Journal of Neurological Sciences, 19*, 103–107.

Rajput, A.H. (1993). Environmental causation of Parkinson's disease. *Archives of Neurology, 50*, 651–652.

Rakic, P. (1985). Limits of neurogenesis in primates. *Science, 227*, 1054–1056.

Reading, P.J. (1994). Neural transplantation in the ventral striatum. In S.B. Dunnett & A. Björklund (Eds.), *Functional neural transplantation,* pp. 197–216. New York: Raven Press.

Recanzone, G.H., Merzenich, M.M., Jenkins, W.M., Grajski, K.A., & Dinse, H.R. (1992). Topographic reorganization of the hand representation in cortical area 3b of owl monkeys trained in a frequency-discrimination task. *Journal of Neurophysiology, 67*, 1031–1056.

Redford, E.J., Kapoor, R., & Smith, K.J. (1997). Nitric oxide donors reversibly block axonal conduction: demyelinated axons are especially susceptible. *Brain, 120*, 2149–2157.

Redmond, D.E., Naftolin, F., Collier, T.J., Leranth, C., Robbins, R.J., Sladek, C.D., Roth, R.H., & Sladek, J.R. (1988). Cryopreservation, culture, and transplantation of human fetal mesencephalic tissue into monkeys. *Science, 242*, 768–771.

Redmond, D.E., Leranth, C., Spencer, D.D., Robbins, R.J., Vollmer, T.L., Kim, J.H., Roth, R.H., Dwork, A.J., & Naftolin, F. (1990). Fetal neural graft survival. *Lancet, 336*, 820–822.

Reier, P.J., & Houle, J.D. (1988). The glial scar: its bearing on axonal elongation and transplantation approaches to CNS repair. *Advances in Neurology, 47*, 87–138.

Reisert, I., Schuster, R., Zienecker, R., & Pilgrim, C. (1990). Prenatal development of mesencephalic and diencephalic dopaminergic systems in the male and female rat. *Developmental Brain Research, 53*, 222–229.

Reynolds, B.A., & Weiss, S. (1992). Generation of neurons and astrocytes from isolated cells of the adult mammalian central nervous system. *Science, 255*, 1707–1710.

Reynolds, B.A., Tetzlaff, W., & Weiss, S. (1992). A multipotent EGF-responsive striatal embryonic progenitor cell produces neurons and astrocytes. *Journal of Neuroscience, 12*, 4565–4574.

Rémy, P., Samson, Y., Hantraye, P., Fontaine, A., Defer, G., Mangin, J.F., Fénelon, G., Gény, C., Ricolfi, F., Frouin, V., N'Guyen, J.P., Jeny, R., Degos, J.D., Peschanski, M., & Cesaro, P. (1995). Clinical correlates of [18F]fluorodopa uptake in five grafted Parkinsonian patients. *Annals of Neurology, 38*, 580–588.

Richards, L.J., Kilpatrick, T.J., & Bartlett, P.F. (1992). *De novo* generation of neuronal cells from the adult mouse brain. *Proceedings of the National Academy of Sciences of the United States of America, 89*, 8591–8595.

Richards, S.J., Waters, J.J., Beyreuther, K., Masters, C.L., Wischik, C.M., Sparkman, D.R., White, C.L., Abraham, C.R., & Dunnett, S.B. (1991). Transplants of mouse trisomy 16 hippocampus provide a model of Alzheimer's disease neuropathology. *EMBO Journal, 10*, 297–303.

Ridley, R.M., Baker, H.F., & Fine, A. (1988). Transplantation of fetal tissues. *British Medical Journal, 296*, 1469.

Ridley, R.M., Thornley, H.D., Baker, H.F., & Fine, A. (1991). Cholinergic neural transplants into hippocampus restore learning ability in monkeys with fornix transections. *Experimental Brain Research, 83*, 533–538.

Riopelle, R.J. (1988). Adrenal medulla autografts in Parkinson's disease: a proposed mechanism of action. *Canadian Journal of Neurological Sciences, 15*, 366–370.

Rioux, L., Gaudin, D.P., Bui, L.K., Grégoire, L., DiPaolo, T., & Bédard, P.J. (1991). Correlation of functional recovery after a 6-hydroxydopamine lesion with survival of grafted fetal neurons and release of dopamine in the striatum of the rat. *Neuroscience, 40*, 123–131.

Robertson, H.A. (1992). Dopamine receptor interactions: some implications for the treatment of Parkinson's disease. *Trends in Neurosciences*, 15, 201–206.

Rogers, D.C., & Dunnett, S.B. (1989). Hypersensitivity to a-methyl-p-tyrosine suggests that behavioural recovery of rats receiving neonatal 6-OHDA lesions is mediated by residual catecholamine neurons. *Neuroscience Letters, 102*, 108–113.

Rosenberg, M.B., Friedmann, T., Robertson, R.C., Tuszynski, M., Wolff, J.A., Breakefield, X.O., & Gage, F.H. (1988). Grafting genetically modified cells to the damaged brain: restorative effects of NGF expression. *Science, 242*, 1575–1578.

Rosenblad, C., Martinez-Serrano, A., & Björklund, A. (1997). Intrastriatal glial cell line-derived neurotrophic factor promotes sprouting of spared nigrostriatal dopaminergic afferents and induces recovery of function in a rat model of Parkinson's disease. *Neuroscience, 82*, 129–137.

Rosenstein, J.M. (1987). Adrenal medulla grafts produce blood–brain barrier dysfunction. *Brain Research, 414*, 192–196.

Rosenstein, J.M., & Brightman, M.W. (1983). Circumventing the blood–brain barrier with autonomic ganglion transplants. *Science, 221*, 879–881.

Rosenthal, A. (1998). Auto transplants for Parkinson's disease? *Neuron, 20*, 169–172.

Rosenzweig, M.R., Bennett, E.L., & Diamond, M.C. (1972). Chemical and anatomical plasticity of the brain: replications and extensions. In J. Gaito (Ed.), *Macromolecules and behavior* (pp. 205–278). New York: Appleton-Century-Croft.

Rosvold, H.E. (1972). The frontal lobe system: cortical–subcortical interrelationships. *Acta Neurobiologiae Experimentalis, 32*, 439–460.

Rosvold, H.E., & Delgado, J.M.R. (1956). The effect on delayed alternation test performance of stimulating or destroying electrically structures within the frontal lobes of the monkey's brain. *Journal of Comparative and Physiological Psychology, 49*, 365–372.

Rosvold, H.E., & Szwarcbart, M.K. (1964). Neural structures involved in delayed response performance. In J.M. Warren & K. Akert (Eds.), *The frontal granular cortex and behavior* (pp. 1–15). New York: McGraw-Hill.

Russ, H., Mihatsch, W., Gerlach, M., Riederer, P., & Przuntek, H. (1991). Neurochemical and behavioral features induced by chronic low-dose treatment with 1-methyl-4-phenyl-1,2,3,6-tetrahydropyridine (MPTP) in the common marmoset—implications for Parkinson's disease. *Neuroscience Letters, 123*, 115–118.

Rutherford, A., Garcia-Munoz, M., Dunnett, S.B., & Arbuthnott, G.W. (1987). Electrophysiological demonstration of host cortical inputs to striatal grafts. *Neuroscience Letters, 83*, 275–281.

Sabaté, O., Horellou, P., Vigne, E., Colin, P., Perricaudet, M., Buc-Caron, M.-H., & Mallet, J. (1995). Transplantation to the rat brain of human neural progenitors that were genetically modified using adenoviruses. *Nature Genetics, 9*, 256–260.

Sabel, B.A., Dominiak, P., Häuser, W., During, M.J., & Freese, A. (1990). Levodopa delivery from controlled-release polymer matrix: delivery of more than 600 days *in vitro* and 225 days of elevated plasma levels after subcutaneous implantation in rats. *Journal of Pharmacology and Experimental Therapeutics, 255*, 914–922.

Sagen, J., Pappas, G.D., & Pollard, H. (1986a). Analgesia induced by isolated bovine chromaffin cells implanted in rat spinal cord. *Proceedings of the National Academy of Sciences of the United States of America, 83*, 7552–7556.

Sagen, J., Pappas, G.D., & Perlow, M.J. (1986b). Adrenal medullary tissue transplants in rat spinal cord reduce pain sensitivity. *Brain Research, 384*, 189–194.

Sagen, J., Wang, H., & Pappas, G.D. (1990). Adrenal medullary implants in rat spinal cord reduce nociception in chronic pain model. *Pain, 42*, 69–79.

Sagen, J., Wang, H., Tresco, P.A., & Aebischer, P. (1993). Transplants of immunologically isolated xenogeneic chromaffin cells provide a long-term source of pain-reducing neuroactive substances. *Journal of Neuroscience, 13*, 2415–2423.

Sagot, Y., Tan, S.A., Baetge, E., Schmalbruch, H., Kato, A.C., & Aebischer, P. (1995). Polymer encapsulated cell lines genetically engineered to release ciliary neurotrophic factor can slow down progressive motor neuronopathy in the mouse. *European Journal of Neuroscience, 7*, 1313–1322.

Santana, C., Rodriguez, M., Afonso, D., & Arevalo, R. (1992). Dopaminergic neuron development in rats: biochemical study from prenatal life to adulthood. *Brain Research Bulletin, 29*, 7–13.

Sauer, H., & Brundin, P. (1991). Effects of cool storage on survival and function of intrastriatal ventral mesencephalic grafts. *Restorative Neurology and Neuroscience, 2*, 123–135.

Sauer, H., Rosenblad, C., & Björklund, A. (1995). Glial cell line-derived neurotrophic factor but not transforming growth factor β3 prevents delayed degeneration of nigral dopaminergic neurons following striatal 6-hydroxydopamine lesion. *Proceedings of the National Academy of Sciences of the United States of America, 92*, 8935–8939.

Sautter, J., Strecker, S., Kupsch, A., & Oertel, W.H. (1996). Methylcellulose during cryopreservation of ventral mesencephalic tissue fragments fails to improve survival and function of cell suspension grafts. *Journal of Neuroscience Methods, 64*, 173–179.

Sawle, G.V., & Myers, R. (1993). The role of positron emission tomography in the assessment of human neurotransplantation. *Trends in Neurosciences, 16*, 172–176.

Schapira, A.H.V. (1992). MPTP and other Parkinson-inducing agents. *Current Opinion in Neurology and Neurosurgery, 5*, 396–400.

Schmidt, R.H., Björklund, A., Stenevi, U., Dunnett, S.B., & Gage, F.H. (1983). Intracerebral grafting of neuronal cell suspensions. III. Activity of intrastriatal nigral suspension implants as assessed by measurements of dopamine synthesis and metabolism. *Acta Physiologica Scandinavica, supplementum, 522*, 19–28.

Schneider, J.S., & Rothblat, D.S. (1991). Neurochemical evaluation of the striatum in symptomatic and recovered MPTP-treated cats. *Neuroscience, 44*, 421–429.

Schnell, L., & Schwab, M.E. (1990). Axonal regeneration in the rat spinal cord produced by an antibody against myelin-associated neurite growth inhibitors. *Nature, 343*, 269–272.

Schnell, L., & Schwab, M.E. (1993). Sprouting and regeneration of lesioned cortical tract fibres in the adult rat spinal cord. *European Journal of Neuroscience, 5*, 1156–1171.

Schnell, L., Schneider, R., Kolbeck, R., Barde, Y.-A., & Schwab, M.E. (1994). Neurotrophin-3 enhances sprouting of corticospinal tract during development and after adult spinal cord lesion. *Nature, 367*, 170–173.

Schultzberg, M., Dunnett, S.B., Björklund, A., Stenevi, U., Hökfelt, T., Dockray, G.J., & Goldstein, M. (1984). Dopamine and cholecystokinin immunoreactive neurons in mesencephalic grafts reinnervating the neostriatum: evidence for selective growth regulation. *Neuroscience, 12*, 17–32.

Schvarcz, J.R., Devoto, M., Meiss, R., Torrieri, A., Genero, M., & Armando, I. (1990). Multiloci stereotaxic transplantation of autologous adrenal medullary tissue to the putamen and caudatum in Parkinson's disease—technical note. *Stereotactic and Functional Neurosurgery, 54–5*, 277–281.

Schwab, M.E. (1990). Myelin-associated inhibitors of neurite growth and regeneration in the CNS. *Trends in Neurosciences, 13*, 452–456.

Schwartz, J.P. (1992). Neurotransmitters as neurotrophic factors: a new set of functions. *International Review of Neurobiology, 34*, 1–23.

Scolding, N.J., Rayner, P.J., Sussman, J., Shaw, C.E., & Compston, D.A.S. (1995). A proliferative adult human oligodendrocyte progenitor. *NeuroReport, 6*, 441–445.

Scolding, N.J., Barker, R.A., & Compston, D.A.S. (1998). Immunological and inflammatory damage to the CNS. In A. Crockard, M. Hayward, & J.T. Hoff (Eds.), *Neurosurgery: The scientific basis of clinical practice*, Oxford: Blackwell Science.

Segovia, J., Castro, R., Notario, V., & Gale, K. (1991). Transplants of fetal substantia nigra regulate glutamic acid decarboxylase gene expression in host striatal neurons. *Molecular Brain Research, 10*, 359–362.

Seiger, Å., Nordberg, A., Von Holst, H., Bäckman, L., Ebendal, T., Alafuzoff, I., Amberla, K., Hartvig, P., Herlitz, A., Lilja, A., Lundqvist, H., Långström, B., Meyerson, B., Persson, A., Viitanen, M., Winblad, B., & Olson, L. (1993). Intracranial infusion of purified nerve growth factor to an Alzheimer patient: The first attempt of a possible future treatment strategy. *Behavioural Brain Research, 57*, 255–261.

Sendtner, M., Schchmalbruch, H., Stöckli, K.A., Carroll, P., Kreutzberg, G.W., & Thoenen, H. (1992). Ciliary neurotrophic factor prevents the degeneration of motor neurons in mouse mutant progressive motor neuronopathy. *Nature, 358*, 502–504.

Shihabuddin, L.S., Hertz, J.A., Holets, V.R., & Whittemore, S.R. (1995). The adult CNS retains the potential to direct region-specific differentiation of a transplanted neuronal precursor cell line. *Journal of Neuroscience, 15*, 6666–6678.

Shihabuddin, L.S., Brunschwig, J.P., Holets, V.R., Bunge, M.B., & Whittemore, S.R. (1996). Induction of mature neuronal properties in immortalized neuronal precursor cells following grafting into the neonatal CNS. *Journal of Neurocytology, 25*, 101–111.

Shults, C.W., Hashimoto, R., Brady, R.M., & Gage, F.H. (1990). Dopaminergic cells align along radial glia in the developing mesencephalon of the rat. *Neuroscience, 38*, 427–436.

Shults, C.W., O'Connor, D.T., Baird, A., Hill, R., Goetz, C.G., Watts, R.L., Klawans, H.L., Carvey, P.M., Bakay, R.A.E., Gage, F.H., & U, H.S. (1991). Clinical improvement in Parkinsonian patients undergoing adrenal to caudate transplantation is not reflected by chromogranin-A or basic fibroblast growth factor in ventricular fluid. *Experimental Neurology, 111*, 276–281.

Sieradzan, K., & Vrbová, G. (1994). Replacement of defined neuronal populations in the spinal cord by homotopic neural grafts. In G. Vrbová, G.J. Clowry, A. Nógrádi & K. Sieradzan (Eds.), *Transplantation of neural tissue into the spinal cord* (pp. 1111–1125). Austin, Texas: R.G. Landes.

Silani, V., Falini, A., Strada, O., Pizzuti, A., Pezzoli, G., Motti, E.D.F., Vegeto, A., & Scarlato, G. (1990). Effect of nerve growth factor in adrenal autografts in parkinsonism. *Annals of Neurology, 27*, 341–342.

Silani, V., Mariani, D., Donato, F.M., Mazzucchelli, F., Buscaglia, M., Pardi, G., & Scarlato, G. (1992a). *In vivo* and *in vitro* development of human mesencephalic dopaminergic neurons. *Journal of Neural Transplantation and Plasticity, 3*, 255–256.

Silani, V., Mariani, D., Donato, F.M., Buscaglia, M., Pardi, G., & Scarlato, G. (1992b). Acquisition of the immunophenotype by human adrenal cells. *Journal of Neural Transplantation and Plasticity, 4*, 211–212.

Simonian, N.A., & Coyle, J.T. (1996). Oxidative stress in neurodegenerative diseases. *Annual Review of Pharmacology and Toxicology, 36*, 83–106.

Sinclair, S.R., Svendsen, C.N., Torres, E.M., Fawcett, J.W., & Dunnett, S.B. (1996). The effects of glial cell line-derived neurotrophic factor (GDNF) on embryonic nigral grafts. *NeuroReport, 7*, 2547–2552.

Sinden, J.D., Gray, J.A., & Hodges, H. (1994). Cholinergic grafts and cognitive function. In S.B. Dunnett & A. Björklund (Eds.), *Functional neural transplantation* (pp. 253–293). New York: Raven Press.

Sinden, J.D., Rashid-Doubell, F., Kershaw, T.R., Nelson, A., Chadwick, A., Jat, P.S., Noble, M.D., Hodges, H., & Gray, J.A. (1997). Recovery of spatial learning by grafts of a conditionally immortalized hippocampal neuroepithelial cell line into the ischaemia-lesioned hippocampus. *Neuroscience, 81*, 599–608.

Singaram, C., Ashraf, W., Gaumnitz, E.A., Torbey, C., Sengupta, A., Pfeiffer, R., & Quigley, E.M.M. (1995). Dopaminergic defect of enteric nervous system in Parkinson's disease patients with chronic constipation. *Lancet, 346*, 861–864.

Sirinathsinghji, D.J.S., Dunnett, S.B., Isacson, O., Clarke, D.J., Kendrick, K., & Björklund, A. (1988). Striatal grafts in rats with unilateral neostriatal lesions. II. *In vivo* monitoring of GABA release in globus pallidus and substantia nigra. *Neuroscience, 24*, 803–811.

Sirinathsinghji, D.J.S., & Dunnett, S.B. (1991). Increased proenkephalin mRNA levels in the rat neostriatum following lesion of the ipsilateral nigrostriatal dopamine pathway with 1-methyl-4-phenylpyridinium ion (MPP+): reversal by embryonic nigral dopamine grafts. *Molecular Brain Research, 9*, 263–269.

Snider, W.D., & Johnson, E.M. (1989). Neurotrophic molecules. *Annals of Neurology, 26*, 489–506.

Snyder-Keller, A.M., & Lund, R.D. (1990). Amphetamine sensitization of stress-induced turning in animals given unilateral dopamine transplants in infancy. *Brain Research, 514*, 143–146.

Sofroniew, M.V., & Pearson, R.C.A. (1985). Degeneration of cholinergic neurons in the basal nucleus following kainic acid or N-methyl-D-aspartic acid application to the cerebral cortex in the rat. *Brain Research, 229*, 186–189.

Sofroniew, M.V., Isacson, O., & Björklund, A. (1986). Cortical grafts prevent atrophy of cholinergic basal nucleus neurons induced by excitotoxic cortical damage. *Brain Research, 378*, 409–415.

Sofroniew, M.V., Dunnett, S.B., & Isacson, O. (1990a). Remodeling of intrinsic and afferent systems in neocortex with cortical transplants. *Progress in Brain Research, 82*, 313–320.

Sofroniew, M.V., Galletly, N.P., Isacson, O., & Svendsen, C.N. (1990b). Survival of adult basal forebrain cholinergic neurons after loss of target neurons. *Science, 247*, 338–342.

Spencer, D.D., Robbins, R.J., Naftolin, F., Marek, K.L., Vollmer, T.L., Leranth, C., Roth, R.H., Price, L.H., Gjedde, A., Bunney, B.S., Sass, K.J., Elsworth, J.D., Kier, E.L., Makuch, R., Hoffer, P.B., & Redmond, D.E. (1992). Unilateral transplantation of human fetal mesencephalic tissue into the caudate nucleus of patients with Parkinson's disease. *New England Journal of Medicine, 327*, 1541–1548.

Springer, J.E., Collier, T.J., Sladek, J.R., & Loy, R. (1988). Transplantation of male mouse submaxillary gland increases survival of axotomised basal forebrain neurons. *Journal of Neuroscience Research, 19*, 291–296.

Sramka, M., Rattaj, M., Molina, H., Vojtassak, J., Belan, V., & Ruzicky, E. (1992). Stereotactic technique and pathophysiological mechanisms of neurotransplantation in Huntington's chorea. *Stereotactic and Functional Neurosurgery, 58*, 79–83.

Steece-Collier, K., Collier, T.J., Sladek, C., & Sladek, J.R. (1990). Chronic levodopa impairs morphological development of grafted embryonic dopamine neurons. *Experimental Neurology, 110*, 201–208.

Steece-Collier, K., Yurek, D.M., Collier, T.J., Junn, F.S., & Sladek, J.R. (1995). The detrimental effect of levodopa on behavioral efficacy of fetal dopamine neuron grafts in rats is reversible following prolonged withdrawal of chronic dosing. *Brain Research, 676*, 404–408.

Stenevi, U., Björklund, A., & Svendgaard, N.-A. (1976). Transplantation of central and peripheral monoamine neurons to the adult rat brain: techniques and conditions for survival. *Brain Research, 114*, 1–20.

Stieg, P., Strömberg, I., & Olson, L. (1991). Effects of donor age on superior cervical ganglion transplants: evaluation by Falck–Hillarp histochemistry and immunocytochemistry. *Experimental Brain Research, 85*, 55–65.

Stocchi, F., Nordera, G., & Marsden, C.D. (1997). Strategies for treating patients with advanced Parkinson's disease with disastrous fluctuations and dyskinesias. *Clinical Neuropharmacology, 20*, 95–115.

Stoddard, S.L., Tyce, G.M., Ahlskog, J.E., Zinsmeister, A.R., & Carmichael, S.W. (1989a). Decreased catecholamine content in parkinsonian adrenal medullae. *Experimental Neurology, 104*, 22–27.

Stoddard, S.L., Ahlskog, J.E., Kelly, P.J., Tyce, G.M., Van Heerden, J.A., Zinsmeister, A.R., & Carmichael, S.W. (1989b). Decreased adrenal medullary catecholamines in adrenal transplanted parkinsonian patients compared to nephrectomy patients. *Experimental Neurology, 104*, 218–222.

Strecker, R.E., Sharp, T., Brundin, P., Zetterström, T., Ungerstedt, U., & Björklund, A. (1987). Autoregulation of dopamine release and metabolism by intrastriatal nigral grafts as revealed by intracerebral dialysis. *Neuroscience, 22*, 169–178.

Stricker, E.M., & Zigmond, M.J. (1976). Recovery of function following damage to central catecholamine-containing neurons: a neurochemical model for the lateral hypothalamic syndrome. In J.M. Sprague & A.N. Epstein (Eds.), *Progress in psychobiology and physiological psychology* (pp. 121–189). New York: Academic Press.

Strittmatter, W.J., & Roses, A.D. (1996). Apolipoprotein E and Alzheimer's disease. *Annual Review of Neuroscience, 19*, 53–77.

Strömberg, I., Herrera-Marschitz, M., Hultgren, L., Ungerstedt, U., & Olson, L. (1984). Adrenal medullary implants in the dopamine denervated rat striatum. I. Acute catecholamine levels in grafts and host caudate as determined by HPLC electrochemistry and fluorescence histochemical image analysis. *Brain Research, 297*, 41–51.

Strömberg, I., Herrera-Marschitz, M., Ungerstedt, U., Ebendal, T., & Olson, L. (1985a). Chronic implants of chromaffin tissue into the dopamine-denervated striatum. Effects of NGF on graft survival, fiber growth and rotational behavior. *Experimental Brain Research, 60*, 335–349.

Strömberg, I., Ebendal, T., Seiger, Å., & Olson, L. (1985b). Nerve fiber production by intraocular adrenal medullary grafts: stimulation by nerve growth factor or sympathetic denervation of the host iris. *Cell and Tissue Research, 241*, 241–249.

Strömberg, I., van Horne, C.G., Bygdeman, M., Weiner, N., & Gerhardt, G.A. (1991). Function of intraventricular human mesencephalic xenografts in immunosuppressed rats: an electrophysiological and neurochemical analysis. *Experimental Neurology, 112*, 140–152.

Subrt, O., Tichy, M., Vladyka, V., & Hurt, K. (1991). Grafting of fetal dopamine neurons in Parkinson's disease: the Czech experience with severe akinetic patients. *Acta Neurochirurgica, Supplementum, 52*, 51–53.

Suhonen, J.O., Peterson, D.A., Ray, J., & Gage, F.H. (1996). Differentiation of adult hippocampus-derived progenitors into olfactory neurons *in vivo*. *Nature, 383*, 624–627.

Svendsen, C.N. (1993). Gene therapy: a hard graft for neuroscientists. *Trends in Neurosciences, 16*, 339–340.

Svendsen, C.N., Fawcett, J.W., Bentlage, C., & Dunnett, S.B. (1995). Increased survival of rat EGF-generated CNS progenitor cells using B27 supplemented medium. *Experimental Brain Research, 102*, 407–414.

Svendsen, C.N., & Rosser, A.E. (1995). Neurons from stem cells? *Trends in Neurosciences, 18*, 465–467.

Svendsen, C.N., Clarke, D.J., Rosser, A.E., & Dunnett, S.B. (1996). Survival and differentiation of rat and human EGF responsive precursor cells following grafting into the lesioned adult CNS. *Experimental Neurology, 137*, 376–388.

Svendsen, C.N., Caldwell, M.A., Shen, J., ter Borg, M., Rosser, A.E., Tyers, P., Karmiol, S., & Dunnett, S.B. (1997). Long term survival of human central nervous system progenitor cells transplanted into a rat model of Parkinson's disease. *Experimental Neurology, 148*, 135–146.

Takeuchi, J., Takebe, Y., Sakakura, T., Hara, Y., Yasuda, T., & Imai, T. (1990). Adrenal medulla transplantation into the putamen in Parkinson's disease. *Neurosurgery, 26*, 499–503.

Tan, S.A., & Aebischer, P. (1996). The problems of delivering neuroactive molecules to the CNS. *Ciba Foundation Symposia, 196*, 211–236.

Tanner, C.M., & Goldman, S.M. (1996). Epidemiology of Parkinson's disease. *Neurologic Clinics, 14*, 317.

Thoenen, H., Castren, E., Berzaghi, M.P., Blochl, A., & Lindholm, D. (1994). Neurotrophic factors: possibilities and limitations in the treatment of neurodegenerative disorders. *International Academy of Biomedical and Drug Research, 7*, 197–203.

Thompson, W.G. (1890). Successful brain grafting. *New York Medical Journal, 51*, 701–702.

Tischler, A.S., Perlman, R.L., Nunnemacher, G., Morse, G.M., DeLellis, R., Wolfe, H.J., & Sheard, B.E. (1982). Long-term effects of dexamethasone and nerve growth factor on adrenal medullary cells cultured from young adult rats. *Cell and Tissue Research, 225*, 525–542.

Tkaczuk, J., Bès, J.C., Du, P., Tafani, M., Duplan, H., Abbal, M., Lazorthes, Y., & Ohayon, E. (1997). Intrathecal allograft of chromaffin cells for intractable pain treatment: A model for understanding CNS tolerance mechanisms in humans. *Transplantation Proceedings, 29*, 2356–2357.

Tomlinson, B.E., Blessed, G., & Roth, M. (1970). Observations on the brains of demented old people. *Journal of the Neurological Sciences, 11*, 205–242.

Tomlinson, B.E., & Corsellis, J.A.N. (1984). Aging and the dementias. In A.J. Hume, J.A.N. Corsellis & L.W. Duchken (Eds.), *Greenfield's neuropathology* (pp. 951–1025). London: Edward Arnold.

Tontsch, U., Archer, D.R., Dubois-Dalcq, M., & Duncan, I.D. (1994). Transplantation of an oligodendrocyte cell line leading to extensive myelination. *Proceedings of the National Academy of Sciences of the United States of America, 91*, 11616–11620.

Torres, E.M., Fricker, R.A., Hume, S., Myers, R., Opacka-Juffry, J., Ashworth, S., Brooks, D.J., & Dunnett, S.B. (1995). Assessment of striatal graft viability in the rat *in vivo* using a small diameter PET scanner. *NeuroReport, 6*, 2017–2021.

Trapp, B.D., Peterson, J., Ransohoff, R.M., Rudick, R., Mork, S., & Bo, L. (1998). Axonal transection in the lesions of multiple sclerosis. *New England Journal of Medicine, 338*, 278–285.

Ungerstedt, U. (1971a). Postsynaptic supersensitivity after 6-hydroxydopamine-induced degeneration of the nigro-striatal dopamine system. *Acta Physiologica Scandinavica, Supplementum, 367*, 69–93.

Ungerstedt, U. (1971b). Striatal dopamine release after amphetamine or nerve degeneration revealed by rotational behaviour. *Acta Physiologica Scandinavica, Supplementum, 367*, 49–68.

Ungerstedt, U., & Arbuthnott, G.W. (1970). Quantitative recording of rotational behaviour in rats after 6-hydroxydopamine lesions of the nigrostriatal dopamine system. *Brain Research, 24*, 485–493.

Unsicker, K. (1985). Embryologic development of rat adrenal medulla in transplants to the anterior chamber of the eye. *Developmental Biology, 108*, 259–268.

Unsicker, K. (1986). Differentiation and phenotypical conversion of adrenal medullary cells: the effects of neuronotrophic, neuron-promoting, hormonal and neuronal signals. In P. Panula (Ed.), *Neurohistochemistry: Modern methods and applications* (pp. 183–206). New York: Alan R. Liss.

Unsicker, K. (1993). The trophic cocktail made by adrenal chromaffin cells. *Experimental Neurology, 123*, 167–173.

Unsicker, K., Krisch, B., Otten, U., & Thoenen, H. (1978). Nerve growth factor-induced fiber outgrowth from isolated rat adrenal chromaffin cells: impairment by glucocorticoids. *Proceedings of the National Academy of Sciences of the United States of America, 75*, 3498–3503.

Unsicker, K., Vey, J., Hofmann, H.D., Muller, T.H., & Wilson, A.J. (1984). C6 glioma cell conditioned medium induces neurite outgrowth and survival of rat chromaffin cells *in vitro*: comparison with the effects of nerve growth factor. *Proceedings of the National Academy of Sciences of the United States of America, 81*, 2242–2246.

Utzschneider, D.A., Archer, D.R., Kocsis, J.D., Waxman, S.G., & Duncan, I.D. (1994). Transplantation of glial cells enhances action potential conduction of amyelinated spinal cord axons in the myelin-deficient rat. *Proceedings of the National Academy of Sciences of the United States of America, 91*, 53–57.

Valasco, F., Velasco, M., Cuevas, H.R., Jurado, J., Olivera, J., & Jimenez, F. (1999). Autologous adrenal medullary transplants in advanced Parkinson's disease with particular attention to the selective improvement in symptoms. *Stereotactic and Functional Neurosurgery, 57*, 195–212.

Van den Bosch de Aguilar, P., Langhendries-Weverberg, C., Goemaere-Vanneste, J., Flament-Durand, J., Brion, J.P., & Couck, A.M. (1984). Transplantation of human cortex with Alzheimer's disease into rat occipital cortex: a model for the study of Alzheimer's disease. *Experientia, 40*, 402–403.

Van Muiswinkel, F.L., Drukarch, B., Steinbusch, H.W.M., & Stoof, J.C. (1992). Survival and differentiation of cultured dopaminergic neurons are not impaired by chronic stimulation of DA D-2 receptors. *Journal of Neural Transplantation and Plasticity, 3*, 220–221.

Van Muiswinkel, F.L., Bol, J.G.J.M., Ruijter, J.M., Stoof, J.C., Drukarch, B., & Steinbusch, H.W.M. (1995). Repeated administration of a selective dopamine D2 receptor agonist to 6-OHDA-lesioned rats does not affect the survival and outgrowth of intrastriatal fetal mesencephalic grafts. *Experimental Brain Research, 107*, 52–58.

Vanderwolf, C.H. (1987). Near-total loss of learning and memory as a result of combined cholinergic and serotonergic blockade in the rat. *Behavioural Brain Research, 23*, 43–57.

Varon, S., Manthorpe, M., Davis, G.E., Williams, L.R., & Skaper, S.D. (1988). Growth factors. In S.G. Waxman (Ed.), *Functional recovery in neurological disease* (pp. 493–521). New York: Raven Press.

Verhofstad, A.A.J., Coupland, R.E., Parker, T.R., & Goldstein, M. (1985). Immunohistochemical and biochemical study on the development of the noradrenaline-storing and adrenaline-storing cells of the adrenal medulla of the rat. *Cell and Tissue Research, 242*, 233–243.

Verma, I.M., & Somia, N. (1997). Gene therapy—promises, problems and prospects. *Nature, 389*, 239–242.

Vescovi, A.L., Reynolds, B.A., Fraser, D.D., & Weiss, S. (1993). bFGF regulates the proliferative fate of multipotent (neuronal) and bipotent (neuronal/astroglial) EGF-generated CNS progenitor cells. *Neuron, 11*, 951–966.

Vignais, L., Nait Oumesmar, B., Mellouk, F., Gout, O., Labourdette, G., Baron-Van Evercooren, A., & Gumpel, M. (1993). Transplantation of oligodendrocyte precursors in the adult demyelinated spinal cord: Migration and remyelination. *International Journal of Developmental Neuroscience, 11*, 603–612.

Vonsattel, J.-P., Myers, R.H., & Stevens, T.J. (1985). Neuropathologic classification of Huntington's disease. *Journal of Neuropathology and Experimental Neurology, 44*, 559–577.

Voorn, P., Kalsbeek, A., Jorritsma-Byham, B., & Groenewegen, H.J. (1988). The pre- and postnatal development of the dopaminergic cell groups in the ventral mesencephalon and the dopaminergic innervation of the striatum of the rat. *Neuroscience, 25*, 857–887.

Wang, J., Plunkett, R.J., Sheng, J.G., Oldfield, E.H., & Bankiewicz, K.S. (1991). Recovery in hemiparkinsonian rats after intracaudal implantation of IL-1 containing pellets. *Society for Neuroscience Abstracts, 17*, 348.

Waters, C., Itabashi, H.H., Apuzzo, M.L.J., & Weiner, L.P. (1990). Adrenal to caudate transplantation—postmortem study. *Movement Disorders, 548*, 248–250.

Watts, R.L., Freeman, A., Bakay, R.A.E., Iuvone, P.M., Watts, N., & Graham, S. (1989). Adrenal caudate transplantation in patients with Parkinson's disease (PD). *Neurology, 39*, S127.

Watts, R.L., Bakay, R.A.E., Herring, C.J., Sweeney, K.M., Colbassani, H.J., Mandir, A., Byrd, L.D., & Iuvone, P.M. (1990). Preliminary report on adrenal medullary grafting and co-grafting with sural nerve in the treatment of hemiparkinsonian monkeys. *Progress in Brain Research, 82*, 581–591.

Watts, R.L., Freeman, A., Graham, S., & Bakay, R.A.E. (1992). Early experience with intrastriatal adrenal medulla/nerve cografting in Parkinson's disease. *Restorative Neurology and Neuroscience, 4*, 194.

Watts, R.L., Subramanian, T., Freeman, A., Goetz, C.G., Penn, R.D., Stebbins, G.T., Kordower, J.H., & Bakay, R.A. (1997). Effect of stereotaxic intrastriatal cografts of autologous adrenal medulla and peripheral nerve in Parkinson's disease: Two-year follow-up study. *Experimental Neurology, 147*, 510–517.

Wenning, G.K., Ben, S.Y., Magalhaes, M., Daniel, S.E., & Quinn, N.P. (1994). Clinical features and natural history of multiple system atrophy: an analysis of 100 cases. *Brain, 117*, 835–845.

Wenning, G.K., Granata, R., Laboyrie, P.M., Quinn, N.P., Jenner, P., & Marsden, C.D. (1996). Reversal of behavioural abnormalities by fetal allografts in a novel rat model of striatonigral degeneration. *Movement Disorders, 11*, 522–532.

Wenning, G.K., Odin, P., Morrish, P., Rehncrona, S., Widner, H., Brundin, P., Rothwell, J.C., Brown, R., Gustavii, B., Hagell, P., Jahanshahi, M., Sawle, G., Björklund, A., Brooks, D.J., Marsden, C.D., Quinn, N.P., & Lindvall, O. (1997). Short- and long-term survival and function of unilateral intrastriatal dopaminergic grafts in Parkinson's disease. *Annals of Neurology, 42*, 95–107.

Whishaw, I.Q., Zaborowski, J.A., & Kolb, B. (1984). Postsurgical enrichment aids adult hemidecorticate rats on a spatial navigation task. *Behavioral and Neural Biology, 42*, 183–190.

White, J.K., Auerbach, W., Duyao, M.P., Vonsattel, J.P., Gusella, J.F., Joyner, A.L., & MacDonald, M.E. (1997). Huntingtin is required for neurogenesis and is not impaired by the Huntington's disease CAG expansion. *Nature Genetics, 17*, 404–410.

White, N.M. (1989). A functional hypothesis concerning the striatal matrix and patches: mediation of S–R memory and reward. *Life Sciences, 45*, 1943–1957.

Wictorin, K. (1992). Anatomy and connectivity of intrastriatal striatal transplants. *Progress in Neurobiology, 38*, 611–639.

Widner, H. (1998). The Lund programme for Parkinson's disease and patients with MPTP-induced parkinsonism. In T.B. Freeman & H. Widner (Eds.), *Cell transplantation in neurological disease* (pp. 1–17). Totowa, NJ: Humana Press.

Widner, H., & Brundin, P. (1988). Immunological aspects of grafting in the mammalian central nervous system: a review and speculative synthesis. *Brain Research Reviews, 13*, 287–324.

Widner, H., Tetrud, J., Rehncrona, S., Snow, B., Brundin, P., Gustavii, B., Björklund, A., Lindvall, O., & Langston, J.W. (1992). Bilateral fetal mesencephalic grafting in 2 patients with parkinsonism induced by 1-methyl-4-phenyl-1,2,3,6-tetrahydropyridine (MPTP). *New England Journal of Medicine, 327*, 1556–1563.

Wiesel, T.N. (1982). Postnatal development of the visual cortex and the influence of environment. *Nature, 299*, 583–591.

Wilkinson, G.W.G., Darley, R.L., & Lowenstein, P.R. (1994). Viral vectors for gene therapy. In D.S. Latchman (Ed.), *From genetics to gene therapy: The molecular pathology of human disease* (pp. 161–192). London: Bios Scientific.

Winkler, H., Apps, D.K., & Fischer-Colbrie, R. (1986). The molecular function of adrenal chromaffin granules: established facts and unresolved topics. *Neuroscience, 18*, 261.

Winkler, J., Suhr, S.T., Gage, F.H., Thal, L.J., & Fisher, L.J. (1995). Essential role of acetylcholine in spatial memory. *Nature, 375*, 484–487.

Winn, S.R., Wahlberg, L., Tresco, P.A., & Aebischer, P. (1989). An encapsulated dopamine-releasing polymer alleviates experimental parkinsonism in rats. *Experimental Neurology, 105*, 244–250.

Winnie, A.P., Pappas, G.D., Dasgupta, T.K., Wang, H., Ortega, J.D., & Sagen, J. (1993). Subarachnoid adrenal-medullary transplants for terminal cancer pain—a report of preliminary studies. *Anesthesiology, 79*, 644–653.

Wischik, C.M., Crowther, R.A., Stewart, M., & Roth, M. (1985). Subunit structure of paired helical filaments in Alzheimer's disease. *Journal of Cell Biology, 100*, 1905–1912.

Wolff, J.A., Fisher, L.J., Xu, L., Jinnah, H.A., Langlais, P.J., Iuvone, P.M., O'Malley, K.L., Rosenberg, M.B., Shimohama, S., Friedmann, T., & Gage, F.H. (1989). Grafting fibroblasts genetically modified to produce L-dopa in a rat model of Parkinson disease. *Proceedings of the National Academy of Sciences of the United States of America, 86*, 9011–9014.

Wuerthele, S.M., Freed, W.J., Olson, L., Morihisa, J., Spoor, L., Wyatt, R.J., & Hoffer, B.J. (1981). Effect of dopamine agonists and antagonists on the electrical activity of substantia nigra neurons transplanted into the lateral ventricle of the rat. *Experimental Brain Research, 44*, 1–10.

Wyllie, A.H., Kerr, J.F.R., & Currie, A.R. (1980). Cell death: the significance of apoptosis. *International Review of Cytology, 68*, 251–306.

Xu, X.M., Guenard, V., Kleitman, N., Aebischer, P., & Bunge, M.B. (1995). Combination of BDNF and NT-3 promotes supraspinal axonal regeneration into Schwann cell grafts in adult rat thoracic spinal cord. *Experimental Neurology, 134*, 261–272.

Xu, X.M., Chen, A., Guénard, V., Kleitman, N., & Bunge, M.B. (1997). Bridging Schwann cell transplants promote axonal regeneration from both the rostral and caudal stumps of transected adult rat spinal cord. *Journal of Neurocytology, 26*, 1–16.

Xu, Z.C., Wilson, C.J., & Emson, P.C. (1991). Synaptic potentials evoked in spiny neurons in rat neostriatal grafts by cortical and thalamic stimulation. *Journal of Neurophysiology, 65*, 477–493.

Yakovleff, A., Roby-Brami, A., Guezzard, B., Mansour, H., Bussel, B., & Privat, A. (1989). Locomotion in rats with transplanted noradrenergic neurons. *Brain Research Bulletin, 22*, 115–121.

Yakovleff, A., Cabelguen, J.M., Orsal, D., Ribotta, M.G.Y., Rajaofetra, N., Drian, M.J., Bussel, B., & Privat, A. (1995). Fictive motor activities in adult chronic spinal rats transplanted with embryonic brainstem neurons. *Experimental Brain Research, 106*, 69–78.

Yamaguchi, F., Richards, S.J., Beyreuther, K., Salbaum, M., Carlson, G.A., & Dunnett, S.B. (1991). Transgenic mice for the amyloid precursor protein 695 isoform have impaired spatial memory. *NeuroReport, 2*, 781–784.

Yong, V.W., Horie, H., & Kim, S.U. (1989). Comparison of 6 different substrata on the plating efficiency, differentiation and survival of human dorsal root ganglion neurons in culture. *Developmental Neuroscience, 10*, 222–230.

Yurek, D.M., Steece-Collier, K., Collier, T.J., & Sladek, J.R. (1991). Chronic levodopa impairs the recovery of dopamine agonist-induced rotational behavior following neural grafting. *Experimental Brain Research, 86*, 97–107.

Yurek, D.M., Lu, W., Hipkens, S., & Wiegand, S.J. (1996). BDNF enhances the functional reinnervation of the striatum by grafted fetal dopamine neurons. *Experimental Neurology, 137*, 105–118.

Zabek, M., Mazurowski, W., Dymecki, J., Stelmachów, J., & Zawada, E. (1994). A long term follow-up of fetal dopaminergic neurons transplantation into the brain of three parkinsonian patients. *Restorative Neurology and Neuroscience, 6*, 97–106.

Zetterström, T., Brundin, P., Gage, F.H., Sharp, T., Isacson, O., Dunnett, S.B., Ungerstedt, U., & Björklund, A. (1986). *In vivo* measurement of spontaneous release and metabolism of dopamine from intrastriatal nigral grafts using intracerebral dialysis. *Brain Research, 362*, 344–349.

Zhang, W.C., Ding, Y.J., Cao, J.K., Du, J.X., Zhang, G.F., & Liu, Y.J. (1994). Intracerebral co-grafting of Schwann cells and fetal adrenal medulla in the treatment of Parkinson's disease. *Chinese Medical Journal, 107*, 583–588.

Zhou, F.C., & Azmitia, E.C. (1988). Laminin facilitated and guides fiber growth of transplanted neurons in adult brain. *Journal of Chemical Neuroanatomy, 1*, 133–146.

Zhou, F.C., & Chiang, Y.H. (1995). Excitochemical-induced trophic bridging directs axonal growth of transplanted neurons to distal target. *Cell Transplantation, 4*, 103–112.

Zigmond, M.J., Acheson, A.L., Stachowiak, M.K., & Stricker, E.M. (1984). Neurochemical compensation after nigrostriatal bundle injury in an animal model of preclinical parkinsonism. *Archives of Neurology, 41*, 856–861.

Zigmond, M.J., & Stricker, E.M. (1972). Deficits in feeding behavior after intraventricular injection of 6-hydroxydopamine in rats. *Science, 177*, 1211–1214.

Zigmond, M.J., Abercrombie, E.D., Berger, T.W., Grace, A.A., & Stricker, E.M. (1990). Compensations after lesions of central dopaminergic neurons: some clinical and basic implications. *Trends in Neurosciences, 13*, 290–296.

Glossary

Acetylcholine: a classical neurotransmitter; found both in the *central* and *peripheral nervous systems*. In the PNS it is the neurotransmitter at the neuromuscular junction and within the autonomic nervous system, whilst in the CNS it is found in the basal forebrain projections to cortex and *hippocampus* as well as in interneurones of the neostriatum.

Adeno-associated virus (AAV): a class of virus used as a vector for gene transfer into neural cells.

Adenovirus: a class of virus used as a vector for gene transfer into neural cells.

Adrenal medulla: the core of the adrenal gland, a neuroendocrine organ lying above the kidney. Cells of the adrenal medulla secrete adrenaline in the "fight–flight" response to stress. It has been considered as a possible source of graft tissue to replace *dopamine* loss in *Parkinson's disease*.

Allocortex: evolutionarily older areas of cortex characterised by less than six cell layers. Associated with the limbic system, allocortex includes the cingulate cortex, piriform cortex, and *hippocampus*.

Allograft: a graft between unrelated individuals of the same species.

Alzet® pump: a capsule that is implanted subcutaneously in experimental animals to provide slow stable delivery of drug solutions over several weeks, either by diffusion into the periphery or via an implanted cannula into the brain or a blood vessel.

Alzheimer's disease (AD): a neurodegenerative disease that is the commonest cause of dementia in man, identified by a characteristic neuropathology involving *senile plaques* and *neurofibrillary tangles* in *hippocampus* and *neocortex*. Forebrain cholinergic neurones also undergo marked degeneration, although the primacy of this aspect of the pathology is disputed.

Amygdala: a nucleus of the limbic system, involved in the response to reward and evaluation of the motivational significance of stimuli.

Amyloid: an extracellular deposit in many tissues, defined by its particular optical properties when viewed under polarised light. The "*ß/A4*" type of *amyloid* has been identified as the major protein constituent of *Alzheimer's disease* plaques and is an abnormal cleavage product of the amyloid precursor protein, a cell surface molecule the normal function of which is still unclear.

Amyloid precursor protein (APP): cloning of the *ß/A4* protein has enabled sequencing of the full amyloid precursor protein. There are three isoforms in brain, 695, 751, and 770 amino acids long. APP is believed to be a membrane-bound protein with the *ß/A4* protein located close to its C-terminal end, in the region thought to span the membrane. The function of APP in the intact *CNS* is at present unknown.

Amyotrophic lateral sclerosis: a form of motor neurone disease involving degeneration of the *motor neurones* of the *CNS*. It has been considered as a possible candidate for motor neurone transplantation as well as for neurotropic therapy with *ciliary neurotrophic factor*.

Apoptosis: an active programmed form of cell death, including that seen in the mature adult.

Association cortex: areas of the cortex that are neither primary sensory nor motor in nature. These areas of cortex include the prefrontal, posterior parietal, and temporal cortices, and are involved in higher integrating functions.

Astrocytes: *glial cells* of the central nervous system, the functions of which include providing a structural and growth substrate for neurones, nourishment of neurones, and regulation of the blood–brain barrier, removal of debris and structural changes in response to injury.

Atropine: a drug that, like *scopolamine*, is an antagonist of the cholinergic muscarinic receptor.

Autograft: a graft back into the same individual.

β/A4 amyloid protein: the particular form of *amyloid* that is deposited in extracellular spaces and around blood vessels in *Alzheimer's disease*. It is thought to be an abnormal product of the amyloid precursor protein.

Baby hamster kidney (BHK) cells: a well-characterised stable type of cell widely used for genetic engineering.

Basal ganglia: a group of nuclei in the depths of the forebrain hemispheres, including *caudate nucleus*, *putamen*, *globus pallidus*, *subthalamic nucleus*, and *substantia nigra*.

Brain-derived neurotrophic factor (BDNF): a *neurotrophic factor* originally isolated from the bovine brain. It was the second member of the neurotrophin family of growth factors to be discovered, based on structural homologies to the previously known *nerve growth factor*. It promotes the survival of *CNS* cholinergic and dopaminergic neurones in culture.

Brattleboro rat: a mutant strain of rats that have diabetes insipidus as a result of producing no antidiuretic hormone (*vasopressin*).

Bridge graft: a graft of cells or other material that provides a good substrate for axon growth, and which thereby supports long-distance regrowth of axons to distance targets in the mature *CNS*.

Bromodeoxyuridine (BrDU): a labelled form of uridine that can replace normal uridine in the DNA of cells during cell division, and hence provide a permanent label of cells that divide at the time BrDU was present (see *thymidine*).

CA1, 3, etc.: sub-fields of the *hippocampus*, connected in a sequential circuit. The different sub-fields are sensitive to different insults such as *ischaemia*, *excitotoxins*, etc.

CAG repeats: the three nucleotide bases cysteine-adenosine-guanine in DNA encode the protein glutamine. Long stretches of CAG repeats result in polyglutamine sequences in the protein. Expanded CAG repeats in different structural proteins are associated with a range of different inherited neurological diseases, including *Huntington's disease* and several forms of spinocerebellar ataxia.

CAPIT: Core Assessment Protocol for Intracerebral Transplantation. An agreed battery and schedule of neurological, neuropsychological, psychiatric, and imaging tests to provide comparability across multi-centre trials of neural transplantation. Different forms exist for trials in *Parkinson's disease* and in *Huntington's disease*.

Carotid ganglion: a peripheral ganglion in the neck, comprising sympathetic neurones using dopamine (rather than noradrenaline) as their primary transmitter.

Caudate nucleus: a major nucleus of the basal ganglia, which together with the *putamen* composes the *neostriatum*.

Central nervous system (CNS): that part of the nervous system that maintains a specialised environment with a dedicated blood supply and its own cerebrospinal fluid drainage, all encased within the protective bony mantle of the cranium and spinal vertebrae. The CNS has a distinctive population of glial cells—*astrocytes* and *oligodendrocytes*—that are considerably less supportive of axon regeneration than the *Schwann cells* of the *peripheral nervous system*.

Cholecystokinin: a peptide neurotransmitter, localised in a small corticostriatal projection and co-localised with dopamine in the innervation of the ventral tegmental area projection to the *ventral striatum*.

Choline acetyl transferase (ChAT): the rate-limiting enzyme in *acetylcholine* synthesis, used as a convenient biochemical marker for the integrity of cholinergic neurones.

Chromaffin cells: the primary adrenaline-secreting cell of the *adrenal medulla*.

Ciliary neurotrophic factor (CNTF): a neurotrophic factor that, among other actions, promotes survival of motor neurones.

Cyclosporin A: an "immunosuppression" drug used to block the rejection of grafts in the brain and elsewhere by inhibiting T-lymphocyte function.

D1 receptors: one major class of dopamine receptors, which stimulate adenylate cyclase activity, with mixed excitatory and inhibitory actions electrophysiologically, and located presynaptically on *dopamine* dendrites and axon terminals as well as on postsynaptic neurones. The drugs SKF 38393 and SCH 23390 are selective agonists and antagonists, respectively.

D2 receptors: a second main class of dopamine receptor independent or inhibitory of adenylate cyclase, and primarily located on postsynaptic neurones. In the *striatum* it is considered the main inhibitory receptor driving the indirect output pathway of the striatum. The drugs apomorphine and quinpirole are selective agonists, and haloperidol, sulpiride, and raclopride are selective antagonists.

DARPP-32: *dopamine* and adenosine receptor phosphoprotein of 32 kDa molecular weight. DARPP-32 antibodies provide good immunohistochemical markers of basal ganglia neurones, in particular in the *neostriatum*, *ventral striatum* and *substantia nigra*.

Delayed alternation: a task in which the animal is required to alternate its responses between two alternatives (e.g. spatial alternation, object alternation) requiring short-term memory of the last response over the delay interval that separates each trial. It is a classic test of prefrontal cortex integrity, but is also markedly disrupted by striatal and hippocampal lesions.

Delayed response: a task in which the animal is first shown the location of a reward, but only has the opportunity to respond after a variable delay. The task requires efficient short-term memory of the correct location over the delay interval, and is another classic test of *dementia*.

Dementia: a class of diseases, predominantly of old age, associated with widespread neuronal degeneration in the higher levels of the forebrain, and resulting in progressive functional deterioration of cognition, attention, learning, language and memory. Diagnosis is based on the presence post mortem of specific neuropathological hallmarks, e.g. *neurofibrillary tangles* and *senile plaques* in the *neocortex* and hippocampus with *Alzheimer's disease*.

Demyelination: the loss of the *myelin* sheath around axons, thereby impairing their conduction of action potentials. In the *CNS* this type of pathology is seen with *multiple sclerosis*.

Dentate gyrus: a major sub-field of the hippocampal formation (see *CA1,3* etc.).

2-deoxyglucose (2-DG): an analogue of glucose, taken up by cells in response to their energy requirements, but not then further metabolised; consequently, accumulation of 2-DG provides a direct marker of the energy requirements of cells under particular conditions, which can be visualised either histochemically or by *in vivo PET* scans.

Disconnection syndromes: functional deficits arising from damage to axons connecting related centres rather than to neuronal or nuclear damage *per se*.

The idea of disconnection syndromes is related to the concept that the nervous system is organised in interconnected neural systems rather than discrete functions controlled by discrete nuclei.

Dopamine: a classical monoamine neurotransmitter, located in a number of forebrain systems including the nigrostriatal pathway, which degenerates in *Parkinson's disease.*

Dorsal column: a major ascending sensory pathway in the white matter of the dorsal midline of the spinal cord.

Dorsal horn: cell nuclei in the dorsal half of the grey matter at the core of the spinal cord, providing the first central level of cell bodies relaying afferent sensory information.

Dorsal root: the main fibre bundles relaying afferent sensory information from the periphery into the *CNS* at the level of the spinal cord.

Dorsal root ganglia: the primary sensory neurones of the somatosensory nervous system are located outside of the *CNS*, in ganglia positioned within the dorsal roots on either side of the spinal cord.

Down's syndrome: a developmental disorder due to *trisomy 21* in humans. Recently research on this condition has grown, as affected individuals develop *dementia* and neuropathological features of *Alzheimer's disease* in middle life, suggesting a link of Alzheimer's disease pathogenesis to chromosome 21.

DRL: differential reinforcement of low rates of responding; a popular schedule in operant conditioning typically used with rats in a *Skinner box*; used to assess perseveration and an animal's ability to inhibit prepotent responses.

Ectopic placement: graft placement into a site other than the normal location of the populations of cells being transplanted, e.g. implantation of *dopamine* cells into the *striatum* rather than into the *substantia nigra* itself. Contrast with *homotopic placement* of grafts.

Encapsulation: a technique for packaging cells in a semi-permeable capsule followed by implantation into a host animal. The capsule membrane allows free diffusion of nutrients in and soluble cell products out but protects the implanted cells from attack by the host immune system and protects the host from tumour formation or overgrowth of the grafts.

Enkephalin: an opiate peptide neurotransmitter, co-localised with *GABA* in striatal output neurones projecting to the *globus pallidus.*

Epidermal growth factor (EGF): a neurotrophic factor that has attracted particular interest for its capacity to promote proliferation (expansion and self-replication) of *stem cells* and neuronal *precursor cells.*

Ethidium bromide: a cytotoxin used to lesion *glial cells*, producing experimental demyelination in the spinal cord.

Excitotoxins: a class of neurotoxic glutamate receptor agonists that kill neurones carrying glutamate receptors by excessive stimulation, depolarisation, and membrane collapse. The most popular excitotoxins include *kainic acid, ibotenic acid, quinolinic acid*, and NMDA.

***Ex vivo* gene transfer**: the process of transfer of genes into the CNS by inserting the genes into neutral cells *in vitro* (i.e. *ex vivo*: outside the animal), followed by transplantation of the engineered cells into the host brain.

Fibroblasts: one of the primary cell types throughout the body including skin. They can be readily grown, expanded, and genetically engineered in culture for subsequent implantation, potentially as *autografts* (see *ex vivo gene transfer*).

Fibroblast growth factor (FGF): a neurotrophic factor with relatively broad and non-selective survival promoting action on all neuronal (and some non-neuronal) populations, possibly mediated via action on *astrocytes*. Also promotes proliferation of *stem cells* both *in vitro* and *in vivo*.

Fimbria–fornix: a major fibre pathway of the forebrain connecting the hippocampus to the septum and other subcortical sites. The pathway is a major relay for cholinergic, serotonergic, noradrenergic, and *GABA* inputs to the hippocampus as well as the route for passage of its major outputs.

Fluorogold: a fluorescent anatomical marker dye that is readily incorporated by axon terminals and retrogradely transported to the cell bodies; fluorescent-labelled cell bodies are readily visualised in microscopy using ultraviolet illumination.

GABA (γ-Amino butyric acid): an amino-acid neurotransmitter, and the major inhibitory transmitter of the nervous system.

β-Galactosidase: the protein product of the *LacZ gene*, undergoes a histochemical reaction with Xgal which labels cells that express the protein deep blue. Widely used as a marker for effective gene transfer and expression in the development of engineering techniques for *in vivo* and *ex vivo* gene transfer.

Ganglionic eminence: a ridge on the floor of the embryonic lateral ventricle comprising a germinal cell layer overlying the rudimentary striatum. The area for dissection for *striatal grafts*.

Gene transfer: the process of transfer or insertion of a novel gene into a cell either *in vitro* or in the living brain; achieved by a variety of genetic engineering techniques.

Gene therapy: gene transfer with a therapeutic target or goal. Gene therapy need not involve the replacement or repair of defective genes, but may also involve any transfer of a gene into an organism with the intention of expressing gene products of therapeutic action.

Glial cells: along with neurones, the second main class of cells of the nervous system, including *astrocytes*, *oligodendrocytes*, ependymal cells and microglia.

Glial cell line-derived neurotrophic factor (GDNF): a neurotrophic factor, potent for promoting survival of *dopamine* cells in the *substantia nigra* and of motor neurones in the spinal cord.

Glial fibrillary acid protein (GFAP): a major protein constituent of *astrocytes* in the CNS; antibodies against GFAP are widely used as the primary immunohistochemical marker for astrocytes.

Glial scar: injury or damage in the CNS can cause a proliferation of *glial cells*, particularly reactive *astrocytes*, which provide both a physical and a molecular barrier to regrowth of axons through the area of damage.

Globus pallidus: a nucleus of the *basal ganglia*, being the main target of outputs of the *neostriatum* (*caudate nucleus* and *putamen*), and which in turn projects to the thalamus, *subthalamic nucleus* and *substantia nigra*.

Glutamate: an amino-acid neurotransmitter, and the major excitatory transmitter of the nervous system. In excess, glutamate and its agonists can be toxic.

Glutamic acid decarboxylase (GAD): the rate-limiting enzyme in *glutamate* and *GABA* synthesis, used as a convenient biochemical marker for the integrity of, for example, intrinsic striatal neurones.

Golgi stain: a classical anatomical technique involving staining neurones with silver salts, producing a dense black reaction product and allowing detailed description and analysis of cell morphology.

Graft: an implant of living cells into the host animal (into the CNS in the present context). Includes implantation of cultured and engineered cells and cell lines in addition to direct transplantation of cells between animals.

Growth factors: molecules that are necessary for survival, differentiation, and growth of cells.

Hebb–Williams mazes: a set of mazes of classical design (with walls, corridors, and multiple two-alternative choice points) and varying levels of difficulty; used to study cognitive ability in rats.

Herpes simplex virus: a class of virus used as a vector for gene transfer into neural cells, first used because of its affinity for the nervous system and ability to infect mature cells. In the normal state this virus can cause encephalitis as well as oral and genital ulcers. It is a modified version of the virus that is used for gene transfer.

HiB5 cells: an immortalised cell line derived from embryonic *striatum*, used for *ex vivo* gene transfer.

Hippocampus: a major nucleus of the limbic system, involved in aspects of memory and cognition, and an early site of pathological change in *Alzheimer's disease*.

Hirano bodies: a pathological inclusion seen in the electron microscope, described in axon cytoplasm in dementia.

Homotopic placement: graft placement into the normal location of the populations of cells being transplanted, e.g. implantation of *dopamine* cells into the *substantia nigra*, striatal cells into the *striatum*, or cortical cells into the *neocortex*. Contrast with *ectopic* placement of grants.

Horseradish peroxidase (HRP): a protein that is taken up by neurones and actively transported both anterogradely and retrogradely along the axon. Used as an anatomical tracer of pathways in the nervous system.

Hot plate test: a widely used test of pain sensitivity for rats.

Huntingtin: the protein is coded for on chromosome 4 by the huntingtin gene and has, as yet, an unknown function. In *Huntington's disease* the gene contains an abnormally expanded *CAG repeat* which produces a mutant form of the protein which has a new function linked to neuronal loss, the hallmark of this condition.

Huntington's disease (HD): an inherited neurodegenerative disease involving degeneration of the *neostriatum* and a combination of motor, cognitive, and psychiatric symptoms. Currently being considered as a suitable candidate for striatal cell transplantation.

6-Hydroxydopamine (6-OHDA): a toxic analogue of *dopamine* that selectively kills dopamine and noradrenaline neurones in the vicinity when injected into the CNS.

Ibotenic acid: an excitotoxin, originally derived from the mushroom *Amanita muscaria*.

Immortalisation: engineering a cell with a proto-oncogene so as to make it permanently self-replicating. "Conditional" immortalisation attaches a regulatable switch (e.g. temperature, presence of a hormone) to the *proto-oncogene* so that in one condition the cell replicates, but in the other it enters a state of differentiation into a mature phenotype.

Immunohistochemistry: an anatomical technique for staining brain sections using antibodies raised against specific proteins (transmitters, enzymes, growth factors, structural components of the cell, etc.) and thereby visualising the distribution of those proteins.

Implant: the placement of a substance (not necessarily of living cells) into the host animal. Includes capsules containing cells and slow-release polymers.

IN-1 antibody: an antibody produced by M. Schwab and colleagues against inhibitory components of *myelin*; by blocking the inhibitory activity treatment with IN-1 can disinhibit, to some extent, axon regeneration in the adult CNS.

Internal capsule: the myelinated fibre bundles of ascending and descending projections of the *neocortex* to thalamus and elsewhere, passing through the *neostriatum*.

***In vivo* gene transfer**: transfer of genes directly into the living nervous system, most usually by direct inoculation and infection with a virus carrying the gene.

Ischaemia: loss of blood supply in the CNS; the extent of damage is influenced by the duration and extent of the arterial occlusion.

Kainic acid: an *excitotoxin*, originally derived from certain oriental seaweeds.

Lac Z gene: the gene derived from the bacterium *E. coli* that encodes a bacterial form of *β-galactosidase*, widely used as a marker gene in gene transfer experiments.

L-dopa: the amino acid precursor to *dopamine* in dopaminergic neurones. Unlike dopamine, it crosses the blood–brain barrier, and so can be used as an effective drug therapy in *Parkinson's disease*.

Lentivirus: a class of virus used as a vector for gene transfer into neural cells.

Lewy bodies: an abnormal spherical inclusion seen in the cytoplasm of cell bodies in *Parkinson's disease* and some other types of *dementia*.

Locus coeruleus: a small melanin-pigmented nucleus in the dorsal pons, in which are located the noradrenaline neurones that give rise to the major noradrenergic projections to the neocortex and *hippocampus*.

Magnetic resonance imaging (MRI): a technique for high-resolution structural and functional scanning in the living brain based on the alignment of water molecules in a strong magnetic field and detection of the subsequent collapse of that alignment to changes in the surrounding electromagnetic field.

Matrix: one of the two compartments of the *neostriatum* (the other being the *striosomes*), characterised by high levels of calbindin binding and distinctive patterns of input and output connections. Striatal dysfunction may originate in the matrix neurones in early *Huntington's disease*.

1-Methyl-4-phenyl-1,2,3,6-tetrahydropyridine (MPTP): a pyridine compound that induces a neurological syndrome closely resembling *Parkinson's disease* in mice, monkeys, or man in terms both of the neuropathology—selective death of nigral *dopamine* neurones—and the motor symptoms that result.

Microdialysis: slow perfusion of artificial cerebrospinal fluid through a semi-permeable dialysis membrane implanted into the brain results in diffusion and equilibration of metabolites and other soluble molecules derived from the brain and collected in the perfusate for biochemical analysis. Microdialysis allows biochemical analysis of molecules, such as neurotransmitters and their metabolites, released in the living brain, either under anaesthesia or in the freely moving animal.

Mitogen: a compound which can induce cells to divide (e.g. *epidermal* or *fibroblast growth factor*, or some forms of radiation).

Mitomycin: a drug that inhibits cell *mitosis*.

Mitosis: the process whereby non-germ line cells divide by duplication of their DNA and cytoplasmic division to form two progeny cells.

Morris water maze: a spatial navigation task comprising a large circular tank of water in which rats and mice swim to seek hidden or visible escape platforms onto which they can climb. The task has been found to be particularly sensitive to damage in hippocampal and cortical systems and to cognitive impairments in aged animals.

Motor neurones: large neurones with cell bodies located in the brainstem and *ventral horn* of the spinal cord. These lower motor neurones have axons projecting via the *ventral roots* and peripheral nerves to innervate the skeletal musculature and use *acetylcholine* as their transmitter. The upper motor neurones are found in the motor cortex and project onto the lower motor neurones, which they excite using glutamate at the neurotransmitter. Both these types of motor neurone degenerate in *amyotrophic lateral sclerosis*.

Motor neurone disease: a neurological disease involving degeneration of the motor neurones. It has been considered as a possible candidate for motor neurone transplantation as well as for neurotrophic therapy with *ciliary neurotrophic factor*. See *amyotrophic lateral sclerosis.*

Multi-infarct dementia: the second commonest form of dementia after *Alzheimer's disease,* attributable to accumulation of small vascular infarcts over widespread areas of the brain affecting both cortical and subcortical function.

Multiple sclerosis: a neurological disease involving an autoimmune destruction of the *oligodendrocytes* that are responsible for myelination in the CNS. If progression of the disease can be halted, multiple sclerosis has been considered a possible candidate disease for *glial cell* transplantation.

Multi-system atrophy: a neurodegenerative disease that affects the *basal ganglia,* including the *nigrostriatal dopamine* system as well as other neuronal systems such as the cerebellum and autonomic nervous system. In its early stages it can be mistaken for *Parkinson's disease,* but does not respond well to long-term dopamine replacement therapies.

Muscarine: a drug that is a cholinergic agonist and which defines pharmacologically one of the two main classes of cholinergic receptor (see *nicotine*).

Myelin: the white fatty substance that ensheathes axons to promote accurate, fast action potential conduction. Myelin is made by *oligodendrocytes* in the CNS and by *Schwann cells* in the PNS.

Myoblast: the precursor of a muscle cell.

N-methyl-D-aspartic acid (NMDA): a glutamate agonist. This ligand defines one of the major classes of glutamate receptors, involved in mechanisms of excitotoxicity and cell death.

Necrosis: the classical, passive form of cell death attributable to external damage of cell membranes or fundamental loss of nutrient support (see *apoptosis*).

NECTAR: the European Network of Clinical Transplantation and Restoration, NECTAR is a collaborative and co-ordinated group of all main European centres involved in clinical trials of neural transplantation in the CNS.

Neocortex: the outer mantle of the hemispheres of the mammalian brain, characterised by six distinct cellular layers and a modular columnar organisation throughout; evolutionarily the most recently developed region of the CNS, responsible for the highest level of neuronal function.

Neostriatum: a subgroup of nuclei of the *basal ganglia,* comprising the *caudate nucleus* and *putamen* in primates including man, but that is undifferentiated as the caudate-putamen nucleus in rodents. The neostriatum is the major target of the nigrostriatal dopamine projection.

Nerve growth factor (NGF): the prototypical neurotrophic molecule and first-discovered member of the neurotrophic growth factor family. Promotes survival of CNS cholinergic neurones in culture.

NEST: the European Network of Striatal Transplantation, a subgroup of *NECTAR* with the particular target of developing neural transplantation in *Huntington's disease.*

Neurofibrillary tangles (NFT): a dense accumulation of fibrous deposits within the cytoplasm of neurones, usually visualised in silver-stained brain sections. In *Alzheimer's disease*, NFTs are predominantly in the large pyramidal neurones of the *neocortex* and *hippocampus*.

Neurogenesis: the birth of neurones by *mitosis* from *precursor cells*. Until the last decade neurogenesis in the adult CNS was controversial, but is now established, in particular under the control of *mitogens* such as *fibroblast growth factor*.

Neuropeptide Y: a peptide neurotransmitter, found in interneurones of the *neostriatum*.

Neurospheres: a technique first developed by Reynolds and Weiss for expanding precursor cell populations from the embryonic, neonatal, or adult brain by free-floating culture in the presence of high concentrations of *epidermal* ± *fibroblast growth factor*.

Neurotrophic factors: molecules that are necessary for the division, survival, differentiation, and growth of neurones, both in development and in the degenerative and regenerative responses to injury.

Neurotrophin-3 (NT-3): the third member of the neurotrophin family of growth factors discovered by searching for novel genes containing common sequences of nerve growth factor and *brain-derived neurotrophic factor*. Promotes survival of dopaminergic and other neurones in culture.

Neurotrophins-4 and 5 (NF-4/5): neurotrophin-4 and neurotrophin-5 are homologous molecules first identified in different species; the fourth member of the neurotrophic family of growth factors, discovered like NT-3 by searching for novel genes containing common sequences in other members of the family.

Nicotine: a drug that is a cholinergic agonist and defines pharmacologically the second main class of cholinergic receptors (see *muscarine*).

Nigral grafts: strictly, grafts containing the developing *dopamine* cells of the *substantia nigra*. Typically, nigral grafts involve dissection of the whole embryonic ventral mesencephalon, of which dopamine cells make up only 1–5%.

Nigrostriatal pathway: the dopaminergic projection from the *substantia nigra* to the *neostriatum*, the degeneration of which is the primary neuropathological event in *Parkinson's disease*.

Nissl stain: a classical stain of "Nissl" substance in the cell cytoplasm; provides a good general histological stain of all cells in the nervous system.

3-Nitropropionic acid (3-NPA): a metabolic toxin that disrupts cellular energy metabolism in mitochondria; cells of the *neostriatum* are particularly sensitive to 3-NPA, and peripheral injection produces focal degeneration that may provide an animal model of *Huntington's disease*.

NP-zones: the "non-patch" compartment of *striatal grafts* that does not stain for acetylcholinesterase, DARPP-32, and other markers of striatal neuropil. The NP-zone is presumed to comprise cells that were destined for a non-striatal phenotype, and includes cells with distinct cortical and pallidal morphology.

Nucleus accumbens: the ventral extension of the *caudate nucleus*, a major component of the *ventral striatum*. Contains cell types similar to *neostriatum*, but with some neurochemical differences and major differences in input and output projections.

O-2A progenitor cells: the precursor cell that gives rise to *oligodendrocytes* and type 2 *astrocytes* during the development and maintenance of the nervous system.

Oligodendrocytes: *glial cells* of the central nervous system, the primary function of which is to myelinate and support axons.

Open field test: a simple neurological screening test for rats and mice, monitoring total locomotor activity, time spent in the centre or at the edge, rearing, and defecation when placed in a large open arena.

Operant conditioning: the type of learning first described by Thorndike and developed by B.J. Skinner in which animals learn associations between behaviour and its consequences: Responses that are rewarded in the context of particular discriminative stimuli increase in frequency; whereas responses that are punished or where reward is withheld decrease in frequency. The principles of operant (or "instrumental") conditioning have widespread application to understanding how animals learn to act on their environment to achieve biologically relevant outcomes. There continues to be a debate about whether all operant conditioning can be subsumed under the principles of *Pavlovian conditioning*, or vice versa, or whether the two classes of learning represent essentially distinct processes.

P-zones: the "patch" compartment of striatal grafts that stains for acetylcholinesterase, DARPP-32, and a wide variety of other markers of striatal neuropil. The P-zone comprises the presumptive striatal-like compartment of *striatal grafts* and is necessary for functional recovery.

Paired helical filaments (PHF): electron microscopic studies have shown that the *neurofibrillary tangles* of *Alzheimer's disease* are composed of fine neurofilaments that are twisted together to form regular paired helical structures.

Parkinson's disease (PD): a neurological disease involving primary degeneration of the *nigrostriatal dopamine pathway*. It involves predominantly motor symptoms with a variable cognitive component. There are rare conditions involving known toxic causation, but the aetiology of the idiopathic form is unknown. In spite of many premature and unsuccessful trials, Parkinson's disease has now provided the first convincing cases of successful neural transplantation.

Pavlovian conditioning: the type of learning first described by Ivan Pavlov in which animals learn associations between stimuli, in particular when an initially neutral stimulus predicts a stimulus of biological relevance—when a tone consistently precedes food, the animal learns that the tone predicts food, and the tone comes to elicit responses appropriate for the subsequent delivery of food. The principles of Pavlovian (or "classical") conditioning have widespread application to understanding how animals learn to interpret regularities in a changing environment.

PC12 cells: a cell line originally derived from an adrenal gland tumour—phaeochromocytoma—the cells of which exhibit a predominant catecholamine phenotype.

Peripheral nervous system (PNS): the part of the nervous system lying outside the specialised environment of the CNS; there is a predominance of long-distance myelinated axons projecting in nerve bundles between the CNS centrally and the muscles and sense organs of the periphery; characterised by *Schwann cells* as the primary *glial cell* type; supports a far higher level of nerve regeneration than is observed in the CNS.

Pick's disease: a form of dementia associated with characteristic neuropathological cellular inclusions (Pick's bodies) in the frontal and temporal cortices.

Positron emission tomography (PET): an imaging method based on detection of the pairs of positrons emitted as a radiation breakdown product from injections of radioactive marker compounds. PET allows functional imaging in the living brain but requires the use of radioactive tracers. This imposes safety restrictions on the frequency and variety of scans that can be performed.

Precursor cell: any cell that is not terminally differentiated and precedes other cells in a developmental lineage.

Prefrontal cortex: the association areas of the prefrontal lobe, traditionally associated with higher aspects of intellectual and cognitive function.

Prion: an infectious protein implicated in a range of spongiform neurological diseases including scrapie in sheep, Creutzfeld–Jacob disease (CJD) in man, bovine spongiform encephalopathy (BSE) in cattle, and the "new-variant" form of CJD that may represent transmission of scrapie via cattle to humans.

Progenitor cell: a *precursor cell* that can typically give rise to more than one sort of progeny, although lineage is at least partly restricted, and (unlike a *stem cell*) does not have the capacity for indefinite self-replication.

Progressive supranuclear palsy: a neurodegenerative disease that typically affects elderly patients and is characterised by a progressive loss of voluntary eye movements with parkinsonism and a frontal dementia. It is progressive, incurable, and does not respond to drug therapy. In the early stages it can be mistaken for *Parkinson's disease*.

Promoter gene: a gene that regulates the expression of another adjacent gene. In *gene therapy*, it is important to transfer not only the target genes that are to be inserted or replaced but also relevant promoter genes that regulate when and where the target genes are to be transcribed and the gene products are to be expressed.

Proto-oncogene: a gene that regulates cell division; as well as their obvious relevance to cancer biology, they are used in *gene therapy* to regulate proliferation, immortalisation, and phenotypic differentiation of other gene products.

Pupillary reflex: a simple reflex involving constriction of the dark-adapted pupil in response to light. The neural circuit underlying the reflex is well mapped in the brainstem. This reflex has provided a powerful test of functional connections between transplanted retinae and the host brains.

Push–pull perfusion: a simple way to sample fluids from the brain for biochemical analysis by infusion through one cannula and withdrawal at the same rate through an adjacent cannula. A precursor to *microdialysis.*

Putamen: a major nucleus of the *basal ganglia* which together with the *caudate* makes up the *neostriatum.*

Quinolinic acid: an excitotoxic amino acid that binds to the AMPA class of *glutamate* receptors and is a particularly effective toxin for striatal neurones, mimicking the pattern of cell loss seen in *Huntington's disease.*

Raclopride: a selective *dopamine* antagonist at the D2 receptor. Radio-labelled raclopride is validated as a sensitive ligand for visualising dopamine D2 receptor distribution in post-mortem autoradiography, and is the most sensitive ligand at present available for selective labelling and visualisation of striatal neurones in PET.

Raphé nucleus: cell nucleus running through the core of the brainstem, in which are located the *serotonin* neurones that project widely to forebrain, cerebellum, and spinal cord.

Red nucleus: a brainstem motor nucleus in the pons, which contributes a major projection to the spinal cord.

Retrovirus: a class of virus used as a vector for gene transfer into neural cells. Efficient, but only infects dividing cells.

Robertsonian translocations: the tendency of certain chromosomes to become stuck together in mice, enabling the generation of selective breeding regimes to produce a high incidence of trisomic (and monosomic) offspring (see *trisomy 16*).

Rotation: a behavioural response in which a rat or mouse with unilateral damage in the basal ganglia will turn at a high rate in head to tail circles when activated either by stress or pharmacologically.

Scar: see ***glial scar.***

SCH-23390: a selective *dopamine* antagonist at the D1 receptor. Radio-labelled SCH-23390 has been validated as a sensitive ligand for visualising dopamine D1 receptor distribution in post-mortem autoradiography or *in vivo* PET.

Schwann cell: the major *glial cell* of the *PNS*; Schwann cells provide myelination of peripheral nerve axons, and are the main source of trophic factors and substrate molecules that promote much greater regenerative capacity of axons in the *PNS* than the *CNS.*

Sciatic nerve: one of the main peripheral nerves carrying sensory and motor information to the muscles of the leg. Widely used in the study of regeneration of *PNS* axons *in situ*, and for transplantation of segments of peripheral nerve as *bridge grafts* in the *CNS.*

Scopolamine: a drug that, like *atropine*, is an antagonist of the cholinergic muscarinic receptor.

Scrapie: a *prion* disease of sheep, the infectious nature, principles, and genetics of which have been extensively studied by transmission (via intracerebral inoculation of infected tissue) to mice.

Senile (or neuritic) plaques: extracellular tangles of neurites with a core of *amyloid*. Plaque deposits in the cortex and hippocampus are a second diagnostic neuropathological feature of *Alzheimer's disease*.

Sensitisation: an increase in the behavioural response following repeated exposure to a drug; sensitisation may be attributable either to pharmacological changes in receptor sensitivity or to psychological processes involving conditioning.

Septum: a nucleus of the limbic system involved in aspects of cognition and emotional reactivity. The medial septum is rich in the cholinergic neurones that innervate the *hippocampus*.

Serotonin: a monoamine transmitter of the *CNS*, with cell bodies located in the *raphé nucleus* of the brainstem and projecting widely to the spinal cord, forebrain cortical, limbic, *basal ganglia*, and diencephalic targets.

Skinner box: an automated test apparatus designed by B.J. Skinner, based on the principles of *operant conditioning*; the Skinner box is essentially a test chamber in which stimuli (e.g. lights, tones) can be delivered, responses recorded (e.g. lever press, chain pull, key press), and rewards delivered (e.g. food pellets, water, sucrose), all under automated control. The particular stimulus and response conditions required to produce a reward define the "schedule of reinforcement".

Solid grafts: implantations of cells or tissues as solid chunks into the host brain. The solid graft procedure usually involves identifying a natural cavity (e.g. the lateral or third ventricles) or creating an artificial cavity (e.g. in the cortex) to receive the graft.

Somatostatin: a peptide neurotransmitter, found in a small population of interneurones in the *neostriatum*. These cells are relatively spared in *Huntington's disease*.

Spatial navigation: the ability of animals to find their way and locate goals using spatial cues in a complex environment. Spatial navigation was highlighted in a series of influential reviews by O'Keefe and Nadel as a major function of the *hippocampus*, and tests designed to assess this aspect of function have become a major focus of studies involving grafts in the hippocampus and in aged animals.

SPECT: single photon emission computerised tomography. An *in vivo* scanning technique based on (and cruder but much cheaper than) *PET* scans, allowing detection of single photons rather than pairs of photons in the breakdown of radioactive ligands.

Stem cell: a *precursor cell* originating early in development which can self-renew, proliferating to form multiple copies of itself, and which is multipotential, giving rise to progeny cells of multiple different types. Neural stem cells may continue to exist in the adult brain.

Stereology: a set of microscopy techniques for counting cells and measuring other features of tissues in an unbiased manner.

Stereotactic surgery: a surgical technique in which the head is fixed within a rigid frame so as to permit positioning of an electrode or injection cannula using a geometrical co-ordinates system.

Striatal grafts: strictly grafts containing the developing cells of the *neostriatum*. Typically striatal grafts involve dissection of both medial and lateral ridges of the embryonic *ganglionic eminence* and in addition to primordial striatal neurones include as yet undifferentiated cells of the germinal layer, as well as newly differentiated cells destined for cortical, pallidal, and other forebrain nuclei originating from this common germinal zone.

Striatal mosaic: morphological and neurochemical heterogeneity of the *neostriatum* on the basis of the division of neurones, neuropil, receptors, and connections into two main compartments, the *striosomes* and the *matrix*.

Striatum: major group of nuclei of the *basal ganglia* comprising the *neostriatum* (*caudate nucleus* and *putamen*) and *ventral striatum* (including *nucleus accumbens*). The striatal nuclei receive the major inputs from cortex and elsewhere, and provide the first order of processing in the basal ganglia.

Striosomes: one of two main compartments of the *neostriatum*, characterised by low acetylcholinesterase staining, rich in μ-opiate receptors, and with distinct patterns of input and output connectivity.

Substance P: a peptide neurotransmitter found in several *CNS* sites, including co-localisation with *GABA* in striatal output neurones projecting to the *substantia nigra*.

Substantia nigra: cell group in the ventral mesencephalic area of the midbrain, comprising two parts. *Dopamine* neurones of the "pars compacta", designated as area A9 by Dahlström and Fuxe (1974), are the origin of the *nigrostriatal pathway*, which degenerates in *Parkinson's disease*. GABAergic neurones of the "pars reticulata" are one of the major outputs systems of the basal ganglia, receiving projections from caudate–putamen and *globus pallidus* and in turn projecting to a variety of brainstem motor nuclei.

Subthalamic nucleus (STN): a nucleus of the basal ganglia, receiving direct inputs from the external segment of the *globus pallidus* and the *neocortex*, it projects back to the internal segment of the *globus pallidus* and *substantia nigra* pars reticulata, constituting the "indirect" pathway of striatal outflow. The STN regulates basal ganglia outflow, and is a target for neurosurgical intervention by lesion or stimulation in *Parkinson's disease*.

Subventricular zone: a layer deep in the ventricular wall of the brain in which stem cells remain in a quiescent state throughout life, but can be activated in response to an appropriate signal (e.g. *fibroblast growth factor*). The source of cells of the rostral migratory stream.

Succinate dehydrogenase: an enzyme involved in cellular metabolism, the activity of which can be visualised histochemically as an index of mitochondrial energy metabolism.

Superior cervical ganglion (CCG): a noradrenergic ganglion of the sympathetic branch of the autonomic nervous system, occasionally used as a well-defined source of peripheral noradrenergic neurones for culture or grafting.

Supersensitivity: a change in receptor sensitivity following loss of normal inputs so as to be excessively responsive to any residual transmitter remaining. As part of a normal compensatory response to partial denervation of a system with in-built redundancy (such as the *nigrostriatal dopamine pathway*), it can produce unexpected consequences following experimental probing with low doses of receptor agonist drugs at doses too low to affect normal receptors.

Suspension grafts: implantation of cells or tissues by stereotactic injection of dissociated cell suspensions into the host brain. The suspension graft procedure has the advantage that the surgery is relatively less traumatic, not requiring additional cavities to receive the graft, and multiple grafts can be easily deposited in deep brain sites.

Tail flick test: a widely used test of pain sensitivity for rats.

Tau proteins: the major protein constituents of paired helical filaments. Tau has recently been sequenced, and occurs in six isoforms in the brain.

Thymidine: a DNA base which can be radioactively labelled, and following injection in an animal will be incorporated into the DNA of newly dividing cells. Widely used as a simple method for determining the birthdate of neurones and other cells in developmental studies.

Transgenic mice: a procedure for transferring extra copies of identified genes into the germ line of animals (usually mice) so that subsequent generations can be bred carrying the extra genes, e.g. breeding mice that carry extra copies of the human *amyloid precursor protein*.

Transplant: an implant of living cells derived from one animal and implanted into another.

Treadmill test: a behavioural test to evaluate animals' quadripedal stepping when suspended over a moving floor; treadmill tests can be used to assess automatic spinal locomotor reflexes in the absence of descending control from the forebrain, as well as recovery of both reflexive and voluntary function following spinal injury.

Trisomy 16: triplication of chromosome 16 in mice (equivalent to *trisomy 21*, *Down's syndrome*, in humans).

Trisomy 21: genetic abnormality involving inheritance of an extra copy of chromosome 21. Results in *Down's syndrome* in humans.

Trypsin: a proteolytic enzyme commonly used to aid dissociation of cells during preparation of cell suspensions for grafting.

Tyrosine hydroxylase: the rate-limiting enzyme in the conversion of phenylalanine to tyrosine to *L-dopa* in *dopamine* and noradrenaline neurones. Antibodies against tyrosine hydroxylase provide a widely used *immunohistochemical* marker for the distribution of dopamine and noradrenaline neurones in the normal or parkinsonian brain, or in adrenal and *nigral grafts*.

Ubiquitin: a molecule that is expressed in degenerating neurones in a variety of diseases, and widely used as a marker of cellular pathology.

Ultrastructure: Examination of the structure of cells in the electron microscope, giving detail at a far higher magnification and resolution than can be achieved using conventional light microscopy. Many defining features of cells are only resolvable at the ultrastructural level.

Vasopressin: a peptide neurotransmitter located in particular in the ventral hypothalamus, where it is involved in fluid regulation, and in other areas of the forebrain, where it has (more controversially) been implicated in processes of memory and attention.

Ventral horn: the lower half of grey matter in the core of the spinal cord, in which are located the *motor neurones* controlling the peripheral striate musculature.

Ventral mesencephalon: area in the ventral surface of the developing brainstem. In the embryo, it contains the *dopamine* cells of the developing *substantia nigra* and is the area dissected for "*nigral grafts*".

Ventral root: the peripheral nerve roots along the spinal cord containing bundles of axons projecting from motor neurones in the spinal cord to the peripheral musculature.

Ventral striatum: a ventral extension of the *striatum* in the basal ganglia receiving *dopamine* inputs from the *ventral tegmental area*, projecting to the ventral pallidum, and comprising the *nucleus accumbens* along with other minor cell groups such as the olfactory tubercle.

Ventral tegmental area: a separate group of *dopamine* neurones in the midbrain, designated as area A10, innervating the *striatum* (including *nucleus accumbens*), septum, *amygdala*, and *prefrontal cortex*.

Viral vector: a virus which can infect cells of interest (typically a neurone) and which can accommodate (by genetic engineering) experimental genes of interest into their own genome. Infection of the target cells results in incorporation of both the viral genes and the experimental genes into the host cell. The virus is then said to provide a vector for inserting the experimental gene into the target cell.

Wallerian degeneration: the process in which a cut axon (typically in a peripheral nerve) undergoes progressive retrograde degeneration from the cut stump back towards the cell body.

Water maze: see *Morris water maze*.

Wisconsin Card Sorting Test: a neuropsychology test for evaluating frontal function in humans, based on the subject classifying symbolic cards into categories.

Wisconsin general test apparatus: an experimental apparatus for hand testing cognitive function in monkeys, in which various rules govern the location of food rewards hidden under stimulus objects.

Xenograft: a graft between animals of different species.

Abbreviations

βA4	amyloid protein βA4
A	adrenaline
AAV	adeno-associated virus
ACh	acetylcholine
AChE	acetylcholinesterase
ACTH	adrenocortical trophic hormone
AD	Alzheimer's disease
aFGF	acidic fibroblast growth factor
ALS	amyotrophic lateral sclerosis
AM	adrenal medulla
AMPA	α-amino-3-hydroxy-5-methyl-4-isoxazolepropionic acid
ANS	autonomic nervous system
APP	amyloid precursor protein
ATP	adenosine triphosphate
AV	adenovirus
BBB	blood–brain barrier
BDNF	brain-derived neurotrophic factor
bFGF	basic fibroblast growth factor
BHK	baby hamster kidney (cells)
BrDU	bromodeoxyuridine
CAG	the triplet of DNA nucleotides that encodes the protein glutamine
CAPIT	Core Assessment Protocol for Intracerebral Transplantation
CAT	computerised axial tomography scan
CCK	cholecystokinin
CGRP	calcitonin gene-related polypeptide

ChAT	choline acetyl transferase
CN	caudate nucleus
CNS	central nervous system
CNTF	ciliary neurotrophic factor
CRL	crown–rump length
CSF	cerebrospinal fluid
CS-PG	chondroitin sulphate-proteoglycan
D1	type 1 dopamine receptor
D2	type 2 dopamine receptor
DA	dopamine
DAB	diaminobenzidine
DARPP-32	dopamine- and adenosine-receptor phosphoprotein of 32kD molecular weight
DAT	dementia of the Alzheimer type
DBH	dopamine-β-hydroxylase
DNA	deoxyribose nucleic acid
DRL	differential reinforcement of low rates
E*n*	embryonic age, gestational day *n*
EAA	excitatory amino acid
ECM	extracellular matrix
EGF	epidermal growth factor
FGF	fibroblast growth factor
GABA	γ-amino butyric acid
GAD	glutamic acid decarboxylase
GC	glucocorticoid
GDNF	glial cell line-derived neurotrophic factor
GFAP	glial fibrillany acidic protein
GM-1	ganglioside type 1
3-βHSD	3-β-hydroxysteroid dehydrogenase
HBSS	Hanks balanced saline solution
HD	Huntington's disease
HRP	horseradish peroxidase
HSV	herpes simplex virus
HVA	homovanillic acid
ICSS	intracranial self-stimulation
IGF-*n*	insulin growth factor type *n*
IL-*n*	interleukin type *n*
IN-1	an antibody raised against myelin-derived molecules inhibitory to axon growth
IPD	idiopathic Parkinson's disease
L*n*	lumbar segment *n* of the spinal cord
L-dopa	levodopa
LIF	leukaemia inhibitory factor

LV	lentivirus
MAO	monoamine oxidase
MND	motor neurone disease
MPP+	1-methy-4-phenylpyridium ion
MPTP	1-methyl-4-phenyl-1,2,3,6-tetrahydropyridine
MRI	magnetic resonance imaging
MS	multiple sclerosis
MSA	multi-system atrophy
NA	noradrenaline
NCAM	neural cell adhesion molecule
NECTAR	the European Network for Clinical Transplantation and Restoration
NFT	neurofibrillary tangle
NGF	nerve growth factor
NGS	normal goat serum
NILE	nerve growth factor inducible large external glycoprotein
NMDA	N-methyl-D-aspartic acid
NPY	neuropeptide Y
NP zone	acetylcholine-poor "non-patch" areas of a striatal graft
NT-*n*	neurotrophin-*n*
6-OHDA	6-hydroxydopamine
O-2A	precursor cell to the type 2 oligodendrocyte and astrocyte lineages
P*n*	postnatal day *n*
PBS	phosphate buffered saline
PC12	a phaeochromocytoma cell line
PD	Parkinson's disease
PDGF	platelet-derived growth factor
PET	positron emission tomography
PNMT	phenylethanolamine-N-methyltransferase
PNS	peripheral nervous system
3-NP	3-nitroproprionic acid
Put	putamen
P zone	acetylcholine-rich "patch" areas of a striatal graft
SDNF	striatal-derived neurotrophic factor
SIF	small intensely fluorescent cells of the adrenal medulla
SN	substantia nigra
SNC	substantia nigra pars compacta
SNR	substantia nigra pars reticulata
SP	substance P
S–R	Stimulus–response
SPECT	single positron emission computerised tomography
SVZ	subventricular zone
TGF-α,β	transforming growth factor-α,β

TH	tyrosine hydroxylase
TNF-α,β	tumour necrosis factor-α,β
UPDRS	Unified Parkinson's Disease Rating Scale
VIP	vasoactive intestinal polypeptide
VM	ventral mesencephalon
VTA	ventral tegmental area

Author index

Subject index

For Product Safety Concerns and Information please contact our EU representative GPSR@taylorandfrancis.com
Taylor & Francis Verlag GmbH, Kaufingerstraße 24, 80331 München, Germany

www.ingramcontent.com/pod-product-compliance
Ingram Content Group UK Ltd.
Pitfield, Milton Keynes, MK11 3LW, UK
UKHW022215190926
475702UK00003B/368
* 9 7 8 1 0 4 1 2 4 4 4 9 3 *